Preface

This book has been written principally for doctors working in Primary Care and Community Paediatrics who encounter at first hand the problems and the difficulties of paediatric practice. The contents cover the syllabus for the DCH examination, and we hope that general practitioners will also find the book a useful resource in their day to day work.

The chapters have been written by experienced paediatricians and four general practitioners who are all present or past DCH examiners. The GPs have provided input into the chapters and have constructed the GP overviews, covering some of the common symptoms encountered in the surgery and community clinics. In this way, we hope that we have placed the emphasis of the book in the primary care setting, but have ensured that hospital investigation, management and treatment are also covered. GPs need sound knowledge of secondary care in order to discuss children with their parents and carers in a meaningful way and we hope that this dimension will make the book of value for trainee paediatricians working towards the MRCPCH.

Core knowledge chapters are included, but in addition, important contemporary topics such as informatics, child health surveillance, genetics and child disability are also in the book, all with primary care emphasis.

We have included Internet addresses that we have found useful in the recommended reading section at the end of several chapters and also listed at the end of the book, so that readers can keep up to date in a way that a textbook cannot provide for.

We would like to thank all the contributors for their hard work in compiling their chapters and for their patience with us as editors. In addition, we would like to thank all the staff at Harcourt for their help and input in the preparation of this book and also our wives and families for their support. We wish to record our thanks to Penny Dablin and Tracy Wheelhouse for their expert secretarial help and to Samuel Bellman for drawings.

We hope that doctors will find this book a useful addition to their paediatric library, whether at home, in their surgeries or in their clinics. We would welcome any constructive comments from our readers.

2000

Martin Bellman, London
Nigel Kennedy, Aylesbury

Abbreviations used in text

ANA	antinuclear antibody		MCV	mean corpuscular volume
APTT	activated partial thromboplastin time		MLD	moderate learning difficulties
ARF	acute renal failure		NEC	necrotising enterocolitis
AS	aortic stenosis		PCHR	personal (parent-held) child health record
ASD	atrial septal defect			
A/VSD	atrioventricular septal defect		PDA	patent ductus arteriosus
CDC	Child Development Centre		PEEP	positive end expiratory pressure
CDH	congenital dislocation of the hip		PS	pulmonary stenosis
CDT	Child Development Team		PT	prothrombin time
CHD	congenital heart disease		RDS	respiratory distress syndrome
CPAP	constant positive airways pressure		RSV	respiratory syncytial virus
CPR	cardiopulmonary resuscitation/Child Protection Register		SCD	sickle cell disorders
			SEN	special educational needs
CRP	C-reactive protein		SGA	small for gestational age
CSA	child sexual abuse		SIDS	sudden infant death syndrome
DMD	Duchenne muscular dystrophy		SLD	severe learning difficulties
ESR	erythrocyte sedimentation rate		SLT	speech and learning therapist
FC	febrile convulsion		SLE	systemic lupus erythematosus
FH	familial hypercholesterolaemia		SMA	spinal muscular atrophy
GBS	group B haemolytic streptococcus		SSD	Social Services Department
GFR	glomerular filtration rate		STD	sexually transmitted diseases
GH	growth hormone		SVT	supraventricular tachycardia
HCT	haematocrit		URTI	upper respiratory tract infection
HOCM	hypertrophic obstructive cardiomyopathy		UTI	urinary tract infection
			VLBW	very low birth weight
INS	idiopathic nephrotic syndrome		VSD	ventricular septal defect
LBW	low birth weight		VT	ventricular tachycardia

Contributors

Michael F M Bamford MA FRCP FRCPCH DCH
Consultant Paediatrician, Ipswich NHS Trust,
UK

Jeffrey Bissenden MA FRCP FRCPCH
Consultant Paediatrician, City Hospital Trust,
Birmingham, UK

Andrew W Boon MD FRCP FRCPCH DCH
Consultant Paediatrician, Royal Berkshire
Hospital, Reading, UK

Peter D Campion PhD FRCGP MRCP(UK) DCCH
Professor of Primary Care Medicine, University
of Hull, Hull, UK

S N J Capps BSc MBBS FRCS
Consultant Paediatric Surgeon, Queen Mary's
Hospital for Children, Carshalton and St
George's Hospital, London, UK

John Cohen MA MSc MBBS FRCGP
Professor and Director of the Centre for
Community Care and Primary Health,
University of Westminster; Senior Lecturer in
Primary Care, Royal Free Hospital and
University College London Medical School;
General Practitioner, London, UK

David Cottrell MA MBBS FRCPsych
Professor of Child and Adolescent Psychiatry,
Academic Unit of Child Mental Health, School
of Medicine, University of Leeds, Leeds, UK

Derek I. Johnston MA MD FRCP FRCPCH DCH
Consultant Paediatrician, University Hospital,
Queen's Medical Centre, Nottingham, UK

Michael Modell FRCGP FRCP DCH
Professor of Primary Health Care, Royal Free
and University College Medical School,
Department of Primary Care and Population
Sciences, Archway Campus, London,
UK

Martin W Moncrieff MA BM BCh FRCP
Honorary Consulting Paediatrician, John
Radcliffe Hospital, Oxford, UK

Richard C F Newton MA MB BChir FRCP FRCPCH DCH
DRCOG
Consultant Paediatrician, Ashford and St Peter's
NHS Trust, UK

E Peile MB BS MRCS MRCP(UK) FRCGP DCH DRCOG
Senior Partner, Ashton Clinton Surgery,
Buckinghamshire, UK

A K M Raffles MBBS FRCP FRCPCH DCH
Consultant Paediatrican, East Hertfordshire
NHS Trust, Queen Elizabeth II Hospital,
Welwyn Garden City, UK

Anthony Robinson MD FRCPCH FRCP DCH
Consultant Paediatrician, South Manchester
University Hospitals NHS Trust, Manchester,
UK

Brent Taylor PhD MBChB FRCP FRCP FRACP FRCPCH
Professor of Community Child Health, Royal
Free and University College Medical School of
University College London, Royal Free Campus,
UK; Chairman National Child health
Informatics Consortium

Tony Waterston MD FRCP FRCPCH DCH DRCOG
Consultant Paediatrician (Community Child
Health), Newcastle General Hospital,
Newcastle-upon-Tyne, UK

Michael J H Williams MBBS LRCS FRCP FRCPCH DCH
Consultant Paediatrician and Director of
Children's Services, West Hertfordshire
Community NHS Trust, UK

Jane Wynne MBChB FRCP FRCPCH DM(Hons)
Consultant Community Paediatrician, Leeds, UK

Contents

1

Epidemiology and social paediatrics

Tony Waterston

INTRODUCTION

One of the main concerns of doctors who practise with children is the patient as a whole person, and the relationship between their patient and society at large. Two examples will show why a study of epidemiology and social paediatrics is central to an understanding of paediatrics and child health.

Example 1: Sudden infant death

Sudden infant death (SIDS) or 'cot death' as it used to be called, is the most common cause of death in infants between the age of a week and a year. For many years the cause was unexplained and many theories were investigated, from cardiac arrhythmias to allergy or infections. None proved hopeful and the possibility of prevention seemed remote. Then the observation was made by an epidemiologist that the incidence varied considerably between countries, notably Hong Kong (low incidence) and the UK (high incidence). What customs differed between these countries, enquired the social paediatrician? A notable one was sleeping position: children were laid down to sleep on their backs in Hong Kong, on the front in the UK. Indeed, paediatricians had long advocated the front sleeping position because it was thought to reduce the likelihood of aspiration and promote muscular development. A 'back to sleep' campaign had been effective in New Zealand in reducing SIDS incidence and was instituted in the UK with very

1

good effect—there has been a dramatic fall in deaths from this cause.

Example 2: Undernutrition in children

It has long been known that children growing up in disadvantaged and low income families have a poor state of nutrition: this can take the form of unbalanced nutrition (e.g. too much sugar and fat), failure to thrive, obesity, short stature and iron deficiency anaemia. It is often suggested that the reason is ignorance—lack of education and awareness of what constitutes a healthy diet—which could be corrected by good advice and cooking lessons. Closer examination of the cost of a healthy diet, however, shows that in fact it is much cheaper to provide calories from chips, sausages, pies, crisps and potatoes than from vegetables, meat or fruit (Table 1.1). Children demand filling food and require calories first. If money is short and children decline food they don't like, then there may be no money for alternatives. Hence parents will spend their money on food that is filling and that they know their children like. Families on higher incomes will be much more prepared to experiment and intro-

duce a wider variety of foods on a regular basis. A socially aware paediatrician will realise that income is all important in ensuring good nutrition and will address social as well as dietary factors in countering malnutrition in low income patients.

Put simply, epidemiology is the study of populations and social paediatrics is the study of children in relation to society. Both disciplines are exciting, challenging and absorbing, and their application is needed for the problems which clinicians encounter every day (see Case studies 1.1–1.7).

In addition to these clinical situations, a GP will need access to epidemiological skills for the following work that is being carried out by the practice:

Table 1.1 Cost/100 kcal of 'healthy' and 'unhealthy' foods in the UK in the 1980s. Source: Lobstein T 1988 Poor children and cheap calories. Community Paediatric Group Newsletter. British Paediatric Association, London.

	Cost (pence)/100 kcal
Lean beef	40
Cod fillet	50
Lean pork	23
Chicken leg	18
Meat pies	7
Sausages	6
Tomatoes	70
Cabbage	15
Potatoes	6
Chips	6
Crisps	9
Oranges	25
Apples	14
Mars Bar	8
Fruit juice	20
Cola drink	16
Lard	1
Sugar	2
White bread	2
Wholemeal bread	3

Case study 1.1 John, a 4-year-old, has acute otitis media. The parents ask whether antibiotics are needed.

The doctor needs to know the results of trials of treatment in otitis media. This requires an ability to assess the value of different trials: the best kind is a randomised controlled trial, in which treatment is given to one group of patients and not the other and the outcome compared, with neither the patient nor the doctor being aware of who is in each group (double blind). The current consensus is that antibiotics are not of benefit in most cases of otitis media.

Case study 1.2 Sarah is a wheezy baby of 6 months whose parents smoke. Her parents ask if she will have asthma.

Here an understanding is needed of the natural history of wheezy babies, and of the effects of passive smoking on babies. Both are supplied by epidemiology. Wheezy babies seem to fall into two groups: those with atopic family and personal histories may go on to have asthma, those without such a history may wheeze only with a viral upper respiratory infection. Passive smoking causes respiratory symptoms in infants and exacerbates asthma, and it is important that parents are made aware of this. Social paediatrics gives us an understanding that parents living in poverty who smoke do so to relieve stress in their lives; for women in particular it may be the only source of pleasure. Advice on stopping smoking should therefore be offered in a non-judgemental way.

Case study 1.3 William is a 6-year-old with asthma. The school will not let him use his inhaler without help from his parents so he generally has to miss school when he is wheezy. The parents ask the GP to intercede.

This illustrates the close connection between childhood illness and the educational system. In a child with a chronic illness the co-operation of the school is essential, and the doctor may be asked to facilitate the provision of information to school teachers. In this case advocacy is needed to take up the child's needs with the school staff: if the child is capable of using his inhaler at home then he should be allowed to use it at school.

Case study 1.4 Lianne is a 7-year-old with cerebral palsy. She has to attend four different clinics to see specialists in hospital; the parents find this very difficult as they have limited finances and the transport costs are high. Can social services help?

It is necessary to see this situation from the point of view of the family. The clinics should be better planned and, ideally, the consultants should see the child in a joint clinic. It is the responsibility of the paediatrician to co-ordinate care and improve the way in which different professionals work together. If there are financial problems it may be possible to obtain assistance, either from Children Act funding held by the local authority or from the Disability Living Allowance.

Case study 1.5 Jill is a 9-month-old baby who has failed her distraction hearing test but her parents think that she can hear quite well. They ask, is it a reliable test?

Here the doctor needs to know how effective the distraction hearing test is as a screening test for hearing loss. What is its sensitivity and specificity (see below)? The answer is that a lot depends on the test conditions and the state of the baby: if the room was noisy or the baby had a cold then she might have failed the test despite having good hearing. This is epidemiology in practice.

Case study 1.6 The parents of a very small pre-term baby, who was born at 28 weeks' gestation and is now 3 months old, come to obtain some prescriptions and ask what are her chances of entering normal school?

This situation requires both epidemiology and social paediatrics! Data on outcome of low birth weight babies have been obtained from follow-up studies. In general, babies born at over 30 weeks who have no neonatal complications have a good chance of surviving unscathed. Risks increase with reducing birth weight and with hypoxia and infections. In communicating with the parents it is important to judge their ability to accept hypothetical information, and to avoid long-term prognostication at such an early age.

Case study 1.7 Trevor is a 3-year-old whose mother brings him because of a cough and temperature. You notice a bruise on the side of his head and another on his neck; his mother does not have an adequate explanation. His mother lives alone but is often visited by her sometimes violent partner. How are you going to assess this situation?

This is a situation of potential child abuse, one of the central problems of social paediatrics. Here the practitioner must put the interests of the child first but be open with the parent about the nature of the concerns. Child abuse is a multidisciplinary problem and one in which there are local guidelines which the doctor needs to be aware of and follow. These include discussing the case with a colleague and informing social services who will convene a case conference, having investigated the family dynamics. In this case the mother's partner may have been responsible for the bruises and separation may be desirable, perhaps with police protection.

- audit of screening tests in pre-school children
- feeding survey with the aim of improving breast feeding rates
- accidental injury survey to determine where education should be targeted
- health needs assessment in relation to the ethnic minority population.

Definitions

Advocacy means speaking out on behalf of a child, a family or a public policy issue such as legislation on tobacco advertising. It may be undertaken on behalf of individuals or communities, or nationally. Effective advocacy requires a good case supported by data, persistence and the avoidance of party political bias, together with an awareness of how the political system and the media operate.

Community development is the process by which local people define their own health needs and organise to make these needs known to service providers, or take action themselves to bring about change. The process may be facilitated by health professionals but should not be dependent on them.

Epidemiology. The study of disease occurrence in human populations.

Incidence. The risk of acquiring the disease or a characteristic thereof. The numerator consists of new cases developing the disease in a specified time period; the denominator is the population or sample from which this information was collected.

Prevalence. The risk of having the disease or a characteristic thereof at any given point or within a given time period; the former is called point prevalence and the latter period prevalence.

Health education is any activity which promotes health through learning.

Health promotion. Any planned and informed intervention which is designed to improve physical or mental health or to prevent disease, disability and premature death.

Prevention of disease is conventionally divided into three categories:

- *Primary prevention* means reduction in the number of new cases of a disease, disorder or condition, i.e. reduction of the incidence. Examples include immunisation and the prevention of accidental injury.
- *Secondary prevention* is aimed at reducing the prevalence of disease by shortening its duration or diminishing its impact through early detection, e.g. by screening programmes.
- *Tertiary prevention* is aimed at reducing impairment and disability and helping adjustment through effective treatment and information provision.

Public health is the science and art of preventing disease, prolonging life and promoting health through the organised efforts of society.

Screening has been defined as the presumptive identification of unrecognised disease or defect by the application of tests, examinations and other procedures which can be applied rapidly (see Box 1.1).

Screening tests (Box 1.2) sort out apparently well persons who may have a disease from those

---

Box 1.1 Wilson & Jungner: criteria for screening programmes

- The condition sought should be an important public health problem
- There should be an accepted treatment for patients with recognised disease
- Facilities for diagnosis and treatment should be available
- There should be a latent or early symptomatic stage
- There should be a suitable test or examination
- The natural history of the condition should be understood
- There should be an agreed definition of what is meant by a case of the target condition
- Treatment at the early, latent or pre-symptomatic stage should favourably influence prognosis
- The cost of screening should be economically balanced in relation to expenditure on the care and treatment of persons with the disorder and to medical care as a whole
- Case finding is a continuous process and not a once and for all project

---

Box 1.2 Cochrane and Holland characteristics of the ideal screening test

- Simple, quick and easy to interpret: capable of being performed by paramedics and other personnel
- Acceptable to the public, since participation in screening procedures is voluntary
- Accurate, i.e. giving a true measurement of the attribute under investigation
- Repeatable
- Sensitive: this is the ability of the test to give a positive finding when the individual screened has the disease or abnormality under investigation
- Specific: this is the ability of the test to give a negative finding when the individual being screened does not have the disease or abnormality

---

who do not. A screening test is not intended to be diagnostic.

- *Sensitivity* is the capacity of a test to detect all those who are truly affected by the condition or disorder.
- *Specificity* is the capacity of a test to identify correctly all those who are truly not affected by the condition or disorder.
- *Coverage*: the proportion of the population offered a screening test who have actually had the test. Coverage must be high (over 80%) for

screening to be effective because the healthier members of the population tend to present first for screening tests. (*Inverse care law*: those whose needs are greatest are least likely to access medical services, and those in least need of them are most likely to get them.)

- *Yield:* the number of new previously unsuspected cases detected per 100 individuals screened.

WHAT DO CHILDREN DIE FROM IN THE UK?

The current causes of death of children aged between 1 and 19 years in the UK are shown in Figure 1.1; selected age breakdowns are shown in Figures 1.2–1.4. Data sources for childhood mortality and morbidity are listed in Box 1.3. There have been major changes in recent years: the trends are shown in Figure 1.5. The remark-

able decline in mortality has occurred mainly as a result of improved living conditions, particularly nutrition, housing and sanitation. The impact of health care has been important but is

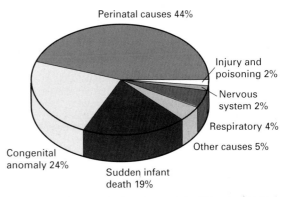

Figure 1.2 Causes of infant death, United Kingdom 1990. Source: OPCSS DH2/17, DH6/4; RG Scotland 1990; RG N Ireland 1991. Total 6292 deaths.

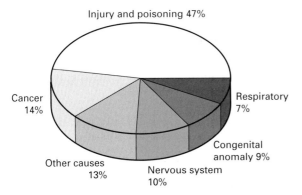

Figure 1.1 Causes of death age 1–19 years, United Kingdom 1990. Source: OPCSS DH2/17, DH6/4; RG Scotland 1990; RG N Ireland 1991. Total 4488 deaths.

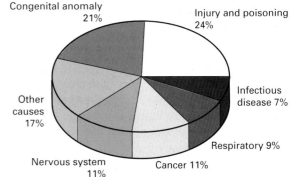

Figure 1.3 Causes of death age 1–4 years, United Kingdom 1990. Source: OPCSS DH2/17, DH6/4; RG Scotland 1990; RG N Ireland 1991. Total 1163 deaths.

Box 1.3 Sources of data	
Registration of Births, Marriages and Deaths:	Registrar General and Office of National Statistics
National Census: carried out every 10 years	As above
Notification of congenital anomalies	Office of National Statistics
Regular sample surveys:	Office of National Statistics
General Household Survey, National	
Food Survey, disability surveys	
National birth cohort studies: children born in 1946, 1958 and 1970	
National registers: e.g. cancer	
Hospital activity statistics	
General practice surveys	

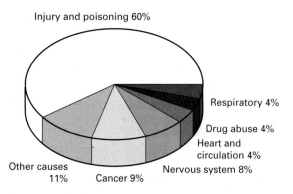

Figure 1.4 Causes of death age 15–19 years, United Kingdom 1990. Source: OPCSS DH2/17, DH6/4; RG Scotland 1990; RG N Ireland 1991. Total 2021 deaths.

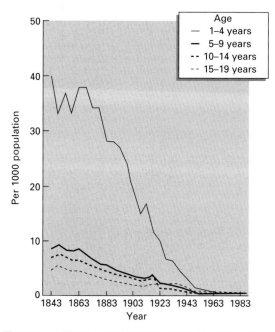

Figure 1.5 Trend in mortality under 20 years 1841–45 to 1986–90, England and Wales. Source: OPCS DH1/19 and DH2/17. 5-year averages.

generally considered to be secondary to factors outside the health care system. In health care, immunisation and the development of antibiotics have been the most significant advances in reducing the burden of infectious disease mortality and morbidity.

In the neonatal period, the main causes of death are congenital anomalies and prematurity (Fig. 1.2). Advances in antenatal diagnosis and genetic manipulation together with improved intensive care and the effective treatment of respiratory distress syndrome are likely to reduce these conditions further in coming years. During the first year of life, SIDS contributes nearly half of all deaths despite the drop following the 'back to sleep' campaign. This was a good example of an effective health education campaign whereby national publicity encouraged parents to alter their habits in relation to placing infants in the supine sleeping position instead of prone. Research continues into other causes of SIDS and further falls in the death rate are anticipated.

In children over one year, injury and poisoning form the largest group of causes of death, followed by cancer for the over 5s. Infectious diseases, including meningitis, still make a significant contribution. There are marked differences between boys and girls in relation to accidents, the death rate between 1 and 4 years being 172 per million boys and 98 per million girls. The scope for prevention in accidental death is considerable and is further considered below.

As well as gender differences in death rates there are very significant social class differences—see below under Inequalities in child health.

WHAT MAKES CHILDREN ILL IN THE UK?

Child health has now improved so much that it is rare for children to die in the UK, but morbidity is increasing. This section considers the burden of illness in British children and also looks at how healthy our children are—not at all the same thing. It is not easy to find accurate, nationwide, up-to-date data. A General Household Survey (GHS) including acute and chronic illness was carried out in 1990, and a disability survey in 1989: these relied on parents' reporting of their children's health. The sources of data on health rather than illness are discussed below.

Acute illness. Episodes of acute illness contribute to morbidity through lost school time and mental health effects on the children, and time off work and additional stress for the parents. If the illness is severe there may be complications which can lead to chronic illness or disability. The General Household Survey revealed that 24% of children 0–4 years old had consulted their GP in the past fortnight. A national study of general practice in 1981–82 showed that a third of all episodes of illness in childhood in which GPs were consulted were for respiratory complaints. Nearly one tenth of children under 5 were admitted to hospital at least once in 1990. 25% of hospital admissions in 0--4-year-olds are for respiratory complaints, and injuries account for almost the same proportion in 5--14-year-olds.

Chronic illness. According to the General Household Survey, chronic illness is increasing in the UK (Fig. 1.6). As the survey depends on parental report, however, this may indicate an increase in awareness. It does appear that asthma prevalence is increasing though the reasons are not well defined: environmental pollutants, particularly car exhaust fumes, are a possible cause. Figure 1.7 illustrates the prevalence of chronic illness and Figure 1.8 shows a breakdown of causes. Mental ill-health (particularly behavioural problems) is probably under-reported; this is further discussed below. The conditions which contribute most to the burden of chronic illness are asthma, eczema and glue ear.

Child abuse could perhaps be considered as a chronic illness but is hard to categorise and

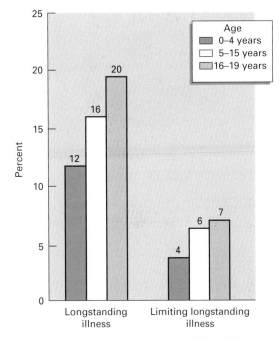

Figure 1.7 Chronic illness: age, Great Britain 1991. Source: OPCS GHS.

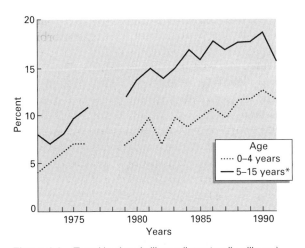

Figure 1.6 Trend in chronic illness (longstanding illness) 1972–91, Great Britain. Source: OPCS GHS 19–21; OPCS Monitor SS GHS 92/1. *Age 5–14 years to 1976.

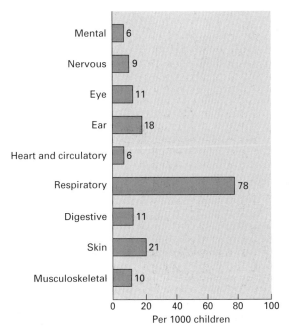

Figure 1.8 Longstanding illness age 0–15 years: type of illness, Great Britain 1989. Source: OPCS GHS 20. Mean 1.2 conditions per child.

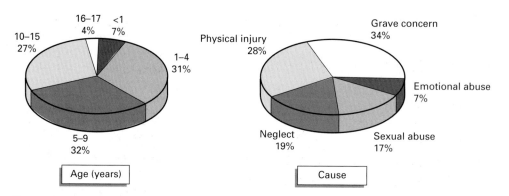

Figure 1.9   Children on child protection registers: age and cause, England 31 March 1992. Source DH 1993. Total of percentages exceed 100 because some children are counted in more than one category.

even harder to measure (see Chapter 17). Figure 1.9 shows the percentage of children on child protection registers for different causes in 1992. The number of children registered increased from 41 200 in 1989 to 45 300 in 1991.

Disability. As acute illness becomes less common and less serious, so more emphasis is placed on disability and the quality of life of children with a disability (see also Chapter 4). Figure 1.10

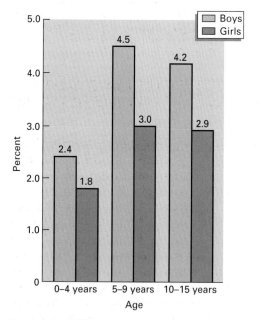

Figure 1.10   Children with a disability: age and sex, Great Britain 1985–88. Source: Bone M, Melzer H 1989 The prevalence of disability among children. OPCS Surveys of disability in Great Britain. Report 3. HMSO, London.

shows the prevalence of children with disability in the UK; Figure 1.11 illustrates their functional categories. Overall, 3% of children under 15 years in the UK have a disability; note that behavioural problems are the most common category of functional disability. Another means of measuring the extent of disability is through the number of statements of special educational need, which amounted to 148 300 children aged 5–16 years in 1991 (2% of the population).

Hall and Hill divide disabilities into three groups: those which are of high severity and low prevalence, usually of organic origin (blindness, deafness, cerebral palsy and intellectual impairment); those which are common but more minor and organic (e.g. squint, myopia, conductive hearing loss); and the low severity, high prevalence developmental disorders (speech delay, clumsiness, reading difficulty).

Health. The well-known and unfairly disparaged World Health Organization (WHO) definition of health is 'complete physical, mental and social well-being and not simply an absence of disease'. Well-being is very hard to measure but it is important not to draw the conclusion that measuring illness is a sufficient measure of health: a holistic view of health must include some other measures (Box 1.4). Among the possible candidates for measures of health are self-esteem, happiness, relationships, dietary habits, smoking, risk taking behaviour, immunisation uptake, and growth and nutrition indices. There is only a limited relationship between health and health services activities.

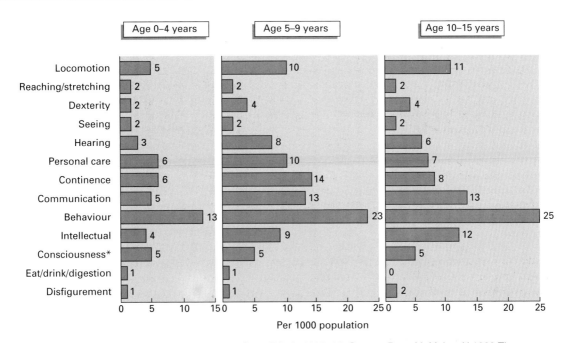

Figure 1.11   Disabilities: functional categories, Great Britain 1985–88. Source: Bone M, Melzer H 1989 The prevalence of disability among children. OPCS Surveys of disability in Great Britain. Report 3. HMSO, London. *Includes fits and convulsions.

Box 1.4	Possible measures of health
Self-esteem	An objective measure of mental health
Self-assessed health	A self-assessment measure
Growth data	An overall index of long-term health in children
Risk factor prevalence	Measures specific factors associated with illness
Exercise levels	Contributes to mental and physical health
Immunisation uptake	Indicates degree of protection from infectious disease

Much of the above information requires self-report by children and young people themselves. The WHO carries out a 4-yearly survey of health behaviour in school children in Canada and 24 European countries, which include Scotland and Wales but not England. Some of the key results of this survey are shown in Table 1.2.

Growth and nutrition are often used as measures of health. Where does the UK stand on this score? Do we have malnutrition or undernutrition, which are so prevalent throughout the world? The answer is almost certainly yes, but there is greater evidence for poor dietary intake than for poor nutritional status. Table 1.3 shows some of the current findings.

CURRENT TRENDS IN MORTALITY AND MORBIDITY AND THE REASONS FOR THEM

Infectious disease. Remarkable reductions have occurred over the past few decades in the incidence of major infectious diseases, particularly tuberculosis, measles, pertussis, diphtheria, streptococcal infections and *Haemophilus influenzae* (see Figures 1.12–1.14). Those diseases which were responsible for most child deaths up to 50 years ago are now within reach of eradication. The reduction was initially caused by improvements in nutrition, housing and sanitation, and more latterly by immunisation: the dramatic response to Hib vaccine is especially notable. Infections are still with us, however, and cause a great deal of morbidity and some mortality. In early childhood, rotavirus and respiratory

Table 1.2 Health behaviour of school-aged children. Figures are for Scotland. Source: WHO 1996

Children who smoked cigarettes once a week or more:
aged 11 years	2%	(both sexes)
aged 15 years	26%	(female)
	21%	(male)

Children who drank alcoholic beverages at least once weekly:
aged 11 years	11%	(male)
	5%	(female)
aged 15 years	41%	(male)
	32%	(female)

Children who watched TV for at least 4 hours a day:
aged 15 years	31%	(mean)

Children who ate hamburgers or hot dogs daily or more often:
aged 15 years	23%	(male)
	9%	(female)

Students who were on a diet or felt the need to lose weight:
aged 15 years	53%	(female)
	22%	(male)

Students who felt very healthy:
aged 15 years	9%	(female)
	28%	(male)

Students who felt very happy about their life:
aged 15 years	22%	(female)
	34%	(male)

Students who felt low or depressed once a week or more:
aged 15 years	31%	(female)
	17%	(male)

Students who reported serious injuries during the past year:
aged 13 years	21%	(female)
	32%	(male)

Students who were bullied at least once this school term:
aged 11 years	30%	(mean)

Table 1.3 Nutrition of children in the UK

Infants breast fed at birth (1990)	64%
Infants breast fed at 6 months (1990)	21%
Iron deficiency anaemia—toddlers	13–20%
Iron deficiency	
boys 12–14 years	3.5%
girls 12–14 years	10.5%
Dental caries	
Scottish children	50–59%
North of England children	40–49%

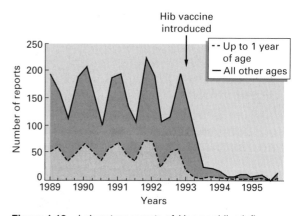

Figure 1.12 Laboratory reports of *Haemophilus influenzae* type B by age. England and Wales 1989–95. Source: PHLS, CDSC.

syncytial virus (RSV) are major pathogens that will continue to be responsible for many hospital admissions until a vaccine is available. New pathogens are emerging in the form of human immunodeficiency virus (HIV), Campylobacter and Pneumocystis, while tuberculosis is showing a resurgence, possibly associated with increasing poverty in the UK as well as increasing HIV prevalence. Drug resistance is being observed in some well known bacteria, including streptococcus. We are moving towards a situation where it is the vulnerable (whether from poor environment or immunodeficiency) who are more likely to contract a severe infectious disease in childhood.

Congenital disorders. As infectious disease plays a smaller part in the toll of mortality and morbidity, so congenital disorders become more important, particularly in their contribution to lifelong illness and disability. The congenital disorder most commonly leading to chronic illness is cystic fibrosis; the most common disorders associated with disability are Down's syndrome and cerebral palsy. The frequency of the two latter conditions is shown in Figure 1.15.

Cancer. As with congenital anomalies, cancer becomes a relatively more frequent cause of death as infectious disease is controlled by better health care and environmental improvements. The relative frequency of childhood cancers is shown in Table 1.4. The amenability of childhood cancer to drug treatment has improved radically in recent years, and many cancers including leukaemia and cerebral tumours are highly curable: the 5-year survival for lymphoblastic leukaemia is over 70% and for medulloblastoma

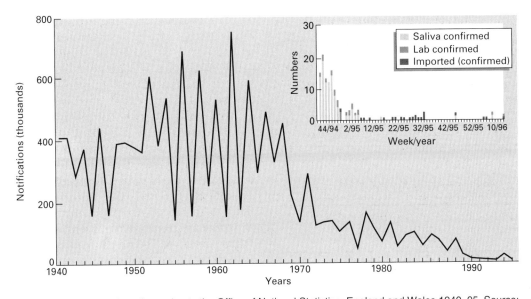

Figure 1.13   Notification of measles to the Office of National Statistics. England and Wales 1940–95. Source: PHLS, CDSC.

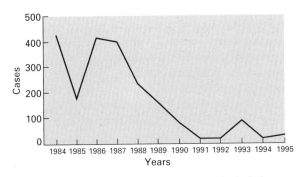

Figure 1.14   Laboratory confirmed reports of rubella in children age 1–14 years. England and Wales 1984–95. Source: PHLS, CDSC.

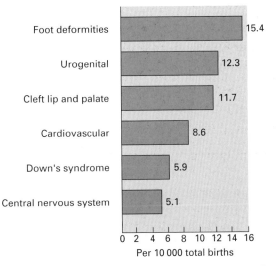

Figure 1.15   Notifications of selected congenital anomalies. England and Wales 1990. Notified within 10 days of birth. Source: OPCS MB3/6.

over 40%. Cancer is still rare—only one child in 650 will develop cancer by 15 years of age.

Prematurity. As a result of improved maternal nutrition and antenatal care fewer babies are being born before term, and those babies who are born earlier are surviving for longer. Owing to improved neonatal intensive care the burden of disability in surviving very low birth weight babies is not increasing markedly. Table 1.5 shows the outcome at follow-up of babies born at less than 28 weeks' gestation.

Accidents. In England and Wales the mortality

from injuries in childhood has fallen by a quarter over the last 40 years. This improvement is rather less than the decrease in mortality from other causes, which fell by nearly three quarters over the same period. The drop in mortality may be partly due to more effective management

Table 1.4 Frequency of different types of childhood cancer in the UK

Cancer	% of all childhood cancers
Leukaemia	35
Brain tumour	23
Lymphoma	12
Wilms' tumour	7
Neuroblastoma	7
Bone tumours	6

Table 1.5 Follow-up at 3 years of age of babies of less than 28 weeks' gestation

Normal	72%
Lesser disability	9%
Moderate or severe disability	19%

of children following trauma, and there may be more children surviving with a disability. It is likely that safety measures in the home have also been partly responsible. There has been a steeper drop in road traffic accident deaths despite the increased number of motor vehicles (see Fig. 1.16). Injuries to children in cars have been prevented by the adoption of seat belt legislation. Another reason for the drop, but a more concerning one, is that fewer children walk

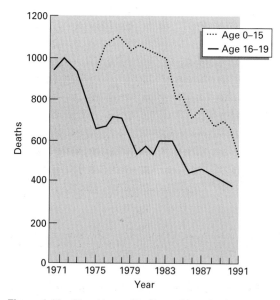

Figure 1.16 Trend in road traffic accident deaths: age, Great Britain 1970–91. Source: DoT.

or cycle to school, i.e. the exposure to accident risk is less because more children are transported by car. This is beneficial from the accident prevention point of view, but the trend to less exercise has contributed to increasing obesity in children, and increased car traffic results in higher levels of atmospheric pollution. Increasing social class disparity is evident in road accident deaths since many more social class I than social class V families own a car, and those without a car are more likely to be a victim of one.

Nutrition. Overall, the nutritional state of children in the UK is improving but a number of worrying trends have been highlighted by dietary surveys. The breast feeding rate is static despite much promotional activity over recent years. At present the proportion of babies who are initially breast fed is around 55% but there is much regional variation and rates are closely related with socio-economic class.

Undernutrition presents in the UK as failure to thrive (see p. 141) and iron deficiency anaemia (see p. 278). The prevalence of failure to thrive in community surveys varies from 5–20% and is generally associated with low income; it also presents in well-off families, however, often because high fibre, low fat, low energy diets are used inappropriately in toddlers. Iron deficiency is present in 13–20% of toddlers in inner cities and is caused by the early introduction of unfortified cow's milk and the use of diets low in iron. Even at the age of 12–14 years 3.5% of boys and 10.5% of girls are anaemic.

Overnutrition is becoming more common in the UK. Using a definition of body mass index (BMI) of 25–30 as overweight and over 30 as obese, 18% of young men and 17% of young women were overweight in 1986–87, an increase over the previous 6 years. The proportion of obese young women doubled (from 3–6%) over this period. The main reason for the increase in obesity is reduction in exercise, as overall calorie intake has not markedly increased.

'New morbidity'

This is the term given to conditions which are increasingly common in young people and are recognised to be major contributors to morbidity whilst intimately associated with the changes occurring in modern society.

Smoking. A quarter of 15-year-olds smoke at least one cigarette a week; only a third of 15-year-olds have never smoked. The trend at present (see Figure 1.17) is for smoking to decline in young people but the decline has levelled off in recent years and there may be an increase in young women smoking. Young people are targeted by tobacco advertising and it is generally considered by health professionals that a complete ban on tobacco advertising and sponsorship of sport by tobacco companies is desirable; the first of these is agreed policy of the UK government.

Drug abuse. Figure 1.18 illustrates drug use by 15--16-year-olds in Wales in 1990. The figures are likely to have increased considerably since then. Deaths from drug abuse are rising: those following ingestion of Ecstasy have received much publicity, though deaths from glue sniffing may be more common—see Figure 1.19.

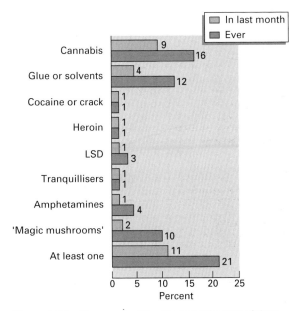

Figure 1.18 Drug use by 15--16-year-olds: type of drug, Wales 1990. Source: Smith & Nutbeam 1992.

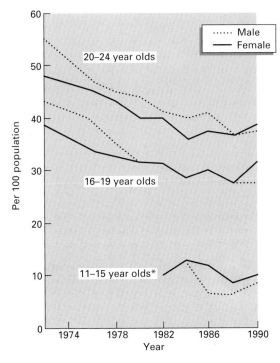

Figure 1.17 Trends in smoking: age, Great Britain 1972–90. Source: OPCS GHS 21; Lader & Matheson 1991. *England only.

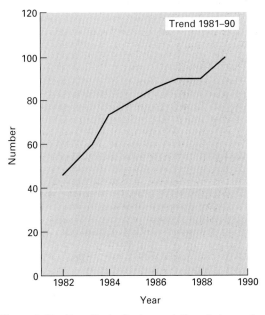

Figure 1.19 Trend in deaths from volatile substance abuse, age 9–20 years, United Kingdom 1981–90. 3-year averages.

Alcohol. Alcohol abuse by young people is also on the increase and there is much concern over the marketing of 'alcopops' or alcoholic lemonades which are likely to be particularly attractive to teenagers. In 1997 the alcoholic milk drink 'Moo' was introduced. In England, in 1990, 42% of boys aged 15 and 39% of girls questioned had had an alcoholic drink in the previous week. 26% of 16--17-year-old boys who had had a drink in the last week admitted to 'binge' drinking (more than 8 units on one occasion).

Sexual health. In England and Wales in 1990 there were 55 500 births to mothers under 20, and 1300 to under 16s. Figure 1.20 shows the trend in teenage birth rate up to 1991. Over half of pregnant 14--15-year-olds in England and Wales choose termination if they become pregnant, whereas nearly 70% of pregnant 19-year-olds continue with the pregnancy.

INEQUALITIES IN CHILD HEALTH

The term 'inequality' describes the variation in health status by social class across the population. Social class data have been collected for many years in the UK, making it easy to compare mortality and morbidity in different socioeconomic groups. The most important factor

Table 1.6   Measures used as indices of deprivation

Jarman Index	Townsend Index
Elderly living alone	Unemployment
Children aged under 5 years	Overcrowding
Unskilled (social class V)	Car ownership
Unemployed	Home ownership
Single parent families	
Overcrowded (> 1 person per room)	
Mobility (changing house in a year)	
Ethnic (New Commonwealth and Pakistan)	

which separates the classes is income, yet social class does not measure income well (nor environmental factors such as housing). The Townsend Deprivation Index is a measure of material deprivation which relies on demographic data collected in the census; this measure is best applied to a small geographic area which is likely to be socially homogeneous. Areas can then be compared and analysed according to their degree of deprivation. Social class is intended to be applied to individuals whereas the Townsend Index is normally applied to populations. Another measure of material deprivation is the Jarman Index or Under-privileged Area Score which uses eight variables (see Table 1.6) to give a deprivation ranking to an area or practice population.

Extent of inequalities. Child mortality at all ages shows a social class gradient. Figure 1.21 shows mortality aged 1–14 years by social class. The variation is much greater for specific causes and is highest for accidents: Figure 1.22 shows the mortality for traffic collisions for 1--14-year-olds, where there is a five-fold difference between class I and class V mortality. There is a 9-fold difference in fire deaths, 2.5-fold for congenital anomalies and 2-fold for deaths from respiratory conditions between these classes. Similar differences are seen for morbidity, with marked variations in low birth weight, pneumonia, bronchiolitis, otitis media, asthma, gastroenteritis, cerebral palsy, child nutrition, dental caries, accidents, behavioural problems, smoking, drug use and teenage pregnancy.

Reasons for inequality. Four possible reasons for the health inequalities described above are shown in Box 1.5.

Artefact is excluded because of the consistency

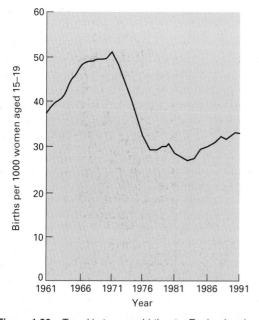

Figure 1.20   Trend in teenage birth rate, England and Wales 1961–91. Births per 1000 women age 15–19. Source: OPCS FMI, Population Trends.

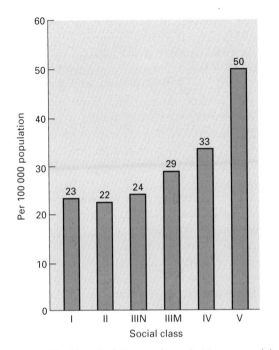

Figure 1.21 Mortality (all causes) age 1–14 years: social class, England and Wales 1979–80 and 1982–83. Source: OPCS DS 8. 4-year averages.

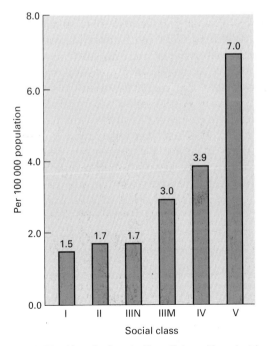

Figure 1.22 Mortality from traffic collision with pedestrian age 1–14 years: social class, England and Wales 1979–80 and 1982–83. Source: OPCS DS 8. 4-year averages.

> **Box 1.5** Possible reasons for health inequalities (Black Report, 1980)
>
> - Artefact of measurement (e.g. bias of class measurement)
> - Social selection (i.e. health determines social position rather than vice versa)
> - Behavioural and cultural differences (e.g. smoking, ignorance about diet)
> - Structural (e.g. income level, housing circumstances)

of the findings whatever measures are used and because of the differences found between countries as well as within countries. Social selection has been shown in longitudinal studies to explain little of the difference between socio-economic groups; social mobility is a relatively recent phenomenon whereas social class differences in health were seen in the nineteenth century.

Behavioural and cultural factors are very closely linked to income differences. Smoking, for example, is common in low income families because it is stress relieving and a ready source of pleasurable experience when few other leisure activities are available. A 'healthy diet' is more expensive than one based on cheap calories, and food costs are a major factor for poor families. Whilst education and lack of knowledge about health are important, they are outweighed as causes of the inequalities by economic and environmental factors. Although education is important in remedying the variations, it will not be effective without action on the economic disparities, which are paramount (see below). There is further valuable discussion on the socio-economic determinants of health inequalities, and presentation of interventions to reduce these inequalities, in the Acheson report commissioned by the government in 1997.

CHILDREN IN SOCIETY

This section covers the changes which have taken place in society in recent years and their effects on children's health. Mortality and morbidity statistics show that children are very much healthier now than they have ever been in the past, but there is no cause for complacency as certain conditions are increasing in prevalence

Table 1.7 Effects of poverty on child health

Factor	Effect
High food costs	Poor nutrition
Poor housing	Asthma, respiratory infections, accidents, burns
Lack of safe play space	Accidents
Stress	Emotional distress, behavioural problems

and the gap in health between the poor and the well-off appears to be widening.

Poverty. The effects of poverty on child health are listed in Table 1.7. There is no official definition of poverty in the UK. The most widely accepted criterion is that poverty is below half the national mean household income, as used in the European Union. Table 1.8 shows the number and trend for children in the UK since 1979, showing the steady year-on-year increase which has taken place over this period. Figures from the European statistics agency show that the current figure, 32%, is the highest in Europe (Figure 1.23). According to Spencer (see Further reading), the reasons for the increase in child poverty are rising unemployment, the increase in lone-parent families and changes in the tax and benefit structure.

Family structure. The number of children living in lone-parent families is rapidly rising, see Figure 1.24. Divorce is the most common reason for lone-parenthood, but there has been a steep increase in the number of mothers who have never married. It is quite possible for a lone parent to provide for all a child's needs but the additional stresses are considerable; without outside support in the form of finance or good child care the child becomes vulnerable to physical and emotional ill-health.

Diet. Children's diets have changed considerably over the past 20 years as a result of increased income, pocket money and food marketing, particularly on television. Whilst it is difficult for families on low income to provide a healthy diet (see Table 1.1) consumption of high sugar, high fat snacks and convenience foods has increased greatly among those with disposable income. The consumption of high sugar soft drinks has rocketed. This has skewed nutritional intake away from Health of the Nation targets and contributes to the rising levels of obesity seen in young people.

Exercise. Children are taking exercise less than in the past because of greater car usage (particularly for journeys to school), more time spent watching television and reduced emphasis on sport in school. In 1990 a third of males and over half of females aged 16–24 took moderate exercise on less than 12 20-minute occasions in four weeks. This reduction in exercise is likely to persist into adulthood and will lead to increased obesity and a greater risk of coronary heart disease at a younger age. The well known stress-reducing effects of exercise are also missed.

Traffic. Car usage in the UK is increasing dramatically. Car travel has doubled since 1970 to an average of 6500 miles per person per year, while travel on other passenger vehicles (mainly buses and coaches) has fallen by a quarter, to less than 600 miles per person per year. 7% of car journeys are less than half a mile and 24% are between half and one mile. The percentage of 7–8-year-olds travelling to school alone (on

Table 1.8 Numbers below the poverty line. Source: Households below average income. A statistical analysis 1979–1993/4. 1996 The Stationery Office, London.

	Total numbers below poverty line	% Total population below poverty line	Total numbers of children below poverty line	% Total child population below poverty line
1979	5.0 m	9	1.4 m	10
1988/89	12.0 m	22	3.1 m	25
1991/92	13.9 m	25	4.1 m	32
1992/93	14.1 m	25	4.3 m	33
1993/94	13.7 m	24	4.2 m	32

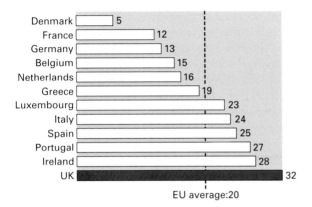

Figure 1.23 Proportion of children living in poor households 1993. Source: Eurostat.

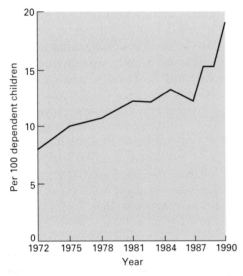

Figure 1.24 Trend in children living in lone-parent families 1972–90. Source: Haskey 1991; OPCS GHS 21.

foot or by bicycle) dropped from 80% in 1971 to only 9% in 1990. The more cars congest the roads, the less parents trust their children to travel independently.

Increased traffic has three adverse effects on children's health:

1. road accidents, a major cause of children's deaths
2. pollution from car exhausts, which increases respiratory symptoms and asthma attacks
3. reduction in exercise as discussed above.

> **Box 1.6** Methods for reduction of adverse health effects of traffic
>
> * Reduction of road traffic in cities through improved public transport and road pricing schemes
> * Traffic calming in residential neighbourhoods
> * Separation of car traffic from pedestrians and cyclists
> * Production of less polluting cars

Methods for reducing the adverse health effects of traffic are listed in Box 1.6.

Television. Television, video games and computers have had a major impact on children's activities; a considerable amount of time is spent in front of a screen by most children from toddlerhood upwards. Whilst television is an educational medium it is passive—no input is required from the child. The main adverse effects are reduced exercise levels, reduced communication within the family, and an increased tendency to violence among those who are at high risk. Fatty and sugary foods are marketed on TV, resulting in overnutrition. Parents need to be aware of the risks, protect their children from excessive TV watching, and encourage a discriminating approach to viewing habits.

Ethnic minorities. Separate health data are not available in the UK in relation to ethnic origin. Data on birth and death are available only by country of birth, which is of little relevance as ethnic minority populations become established in this country. Children growing up in ethnic minority families face health problems arising from three sources: discrimination, socio-economic factors and heredity. Discrimination against people of a different skin colour and a different culture is widespread in British society and affects the health service as well as other public services. Language differences and ignorance of culture can lead to many problems, one example of which is illustrated in Box 1.7. It behoves health professionals to understand the cultural and religious values of their patients and be familiar with naming systems to ensure that families from different backgrounds are treated with respect.

Ethnic minority families are more likely to be

Box 1.7

'In one of the antenatal clinics where I work they call out the women's names from the files and if the women don't come forward after the second call, they put the file right back to the bottom of the pile. And quite often the way they pronounce the names is completely unrecognisable, and so the women don't go forward and they may wait hours and hours never realising that their names have been called several times.'

Clinic worker

Source: Mares et al 1985

---

poor than the ethnic majority population. It is now thought that the increased prevalence of tuberculosis among people of Asian origin is related to poverty rather than their country of origin.

Certain diseases are more common in particular ethnic groups and this may have implications for screening. Thalassaemia and glucose-6-phosphate dehydrogenase deficiency are more common in people of Mediterranean origin; sickle cell disease is relatively common in families of Afro-Caribbean origin; lactase deficiency occurs in populations originating in many countries in southern Asia and Africa.

Children's rights and consent. Since the adoption of the Convention on the Rights of the Child by the United Nations in 1989 (see Box 1.8), there has been much greater awareness of the

---

Box 1.8   United Nations Convention on the Rights of the Child: key points

- Best interests of the child to have primary consideration
- Children and young people should not be separated from parents or carers
- Children and young people have the right to express their views and have them taken into account
- Children and young people have the right to privacy and confidentiality
- Children and young people have the right to information
- Children should be protected from violence
- Children with disabilities have the right to special services
- Children from minority groups have the right to enjoy their own cultures, religions and languages

---

need to respect children's rights within health care. Health workers should be aware of the Convention and listen to children's views, provide them with adequate information to take decisions, keep their history confidential and consult with them in the planning of services.

Consent in children is legally binding over the age of 16 years; however the so-called Gillick principle, introduced following a court case on the use of contraceptives by young people, established that children under 16 years old can give legally valid consent to medical or surgical treatment, independent of their parents' wishes, provided that they have sufficient understanding of their condition and what is proposed.

Role of health professionals. Doctors and nurses are in a good position to observe the effects on children's health of the changes in society described above and can have considerable influence on policy makers. This is further discussed under Public policy and child health, below.

THE SCOPE FOR PREVENTION

This section covers issues of prevention in child health.

Role of the health service

There is much greater scope for preventive activities outside the health service than within, for example by reduction of poverty and provision of improved housing, child care, education and environmental measures to prevent accidents. Health professionals are, however, in a good position to draw attention to the need for such measures and, on occasion, to co-ordinate their provision. Within the health service itself the scope is more limited but much can be done (Box 1.9).

What should be prevented and what is preventable?

Certain criteria should be applied to decide how resources should be allocated in prevention:

- Importance of the condition in relation to mortality and morbidity.

Box 1.9   Preventive measures within the health service

- *Primary prevention:* prevention of infectious disease by immunisation
- *Secondary prevention:* early detection of congenital disorders by screening
- *Tertiary prevention:* prevention of complications and handicap in chronic disease and disability by effective treatment

Education may also be effective in primary prevention but usually only if it is provided in conjunction with structural change, e.g. loan of home safety equipment offered at the same time as advice/education on avoidance of high risk situations

---

- Is the condition either common and moderately serious (e.g. otitis media) or rare and very serious (e.g. phenylketonuria)?
- Are effective preventive measures available?
- Are the measures cost-effective?

These are similar to the Wilson & Jungner criteria for screening programmes (Box 1.1). Using the first criterion, the top five conditions would be accidents, perinatal causes, congenital anomalies, respiratory disorders and cancer. Effective measures are not available for cancer and respiratory disorders; perinatal causes depend on good obstetric care; congenital disorders require secondary prevention; accidents require action mainly from agencies outside the health service. Hence the scope for effective prevention is not great, but this is partly because there is a dearth of good evidence in relation to effectiveness.

Organisation of programmes for prevention
(see also p. 31)

There are four national programmes for prevention in the UK (Table 1.9), though not all are developed to the same scale of efficiency.

Immunisation programme. This is further described on page 331. The immunisation programme is the only centralised preventive programme for children and is directed by a separate unit in the Department of Health under the professional guidance of the Joint Committee on Vaccination and Immunisation, which sets out immunisation policy. Each district has an Immunisation Co-ordinator who has accountability for the programme; yearly meetings are held for all co-ordinators in London. There are clear targets and strategies, supported by a good data system. This system has been remarkably successful—even though the service is delivered by a wide variety of different professionals working in separate departments, very high uptakes have been achieved across the country to the extent that eradication of certain diseases is being considered possible.

Screening programmes (Table 1.10). See also page 35. Screening programmes for children are much less tightly organised than the immunisation programme, and there is no central structure. The Guthrie test for phenylketonuria, hypothyroidism and certain other inborn errors of metabolism is the best organised and has been subjected to national audit. Collection of specimens is organised regionally and there are procedures to detect missed cases. Other screening tests are discussed in the Joint Working Party report, *Health for All Children*, but there is no central or regional organisation and each district runs its own system with varying degrees of efficiency. The Department of Health has a National Screening Committee which covers all age groups and provides advice to purchasing authorities who commission services from their local providers.

Child health surveillance. See also page 31. This programme is described in the Joint Working

Table 1.9   Programmes of prevention

Programme	Status of co-ordination	Co-ordinator
Immunisation programme	Co-ordinated nationally	Department of Health
Screening programmes (e.g. PKU)	Co-ordinated regionally or in district	Varies
Child Health surveillance/promotion	National working party but co-ordinated in district	Varies
School health surveillance	National working party	Varies

Table 1.10 Conditions screened for in the UK

Condition	Test	Age
Phenylketonuria, hypothyroidism	Guthrie test	10 days
Congenital dislocation of the hips	Ortolani test	birth, 6 weeks
Congenital cataract	Inspection	birth, 6 weeks
Congenital heart disease	Examination	birth, 6 weeks
Undescended testicles	Examination	birth, 6 weeks
Short stature	Height measurement	2 years, 3½ years, 5 years
Hearing loss	Distraction test, audiometry	9 months, 5 years
Squint, poor visual acuity	Orthoptic screen*, vision testing	3 years, 5 years

* Orthoptic screening is not carried out in all districts

Party report, *Health for All Children*. Again, there is no national organisation and little evaluation as yet of the effectiveness of the various schemes used. Health promotion programmes (Box 1.10) are put into practice by health visitors, often with little support from other professionals.

School health promotion. The programme of school health is described in the Joint Working Party report on services for school-aged children (Polnay 1995). Broad recommendations are made in this report but again it is left to districts to determine how they are carried out. The service is in the process of change as the focus moves from medical examination of school children, which has little proven benefit, to focused strategies using school nurses with specific skills and specialist backup from school paediatricians who are part of an integrated child health service. Only a limited amount of 'screening' is now carried out in school—most of the work is divided between 'health promotion' (which includes immunisation, Box 1.11) and support of children with a wide variety of chronic problems.

Public policy and child health

As noted above, the health service has a some-

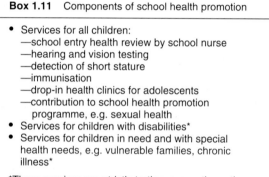

Box 1.11 Components of school health promotion

- Services for all children:
  —school entry health review by school nurse
  —hearing and vision testing
  —detection of short stature
  —immunisation
  —drop-in health clinics for adolescents
  —contribution to school health promotion programme, e.g. sexual health
- Services for children with disabilities*
- Services for children in need and with special health needs, e.g. vulnerable families, chronic illness*

*These services are strictly tertiary prevention rather than health promotion

what limited role in prevention in child health since the solution of many of the problems lies outside its remit. Health workers, however, do have a legitimate role in drawing the attention of policy makers to the problems and influencing both local and national policies to place a greater emphasis on children's needs (Box 1.12). The term 'healthy alliances' is given to the process

Box 1.10 Health promotion programmes for pre-school children (Hall 1996)

- Prevention of sudden infant death syndrome
- Prevention of accidental injury
- Promotion of good nutrition
- Promotion of good parenting and prevention of child abuse
- Prevention of behavioural problems

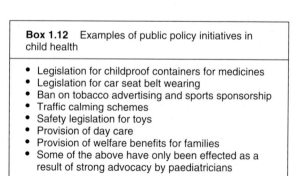

Box 1.12 Examples of public policy initiatives in child health

- Legislation for childproof containers for medicines
- Legislation for car seat belt wearing
- Ban on tobacco advertising and sports sponsorship
- Traffic calming schemes
- Safety legislation for toys
- Provision of day care
- Provision of welfare benefits for families
- Some of the above have only been effected as a result of strong advocacy by paediatricians

of different agencies working together (usually at local level) with the aim of improving health:

- *Child injury prevention groups* at district level bring together health providers, roads, education and health promotion departments, and local parents and voluntary groups.
- *School nutrition action groups* at school level bring together the health service, teachers, providers of school meals, dieticians, the health promotion department, pupils and parents.
- *Food co-operatives* at community level bring together local people, health professionals, dieticians, consumer groups and food marketing agencies.

Health of the Nation

In 1992 the Department of Health laid down a series of health targets in a White Paper entitled *The Health of the Nation*. The targets were selected because of their importance, their achievability and the availability of data to measure progress. More recently a 'Health of the Young Nation' strategy has been adopted to give a higher profile to those aspects of the targets which affect young people. The targets chosen were coronary heart disease and stroke, cancers, accidents, sexually transmitted disease and sexual health, and mental illness (Box 1.13). Limited progress is being made in many of the target areas because they are dependent on factors which require fundamental change across the whole range of government policy, e.g. food policies and marketing.

Box 1.13   Health of the Nation targets for children

- To reduce the proportion of men and women aged 16–64 who are obese by at least 25% and 33% respectively by 2005
- To reduce smoking prevalence of 11- –15-year-olds by at least 33% by 1994 (to less than 6%)
- To reduce the death rate for accidents among children under 15 by at least 33% by 2005
- To reduce the incidence of gonorrhoea by at least 20% by 1995, as an indicator of HIV/AIDS trends
- To reduce the overall suicide rate by at least 15% by the year 2000

Children Act and other legislation for children

The Children Act, introduced in England and Wales in 1989 and Scotland in 1995, brought together much of the legislation for children in line with today's principles of parent partnership and a focus on the child's needs. Its key features:

- define parental responsibilities
- give paramount consideration to welfare of the child
- state that the child's wishes and feelings be respected
- define responsibilities for 'children in need'
- prescribe a register for children with disabilities
- describe court orders in relation to custody and access, to education, and to child protection.

Two other major areas of legislation affect children in the UK: the UN Convention on the Rights of the Child, ratified by the UK government in 1991, which is not binding by law in this country; and the Education Act (1993) which covers issues of special education and children with special educational needs. Features of the Education Act include:

- The emphasis should be on the child's needs rather than on the particular condition which affects them.
- Children's educational needs should be met wherever they are.
- Children with special educational needs should be in mainstream school rather than special school by preference.
- Parents should participate at every stage in the process.
- The wishes and feelings of the child should be ascertained.
- Health and education both contribute to the Statement of Special Educational Need.
- The process of deciding on the child's educational needs (the Code of Practice) is discussed in detail.

ORGANISATION OF SERVICES

This section describes the organisation of services for children in the National Health Service (NHS)

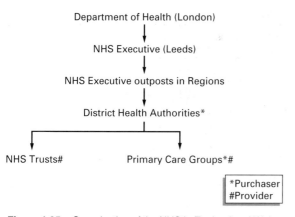

Department of Health (London)

NHS Executive (Leeds)

NHS Executive outposts in Regions

District Health Authorities*

NHS Trusts#   Primary Care Groups*#

*Purchaser
#Provider

Figure 1.25 Organisation of the NHS in England and Wales.

Box 1.14 Primary Care Team	
General practitioner	Self employed, paid by health authority
Receptionist	Employed by GP
Practice nurse	Employed by GP, carries out nursing tasks within surgery
District nurse	Employed by NHS Trust, attached to practice, carries out nursing tasks in patients' homes
Health visitor	Employed by NHS Trust, attached to practice, preventive work primarily with under 5s, sometimes with elderly
Other members may include practice counsellor, psychologist, physiotherapist, dietician	

in England and Wales (see Figure 1.25). Scotland and N. Ireland have separate arrangements.

Primary care teams

Primary health care (PHC) is the first level of care in the health service. It is defined by WHO as:

Essential health care based on practical, scientifically sound and socially acceptable methods and technology made universally accessible to individuals and families in the community through their full participation, and at a cost that the community and country can afford to maintain…Primary health care addresses the main health problems in the community, providing promotive, preventive, curative and rehabilitative services accordingly; PHC includes at least: education concerning prevailing health problems…promotion of food supply and basic nutrition…an adequate supply of safe water and basic sanitation…maternal and child health care including family planning…PHC requires and promotes maximum community and individual self-reliance and participation in the planning, organisation, operation and control of primary health care.

PHC consists of more than medical care and the services in the UK are still far from the WHO ideal, though much progress is being made. The Primary Care Team in the UK is primarily a medical team which provides curative services for its practice population (Box 1.14); prevention is an important part of its work but the scope for health promotion is limited at present and collaboration with agencies outside the health service is virtually non-existent.

Primary care groups. Primary care groups (PCGs) were introduced in the 1997 White Paper on the NHS as a way of ensuring that primary care teams respond to the needs of the localities they serve, and to give primary care more power in the NHS hierarchy. They began working in April 1999. Each group covers a population of approximately 100 000 and may be chaired by a general practitioner; there is a board which includes nurses, a manager and representatives of other agencies. The PCG has a budget and will be responsible for purchasing secondary services as well as developing local services to meet local need. Hence this represents a move towards the ideal of primary health care as originally outlined by the World Health Organization.

Hospital and community services

These services are provided by an NHS Trust—a hospital or community unit which is funded by the health authority (see Purchaser/provider split, below) and has considerable financial autonomy within the NHS. Many Trusts, however, have severe financial restrictions as their funding is related to the local population size; if they provide additional services which are not specially funded (e.g. tertiary services) then they may be subject to cuts. Their leeway for raising money is limited: some do it by seeking drug company or industry sponsorship and some by selling their services to other districts.

Table 1.11 Hospital and community services for children

Hospital services	Community health services
Consultant paediatricians	Consultant paediatricians (community child health)
Consultant paediatric surgeons	Consultant child and family psychiatrists
Consultant paediatric radiologist	Senior clinical medical officer/associate specialist
Consultant paediatric pathologist	Clinical medical officer/staff grade paediatrician
Registrars	Registrars
Senior House Officers	Senior House Officers
Children's nurses	Dental surgeons
Play therapists	Dental nurses
Teachers	Clinical psychologists
Physiotherapists	Community physiotherapists, occupational therapists
Speech therapists	Community speech therapists
	Health education officers
	Audiometricians
	Orthoptists
	Community paediatric nurses
	Health visitors
	School nurses
	Auxiliaries
	Clinic clerks

The development of Trusts has made the provision of an integrated child health service very difficult. This is because community and hospital staff are often included in different trusts with different management structures and hence may appear to be in competition with each other (Table 1.11).

Integrated child health service

The fragmentation of child health services has been criticised for many years because it makes it difficult to deliver services effectively. Until 1974 community health services were administered by local authorities; thereafter they entered the NHS but were distinct from hospital paediatric services as well as from GP services. This situation was addressed by a working party set up by the government in 1973 under the chairmanship of Professor Donald Court, the Professor of Child Health in Newcastle upon Tyne. The committee reported in 1976 under the title *Fit for the Future*; its recommendations were enormously influential and have now been almost fully implemented (Box 1.15).

There has been very widespread appointment of consultant paediatricians (community child health) who have been instrumental in bringing

---

Box 1.15 Key recommendations of the Court Report

- Integrated child health service: 'The organisational structure of the child health services should be changed to provide an integrated 2-tier system based on comprehensive primary care firmly linked with supporting consultant and hospital care'
- General practitioner paediatricians*
- Child health visitors
- Community paediatric nurses
- Consultant community paediatricians
- Multiprofessional district 'handicap' team
- Child health surveillance for all children provided within the primary care team
- Every school to have a nominated school doctor and nurse
- Better facilities for counselling and sex education of young people
- Fluoridation of water
- A national Committee for Children#

*This recommendation was not supported by GP organisations and has not been implemented
#This recommendation was briefly implemented but the committee was later dissolved

---

about integration on the lines recommended by the Court Report. The segregation of services between separate Trusts has made full integration impossible, and a variety of mechanisms such as bridging committees and boards have been used to reduce the separation, not always successfully.

Purchaser/provider split

This was a key policy provision of the Conservative government's NHS reforms; it was intended to reduce costs and place the responsibility for any service cuts on district health authorities rather than the government. It was also intended to bring the perspectives of local people to bear on health service planning.

NHS facilities were classed as either 'purchasers' or 'providers'. District health authorities and primary care groups are purchasers of services; NHS Trusts and GP practices are providers. The purchaser has an obligation to assess the health needs of the community it serves and hence decide what services are required. It then sets up a contract with a provider, which agrees to provide these services. If the provider fails in its task then the contract may be re-allocated. The system has been only partially successful: the spending patterns of many Trusts could not easily be altered as hospitals are essentially demand-led and these demands are continually growing because of the increasing age of the population and the introduction of new and more expensive drugs and investigations. The funding of the NHS will be a major problem for any government and many commentators believe that some form of rationing (sometimes called 'priority setting') will have to be introduced after wide debate with the general public.

Public health

The term 'public health' is used to describe both a function and a specific service. The function is defined at the beginning of this chapter; the service is described below.

Public health within the NHS is led by the Chief Medical Officer (CMO), based in the Department of Health. (There are separate CMOs for England, Wales, Scotland and Northern Ireland.) The CMO is responsible for the Health of the Nation strategy and produces an annual public health report. Each district has a Director of Public Health and several consultants in public health medicine who have specific areas of responsibility. These consultants are based in the

health authority ('purchaser' arm) because they lead the process of assessment of health need which determines the basis of contracts with providers. There is also a consultant in communicable disease control who may be based with a provider and is responsible for the prevention and control of infectious disease outbreaks.

Assessment of health need is a key process in the new system but is difficult to carry out effectively and comprehensively. Sources of information for the assessment are variable in availability and quality (Box 1.16).

Local authority children's services

The local authority provides many services for children which operate alongside those provided by the health service (Box 1.17). Child health is related so closely to education and living conditions that health professionals must collaborate closely with teachers, social workers and others working outside the health service. It is also important that there is a mechanism for joint service planning (see Children's Service Plans, below).

Box 1.16 Assessment of health needs: sources of data

- Epidemiology: mortality and morbidity statistics
- Demographic data: age spread, income, family structure, housing, ethnic mix
- Existing service provision
- Community's expressed needs*

*Specific survey work is required to determine expressed needs

---

Box 1.17 Local authority services for children

- Education department: schools and nursery schools, special schools, support services for special needs, educational welfare officers, educational psychologists, health education co-ordinators for schools
- Social services department: social workers, adoption and fostering service, day nurseries and family centres, family support, home helps, respite care, children's homes, welfare rights, looked after children

Children's service plans

In 1992, local authorities were advised by the government to draw up Children's Service Plans for 'children in need' (see Box 1.18). In 1994 the Audit Commissioner recommended that Children's Service Planning should be mandatory, and in 1996 Parliament amended the Children Act to require local authorities to plan Children's Services in consultation with a number of agencies. The early focus on children in need was extended to all services provided by the local authority and health authority. The intention was to ensure that services provided locally for children were planned and organised jointly, bringing together in particular health, education and social services in addition to voluntary agencies (Box 1.19).

In Newcastle 'children in need' was interpreted by an inter-agency group as including the following groups:

* children living in poverty and at high risk of family breakdown

---

Box 1.18 Definition of children in need (Children Act 1989)

A child is 'in need' if:
* he/she is unlikely to achieve or maintain, or have the opportunity of achieving or maintaining, a reasonable standard of health or development without the provision of services by a local authority
* his/her health or development is likely to be significantly impaired, or further impaired, without the provision of such services
* he/she is disabled

Box 1.19 Selected headings of Newcastle upon Tyne Children's Services Plan 1997–2000

* Overall City Council Strategy for children and young people
* Joint planning and consultation
* Children in need
* Children's rights
* Equal opportunities
* Services action areas including:
  —young carers
  —children under 8
  —children living in poverty
  —children with disabilities
  —children at risk of abuse and neglect

---

* children whose home conditions are unsatisfactory
* children separated from their parents and families
* children not achieving their full health potential
* children whose achievements fall significantly short of their educational potential
* children at risk of abuse and neglect
* children with caring responsibilities
* children at risk of offending
* children with disabilities
* children living on the margins of society.

As an example, one of the targets in the plan is the development of a joint review and planning process for children with disabilities in which children and their parents play the central role. The opportunities provided for improved inter-agency working are great but will require an additional infusion of resources from local authorities and health authorities.

FURTHER READING

Acheson D 1998 Independent inquiry into inequalities in health. The Stationery Office, London

Black D, Morris J, Smith C, Townsend P 1980 Inequalities in health: report of a research working group. Department of Health and Social Security, London

Court SDM 1976 Fit for the future. The report of the Committee on Child Health Services. HMSO, London

Department of Health 1992 Health of the nation. HMSO, London

Hall D 1996 Health for all children. Oxford University Press, Oxford

Hall D, Hill P 1996 The child with a disability. Blackwell Science, London

Mares P, Henley A, Baxter C 1985 Health care in multiracial Britain. Health Education Council, London

Polnay D 1995 Health needs of school age children. British Paediatric Association, London

Rose G, Barker DJP, Coggon D 1997 Epidemiology for the uninitiated, 4th edn. British Medical Association, London

Spencer N 1996 Poverty and child health. Radcliffe Medical Press, Oxford

UN Convention on the Rights of the Child 1989 United Nations, New York

Woodroffe C, Glickman M, Barker M, Power C 1993 Children, teenagers and health—the key data. Open University Press, Milton Keynes

WHO 1996 The health of youth (1993–94 survey). WHO, Geneva

Internet addresses

UK national statistics
http://www.doh.gov.uk/public.stats1.htm

Accidents
http://www.rospa.co.uk

Environmental health
http://www.cehn.org

2

Child health informatics and surveillance

Brent Taylor

INFORMATICS

Good information is an essential accompaniment to a good service—for planning, provision, clinical/financial monitoring and for service development (Box 2.1). The NHS Executive in 1996 acknowledged the importance of accurate and accessible information in child health 'to assess

---

Box 2.1 Good quality data is required in community child health:

- To support the provision of preventive services—immunisation, health promotion and surveillance—which should often be targeted particularly to children in vulnerable families
- To record health information on individual children, such as very pre-term delivery or allergy to medication
- To support children with disabilities, especially children with special educational needs, in co-operation with local education services and to document the use of services by such children
- To identify children in need, in co-operation with local social services
- To assess health needs within a population for the commissioning of health care and to monitor how effectively identified needs are met
- To monitor the development of pre-school children and, for children with persisting health problems or disability, to monitor their progress throughout the school years to handover to adult services
- To support the clinical management and care of children with significant health problems, particularly those with chronic disorders or disabilities
- For public health and audit purposes
- For research purposes, especially epidemiological research, and for service development, e.g. the evaluation of screening programmes and other health care interventions

health needs, to monitor the health and development of children and the performance of providers in delivering child health services'. The fifth report by the Korner Committee to the Secretary of State for Health stated that:

screening and surveillance of children, as well as immunisation, require a level of administration and co-ordination which cannot effectively be undertaken without a computer-based system. As most programmes directed towards children are intended for every child, there is agreement on the need to develop a single integrated administrative system in each district designed to schedule appointments and to ensure an accurate record of immunisation, surveillance, screening tests and action in relation to special education needs.

Terminology and data handling

'Data' and 'information' do not encompass the totality of 'information management and technology' (the term used by the United Kingdom Department of Health). 'Informatics', an awkward word, is increasingly used and encompasses the structure and process of data/information collection, preparation and analysis (Figure 2.1) together with the associated machines and technology. Much data is recorded on paper forms then entered into computer databases by information staff who often work in a central child health administration department. Considerable progress has been made with desktop and handheld equipment to allow the inputting of data directly at the place where it is 'captured', i.e. where a health worker has face-to-face con-

tact with a patient and/or is doing something such as giving an immunisation. This direct inputting, with standard formatting, increases the likelihood of complete, accurate and intelligible recording. Training for field-workers and information/clerical staff and data/system quality control are critical aspects of a successful informatics programme.

Developments needed

Child health information systems are not perfect and are often not optimally used. Much of the information held on computerised child health systems has not been used to full effect: this is in part due to lack of appreciation of the many uses to which such data can be put, including the monitoring of clinical practice and service activities, such as missed appointments, which have considerable resource implications. Improvements can be introduced if the available data is systematically scrutinised for inefficiencies or ineffectiveness. Any changes which have been introduced as a result of this scrutiny can be monitored in their turn.

Areas where improvements need to be made

Data quality. Poor quality input results in poor output (garbage in = garbage out: GIGO). Information must be collected by properly trained staff in a systematic way using standardised terminology, with validity and other checks. Quality control monitoring is essential, but not widely practised. Agreement is required on an essential core data set for child health.

Standardisation. Many different child health systems are in use and there is insufficient standardisation among them. There are some advantages—choice and competition, with associated cost-efficiencies and innovation to capture new customers—however children move between districts which may have different systems; disadvantaged children are most likely to move and are most likely to have health or developmental problems. There is a need for standardised activity coding, e.g. for outpatient/ accident and emergency department attendance,

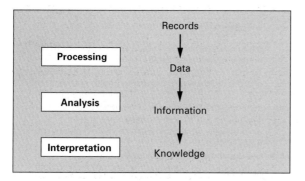

Figure 2.1 The information cascade, from recording to knowledge: data must be analysed and information interpreted in order for it to be useful.

and standardised data collection and recording, e.g. agreed coding for disability in childhood. Health authorities/commissioners should require providers to produce centrally agreed common basic data that is accurate, complete and up-to-date. This should be associated with regular audit of local systems regarding accuracy, completeness and timeliness of data using national accreditation standards and methods, including the ability of the system to make appropriate links with other systems.

Accessibility. The data that is available can be difficult to access. User-friendly interrogation tools are essential; information staff must be accessible and enthusiastic. Systems need commitment and support. Clinicians and managers should become skilled in using information and in developing the uses to which this information can be put.

Linkage. There is often poor or limited communication between the different health service systems: not only between districts, e.g. adjacent child health services, but also within districts, e.g. with other community services, the local hospital, general practices, and the health authority. The need to link systems is a priority. There should be central direction from the government and Department of Health to providers, requiring linked standardised information on a population basis for public health and other monitoring purposes.

Integration. There is in general poor or minimal communication between health service systems and other services dealing with children such as social services, education and voluntary agencies. Some districts have used the 'special needs' module of their child health computing system as the basis for a shared disability register (as required by the Children Act 1989) between health and social services. Child protection and the statementing process for children with special educational needs can also be co-ordinated and made more efficient and accurate by linkage of the health special needs module and local authority systems, with appropriate security and confidentiality safeguards.

Outcomes. There is little routinely-provided outcome information for monitoring, audit or research purposes. Methods need to be developed to record routinely the outcome of referrals made from the pre-school and school surveillance programme. At present a child may be recorded as having a problem but there is no facility to identify if any arrangement was made to assess the problem, whether or not the child attended any appointment made, whether the assessment confirmed a problem (or that the referral was a false positive—the child did not have the suspected problem) or what treatment and/or further follow-up was arranged.

Profiling. Little reliable socio-demographic data is recorded. Ethnic status and socio-economic status—the latter regularly updated—should be routinely documented; additional factors associated with disadvantage, such as maternal educational attainment and parental smoking habit, would further enable the targeting of resources.

Fear of new technology. Information and the tools to deal with it are servants not masters. Luddite attitudes, often associated with inappropriate concerns regarding data access and confidentiality, require sympathetic re-orientation. Those who hold such attitudes should be helped to see and understand the usefulness and necessity of informatics, which can improve the quality of life for patients and health care workers (e.g. by alleviating dull repetitive clerical activity) and dramatically improve efficiency.

Relevance. There is concern that the systems currently employed do not provide useful or appropriate information. The huge investment in systems has not been matched by investment in research, evaluation or training. Systems require on-going development and regular critical review to ensure that the aims of the process are being met and that the aims themselves are appropriate. There is also a need for regular critical research-based review of the usefulness of current child health activities so that change can be instituted when necessary and current activity abandoned if non-productive, with resources directed elsewhere.

The need for standardised data collection and central co-ordination

Children and families frequently move between districts; this particularly affects children in disadvantaged families where health problems are more likely. It is important that the child's computerised record is also transferred to provide continuity for routine monitoring and for any special needs. There is increasing awareness that information should be collected in a standard form to facilitate its interpretation. The National Child Health Informatics Consortium, a co-ordinating body representing some two thirds of NHS child health providers in England, Wales and Northern Ireland, has published a functional specification with a recommended common data set for a child health system to which suppliers of such systems should adhere. This 'gold standard' should be demanded by health service commissioners. Further development of the specification is being undertaken to ensure continuing clinical usefulness.

General practitioner systems and system linkage

General practice has been in the forefront of computer development in British medicine. Most practices provide age/sex data, and some produce very sophisticated information. General practice is increasingly the base for preventive child health care: the associated information flow requires close co-operation between individual general practices and community child health computing systems. The latter are mainly run by community providers but may also be managed by the local health authority. This arrangement facilitates linkage and co-ordination between child health and GP computing systems.

Child health systems can automatically generate appointments for immunisations or health promotion checks. Primary health care team workers usually record preventive health activity data in the (parent-held) personal child health record and send a carbonised slip to the local child health computing department. Some practices and clinics directly input data to the computing system. An interactive system which provides the primary team or field worker with easy access to information on individual children or analysis of the practice population increases enthusiasm, and such feedback promotes accu-

rate and complete data entry. Some feedback—such as regular reports from the child health system—is necessary to maintain co-operation with the systems. Child health systems can link with health authority systems, and immunisation records on the child health system can be the basis for general practice target payments with a reduction in duplication and paperwork. Other intersystem linkage is possible: hospital episode data can be linked with community information to demonstrate relationships between hospital events and the use of child health services, e.g. by the survivors of very pre-term delivery. General practitioner information and accident and emergency/outpatient data is not yet sufficiently standardised or accurate for such linkage, but developments are continuing.

The personal (parent-held) child health record (PCHR)

The PCHR contributes to high quality child health care through the involvement of parents/carers in the delivery of preventive child health programmes. The PCHR provides:

- easily accessible information on the child's development and health service interventions
- a vehicle for conveying health promotion information to families with children
- a priming mechanism for families to identify and inform professionals of any health or developmental problems in the child.
- a permanent record which is less likely to be lost than hospital or clinic based notes.

Pre-school preventive contacts are recorded in the PCHR; a carbonised copy is usually sent to the child health computing department. Some professional notes are required in addition to the computer-based summary. A common professional record used by all community and hospital health care staff is recommended. Over two-thirds of community child health provider services currently use the PCHR and its use is increasing.

Recommendations when the PCHR is introduced to a district are that:

- a single person accepts responsibility for the introduction

- the concept and advantages should be discussed with community doctors and nurses and other child health or paediatric staff
- local general practitioners should be approached in association with the Local Medical Committee and health authority
- local modifications and additions to the national format should be considered although, in general, use of the national format facilitates optimal information exchange, especially for families who move
- the timing of handing the PCHR to the parent should be agreed; options include the health visitor's first visit, the postnatal ward or antenatal class
- decisions be made on funding (allowing for the savings made from phasing out existing records) and ordering
- training sessions be held, particularly regarding the use of the PCHR in cases of concern about child abuse or neglect
- special needs be considered, e.g. special growth charts for children with Turner's or Down's syndrome and the possibility of using the PCHR as a record of therapy for children with chronic disorders such as asthma or epilepsy.

The PCHR should contain a clear statement that data in the record may be used for health services monitoring and research. The record will include health promotion data, information about screening, and growth charts. The PCHR may also include other information such as welfare benefits, leaflets relating to child abuse or cot death, services for special needs children and risk factors for hearing loss and vision defects. The PCHR is not recommended at present for use by the school health service.

Openness with parents is essential. The PCHR plays a role in a true partnership between professionals and parents only if information and opinions are shared. Future developments for the record include translations for ethnic minorities— a library of translations (and of other topics) is maintained in the personal child health record library, Royal College of Paediatrics and Child Health, 50 Hallam Street, London W1N 6DE.

SURVEILLANCE

WHAT IS SURVEILLANCE/HEALTH PROMOTION?

Preventive health care in childhood includes immunisation against infectious diseases, surveillance, and health education and health promotion, together with monitoring of child growth. Box 2.2 provides some definitions of terms used in preventive health care. Surveillance, mainly concerned with monitoring child development, is an unclear process: there are misunderstandings

---

Box 2.2   Definitions in preventive health care.
There is considerable confusion over the many terms used and a need for agreement. The same term may be used for different activities; different terms may be used for essentially similar tasks. For the purposes of this chapter the following definitions (after Butler 1989) will be used.

Preventive child health care
Preventive child health care is an umbrella term describing all the activities of primary care that are concerned with the prevention of disease and the promotion of health in the pre-school child. It includes the more restricted range of activities described below.

Primary prevention
Primary prevention is aimed at the promotion of good health by reducing the incidence of disease and other departures from good health. In the case of the pre-school child, primary preventive measures include: dental and infectious disease prophylaxis (e.g. immunisations); the prevention of accidents; the prevention of child abuse; health education for the child; and education, advice and support to the parents about the health aspects of child-rearing. This heading includes the concept of health promotion involving diverse, community-based activities concerned with enhancing all aspects of child growth and development.

Secondary prevention
Secondary prevention involves actions taken to reduce the prevalence of disease and other departures from good health by shortening the duration or diminishing the impact of the condition. Examples include:

Child health surveillance. This denotes the systematic and ongoing collection, analysis and interpretation of indices of child health, growth and development in order to identify, investigate and, where appropriate, correct deviations from predetermined norms (WHO 1973). Child health surveillance may be of two kinds:

Box 2.2 *(contd)*

1. Population surveillance, which is used in the public health sense to describe the ongoing observation and recording of spatial and temporal incidence of the diseases and conditions of childhood in order to highlight public health problems requiring collective action, and
2. Individual (or clinical) surveillance which is aimed at early detection of abnormality in individual pre-school children to allow prompt and effective intervention. The process involves clinical, laboratory and behavioural tests for specific problems, e.g. vision and hearing disorders. The main purpose of surveillance is the gathering of information to facilitate reaching a diagnosis.

Screening is not intended to be diagnostic but is the presumptive identification of unrecognised disease or defects by the application of tests, examinations and other procedures.

Examination is the action of establishing the clinical state of a child by means of a combination of questioning, testing and observing the child in the context of a professional relationship. It may be diagnostic, preventive, therapeutic or administrative. Consequently, it serves no useful function other than as a description of data collection undertaken by a professional.

Assessment denotes the follow-up of children who are found, through screening, to be positive or in whom there are suspicions regarding the problem being assessed. Assessment is a specialist problem-solving function aimed at reaching a definitive diagnosis and plan of management and leading on to the treatment, care and aftercare of children confirmed as having acute or chronic conditions and handicaps.

Tertiary prevention
Tertiary prevention is aimed at preventing an established condition (disability) from becoming a handicap, i.e. minimising the suffering caused by existing departures from good health and promoting the child's (and the parents') adjustment to conditions that cannot be ameliorated.

United Kingdom Joint Working Party—consisting of paediatricians, general practitioners, public health physicians, health visitors, nurses, representatives from the various health departments/offices and academics—was set up in 1986 to review current surveillance activity. The results of the initial assessment and subsequent reviews have been published with recommendations about what action should be taken in the series of three Hall Reports. They provide a pragmatic 'best buy' for British pre-school surveillance practice, while acknowledging the gaps in present understanding and the continuing need for critical evaluation of much current activity and for further research.

HOW USEFUL IS HEALTH SURVEILLANCE OF PRE-SCHOOL CHILDREN?

Health surveillance programmes for pre-school children are widely regarded as good practice throughout the western world (Hall, 1996), however little scientific evidence exists to justify many of the activities undertaken and there are few data available to indicate whether surveillance programmes reach the appropriate child population or, more importantly, lead to improved health.

There are several unanswered questions about pre-school surveillance:

- is the pre-school surveillance programme clinically effective?
- is it economically worthwhile in relation to its yield, i.e. is it cost-effective?
- are the right procedures being undertaken?

Theory of screening

Screening is a procedure for the early identification of previously undetected disease using a test which is simple, rapid and cheap. The result divides individuals in a population into those with a high likelihood of having the disease in question and those with a low likelihood (Table 2.1). Screening is a primary care activity: individuals who are positive on the screening test must be referred to a secondary service for diagnostic testing.

about what is meant by the term, unclear aims, uncertainties about the process and little definition of what outcomes are to be expected.

Large amounts of public money, estimated to be more than £200 000 000 per year, are spent in the UK on preventive child health care. Immunisation undoubtedly gives value for money but there are many uncertainties, together with a lack of objective evidence of benefit, about other preventive activities, particularly surveillance. A

Table 2.1   Screening results

| Screening test | Disease | | Total |
	Present	Absent	
Positive	a	b	a + b
Negative	c	d	c + d
Total	a + c	b + d	

a = true positives
b = false positives
c = false negatives
d = true negatives

Sensitivity = a / (a + c), i.e. the true positives as a proportion of the population who actually have the disease. It depends on the false negative rate and measures the test's ability to identify the disease

Specificity = d / (b + d), i.e. true negatives as a proportion of the population who do not have the disease. It depends on the false positive rate and is a measure of the test's ability to identify individuals who do not have the disease.

Positive predictive value = a / (a + b), i.e. the true positives as a proportion of the total positive results from the test. It also depends upon the false positive rate.

Is pre-school surveillance clinically effective?

Many health professionals believe that surveillance programmes for pre-school children are valuable in promoting the optimal health and development of children (Box 2.3). Early screening can identify a disorder or departure from normal and hence allow intervention to be introduced at an early stage. A probable cause can be detected and remedied before development becomes frankly abnormal. Early intervention may minimise consequent disability or handicap.

The effectiveness of a child health surveillance programme depends upon the proportion of the population that is covered. For instance, improved coverage of health surveillance in Northumberland to over 90% of eligible children

---

Box 2.3   Benefits of population screening

- Early identification of disease, thus enabling early treatment
- Identification of normal children
- Contact with health professional, thus enabling education, advice and support
- Systematic and continuous case finding in the population

---

reduced the age at which congenital deafness was diagnosed from 25 months in 1973–75 to 9 months in 1983–85. This meant that deaf children were fitted earlier with hearing aids over the same time—at an average age of 15 months compared with 30 months before.

Parents are usually the first people to note abnormal signs in the physical and mental development of the pre-school child, but some defects are unlikely to be recognised even by the most astute parents and may only be detected by health professionals through surveillance programmes. Parents must realise that they have a responsibility to report concerns as professional surveillance alone will inevitably miss some cases.

Despite broad recognition of the value of health surveillance by many health professionals, there is widespread scepticism among many doctors and nurses. The most fundamental objection is simply that the effectiveness and value of surveillance remain unproved. Some health professionals doubt whether many of the 'positive' conditions detected through screening would lead to significant disadvantage or handicap for the child if undetected; others argue the uncertain predictive value of unstandardised and poorly validated screening procedures, and the inadequate training of those who administer the tests and interpret their findings; others again feel that even if a positive or suspicious result is obtained it may not be possible to do anything about it because of the lack of effective treatment.

A high false negative rate (missed cases) has been found in screening during infancy for subsequently identified deafness and visual problems. One report concluded that 'developmental examination has only limited effectiveness when applied during infancy', and that 'medical and paramedical personnel currently engaged in the routine application of this type of developmental examination might not be effectively deployed'.

Is pre-school surveillance economically worthwhile?

There are suggestions that health surveillance programmes for pre-school children are not only effective but also economically worthwhile; costs of the programme can be justified by future savings from the treatment and care that would otherwise have to be provided to children with chronic conditions and handicaps, especially with such 'hard' conditions as phenylketonuria, hypothyroidism, congenital dislocation of hip and maldescent of the testes. For neonatal thyroid screening it is possible to estimate costs with some accuracy and, however the benefits are computed, the ratio has been described as 'overwhelmingly favourable'.

It has been estimated that child health clinics which include primary preventive activities as well as surveillance are less costly when run by general practitioners than by district health authorities. The average cost of a community health clinic session was £93.55 at 1983 prices while the 'allocated' cost for a GP session was £80.85. Such calculations present many difficulties in context and objectivity.

Other health professionals argue that the cost of surveillance is unacceptably high in relation to its yield, and that the financial and other costs may not be justified in terms of benefit accruing to the small number of positive cases detected. A 1974 study in one west country general practice found that the cost of the developmental screening carried out among the 150 children under the age of 5 in the practice amounted to £2250; the process yielded only two speech defects and one squint. The author concluded that 'if one assumes that the children with the speech problems would have presented to the general practitioner, then this leaves one squint which might otherwise have been missed. Therefore, this squint cost the local health authority £2250 for identification'.

The costs would be even higher for screening a condition with an even lower incidence in the population. As a hypothetical example, a condition has a frequency in the population of 0.5%, and a screening test with a 99% level of sensitivity and a 99% level of specificity: in these circumstances, the probability that a child with a positive result will actually have the condition is only 0.33—that is, two out of three children with a positive result on screening will not have the problem. Furthermore, since screening offers no more than a presumptive diagnosis, these children will require follow-up assessments in order to arrive at a definitive diagnosis.

The costs involved in surveillance are by no means confined to those of a direct monetary nature; there will also be the *opportunity costs* of the doctors' and nurses' time and that of the parents. It has been estimated that, in a three-doctor practice of 9000 patients, the workload of the doctor specialising in surveillance could increase by as much as 25%. There are also the probable adverse effects on individual children and family relationships when a normal child 'fails' a developmental or other surveillance check. Such *false positives* can lead to children being unjustifiably regarded as slow or otherwise unsatisfactory.

Thus, the belief that developmental examinations will identify most health problems remains unproved, and more objective reports of the outcomes as well as the methods of screening are needed. The Committee on Child Health Services in 1976 reported that the programme of surveillance recommended at that time 'has only limited research support and a great deal remains to be done in evaluating the effectiveness of various surveillance procedures and in measuring their cost and the benefit that accrues from them'. Little has happened in the intervening years to counter these criticisms.

PATTERN OF SURVEILLANCE PROGRAMMES

Unlike immunisation procedures, there has been no nationally accepted surveillance schedule for the pre-school child dictating the ages at which screening procedures and tests ought to be carried out, with the exception of a limited number of disorders such as phenylketonuria and hypothyroidism. There is a broad consensus but no clear agreement for other conditions such as congenital dislocation of the hip, defects of hearing and vision, squint and even maldescent of the testes.

Large variation has been reported in the age at which screening is carried out for many devel-

Table 2.2 Summary of recommended surveillance procedures at the various recommended ages (after Hall 1996)

Age	Physical	Measure	Hearing/vision	Development	Other
Birth	Congenital dislocated hip (CDH) Heart	Weight (head, length)	Red reflex eyes ?Hearing		Concerns Family history PKU, TSH (Hb electrophoresis)
6 weeks (2 months)	CDH Heart	Weight Head	(eyes) Enquiry (check list)		Concerns
8 months (7–9 months)	CDH Testes Squint	(weight)	Enquiry Distraction testing	Enquiry	Concerns
21 months (18–24 months)	Gait	(length)	Enquiry Speech and understanding	Enquiry (behaviour)	Concerns (Hb)
39 months (36–42 months)	(testes)	Height—Chart!	Enquiry (refer)	Enquiry (special educational problems?)	Concerns
60 months (school entry)	(testes) (heart)	Height—Chart!	Snellen vision Sweep audiogram	Enquiry	Concerns
School years		(height)	Vision 3-yearly	(?enquiry)	Concerns

opmental assessments and in the tests performed to make the assessment. Guidelines from the NHS Management Executive in 1992 suggested a 'core' programme based on the revised second edition of *Health for all children: a programme for child health surveillance* (Hall Report). Most community child health providers and general practices are at present broadly following a programme such as that outlined in Table 2.2.

Surveillance ages

As well as the great variability between localities, professional opinion has varied regarding the ages at which surveillance procedures ought to be carried out. Butler (1989) analysed 35 reports in the literature of programmes for pre-school children and found that there were 14 separate screening ages between 6 weeks and 5 years, utilising no fewer than 24 different combinations of age. Only four ages were mentioned in more than 50% of the reports: 6 weeks, 6–9 months, 16–18 months and 30–36 months. There has been considerable variation between health authorities in England; a 1984 survey found wide variation in the recommended age for surveillance checks, with ten different 'assessment' ages between 2 weeks and 4 years. Only four ages were

common to the policies of half or more of the authorities: 6 weeks (52% of HAs), 6 months (57%), 18 months (61%) and 3 years (63%).

A 1970s survey of 27 child health 'experts' in the United Kingdom on child health surveillance found that, with the exception of the neonatal examination, fewer than half agreed on the desirability of routine surveillance at any of the specified ages, and concluded that 'research is urgently required to test the truths of these assumptions about key age examinations'.

The lack of consensus and the variation in practice regarding target ages for pre-school surveillance have clouded any possible relationship between a disorder for which children are tested and the age at which the test should be carried out. If the main purpose of surveillance is to detect specific disorders or anomalies at the age when they can best be identified and treated, the different combinations of surveillance ages mentioned in the literature cannot be equally appropriate; some ages must be more suitable than others for testing for a particular disorder. The World Health Organization has stated that 'There is clearly little value in detecting disease in advance of the usual time of diagnosis unless such detection precedes the last critical point beyond which treatment would be unsuccessful and/or permanent damage would be done'.

Tests/procedures

There seems to be a small core of agreement that screening for certain conditions or disorders is justified, but considerable disagreement regarding screening for others. There is almost unanimous agreement that babies should be examined at birth, or shortly after, for the presence of physical anomalies, and that they should be screened for metabolic disorders, principally phenylketonuria and hypothyroidism. The Hall Report pointed out that neonatal examination has a high yield, and that 'it is accepted and expected by parents, and there seems little doubt that they value the reassurance of normality at this time'.

A 6-week check was recommended in the second edition of the Hall Report in 1991 to include:

- any parental concerns
- physical examination
- weight and head circumference
- congenital dislocation of the hips
- vision and hearing
- eyes (e.g. squint).

The age appears to have been selected as much to coincide with the recommended 6-week postnatal check for the mother as for any other reason. Earlier surveys had not agreed that 6 weeks was a particularly valuable time, with little agreement about the value of screening at this time. The importance of parental questioning as part of the examination has been stressed but this does not appear in most schedules; perhaps it is taken for granted that such questioning will take place.

Children continue to grow and develop beyond the sixth week, so the number and variety of tests to which they might be subjected expands. As there is little agreement about which screening tests ought to be done at which ages, unclear and ambiguous language used to describe the purpose of the tests in both the literature and practice, and a lack of convincing evidence from evaluation in the field, it is difficult, on the basis of the literature, to formulate a modern programme of pre-school child health surveillance.

The recommended health surveillance programmes, including that of Hall, are far from being 'practical manuals' which can be widely adopted. Explanations for the pronounced variability in surveillance programmes include:

1. that 'the scientific basis of much childhood screening is as yet insufficiently precise to identify the "correct" or "optimal" target ages for different screening tests'
2. that 'in the absence of any objective indicators, screeners select the ages with which they are most familiar, or which correspond most closely to their clinical experience, or which are mandated by the particular test schedules that they, or their health authorities have chosen to adopt'
3. that it 'may be not that the "correct" or "optimal" ages have yet to be established, but that they simply do not exist' (Butler, 1989).

Specific tests

Congenital hip dislocation (see p. 52)

Eyes

Red reflex
- The retina is examined using an ophthalmoscope with the lens set at +10 from a distance of 30 cm.
- The purpose is to observe the red reflection of the light and not to perform fundoscopy.
- A normal red reflex excludes cataract or other serious ocular opacity.
- This test should be done at the neonatal examination and at 6 weeks.

Squint
- Consider:
  —parental concern
  —family history
  —head posture
  —eye movements.
- Torch reflection test. Shine a bright pen torch from a distance of approximately 50 cm and

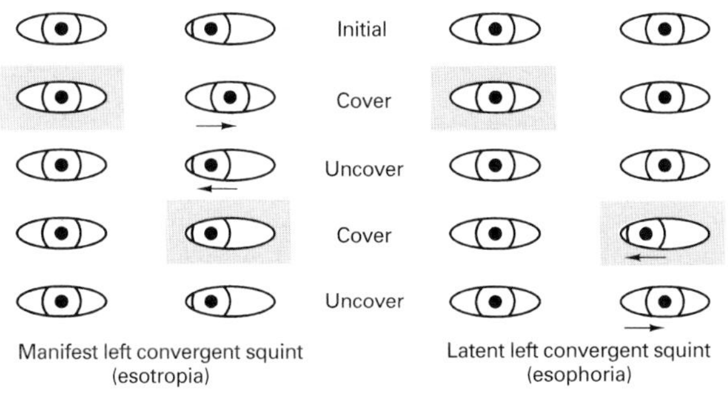

Manifest left convergent squint (esotropia)

Latent left convergent squint (esophoria)

Figure 2.2 The cover test.

observe the corneal reflections. These should be symmetrical in both eyes.

- Cover test (Figure 2.2). This is difficult to perform in young children and should be used with great care and caution by primary health care staff. It is more reliable when done by experienced community orthoptists. Each eye is covered in turn: firstly the uncovered eye is observed for movement in a manifest squint, and secondly the covered eye is watched when the cover is removed as it will move to fixate if it has a latent squint.

Visual acuity. This is also difficult to test in young children.

- Normal visual alertness and responsiveness are the best indicators of normal visual function.
- A useful test in young children is to offer them an object 1–2 mm in diameter (e.g. 'hundreds and thousands' cake decoration) and observe whether they fixate on it or, preferably, reach out to pick it up accurately.
- The STYCAR fixed balls can also be used but rolling balls are not recommended because a moving image is easier to see than a static one.
- These techniques only detect severe visual impairments (visual acuity less than 6/18).

By the age of 3 years most children can usually perform a letter matching test (the child does not need to know the alphabet as it is only the shape of the letter that has to be recognised and matched).

- The simplest are the STYCAR or Sheridan

Gardener single letter optotypes. The single letter cards are shown to the child, preferably at a distance of 6 metres (although they can be administered at 3 metres), and the child points to the same letter on the key card in front of him. Each eye should be occluded in turn so that the individual eye is examined. However, even with patching, the tests underestimate visual loss, and amblyopia can be missed.

- Many children can co-operate with a linear chart test such as the Sonksen–Silver or Egan–Calver tests.
- Because of a crowding phenomenon individual letters in a row are more difficult to identify because of interference by adjacent letters; these tests are more sensitive than single letters.
- The administration technique is the same as for single optotypes.
- By the age of 5 years most children can easily cope with a standard Snellen chart.

Hearing

Infancy

Oto-acoustic emissions (OAEs)

- These have a sensitivity > 90% for a hearing loss of 50 dB or more in the neonatal period.
- They have been widely used for several years in neonatal units on high risk babies; the technique is recommended for universal screening.
- The specificity is approximately 90% and there must be ready access to a secondary audiology service where diagnostic brainstem evoked responses/auditory brainstem responses (BSER/ABR) are available.

Parental observation

- Parents are often the first to notice abnormal hearing responses in their baby.
- Their observations can be enhanced by giving them a structured checklist, e.g. in the PCHR.

Distraction test

- This is best performed between 7 and 9 months of age when it is almost an obligate developmental response. Children up to 18 months old can be persuaded to co-operate but it is more difficult.

- With a high level of training and regular updating and monitoring, the distraction test can be very efficient. However the quality of the test falls if these standards are not maintained. For this reason the distraction test has fallen into disrepute and is not recommended as a national universal screening technique.
- It will still be necessary to test a few children about whom there is concern for their hearing during the second 6 months of life. Hence a small number of professionals working in a secondary audiology service must retain their skills.

Toddler age group

History

- A child with good hearing responses and normal speech and language development is unlikely to have significant deafness.
- Children with recurrent ear infections, glue ear, allergic rhinitis, cleft palate and Down's syndrome have a high risk of conductive deafness.

Speech discrimination tests

- The child is asked to identify common objects when they are named by the examiner.
- The examiner's voice is kept below an intensity of 40 dB using a sound level meter and the mouth is covered.
- Young children can be tested with a small number of familiar objects (e.g. cup, spoon, fork, shoe, doll).
- Older children (> 2½ years) can usually cope with more objects presented in a structured way.
- The McCormick Toy Test consists of 14 toys arranged in pairs with similar sounding names (e.g. house/mouse, plate/plane, duck/cup). Good hearing at specific frequencies is required to distinguish these names. Each toy is produced separately and named as described above.
- The Kendall toy test is similar.
- The E²L test uses objects familiar to children

from families whose first language is not English.

Performance tests

- Children can often be conditioned from the age of 2 years to respond by action to a sound stimulus even though they cannot reply verbally.
- The action must be fun, such as putting toy men in a boat or balls or bricks in a box or bucket.
- Younger children respond best to voice, and the test words are 'Go' (low frequency) and a soft hissed 'ssss' (high frequency).
- The sound is kept to minimal levels (< 40 dB) using a sound level meter and the mouth is covered.
- Older children (> 2½ years) can respond to a free field audiometer which has the advantage of accurately testing different frequencies at varying intensities. This technique is more appropriate for secondary diagnostic testing than primary screening. Speech discrimination and performance tests are very appropriate techniques for testing hearing in surveillance around the age of 3 years.

Audiometry. Over the age of 3 years children become increasingly tolerant of headphones; by the age of the school entry check at 4½ to 5 years old, most children will easily perform a conventional pure tone audiogram which tests varying frequencies in each ear separately. Usually this is done by the school nurse as a 'sweep test' when the audiometer is set to a fixed intensity (e.g. 20 dB) and all frequencies from 0.5 to 4 K are tested in turn.

Growth

Weight

- Baby weighing is a 'sacred' clinic activity which many mothers expect and find very reassuring as long as the gain is satisfactory.
- Weights should always be recorded in the PHCR and plotted on the centile chart.
- Babies must be stripped naked and older children down to underpants.
- Scales must be checked and calibrated regularly.

- Weight should increase steadily along a consistent percentile line, indicating a normal growth velocity.
- A persistent drop below the predicted percentile line suggests pathology (e.g. chronic illness, child abuse) and should be investigated.
- The average weight gain in the first year of life is approximately 150 g per week. Birth weight is roughly doubled by 5 months of age and trebled at 1 year.

Height

- Measurement of length in infants is notoriously inaccurate and is not recommended.
- If there is a good reason to measure length in infancy it should only be done on special equipment with proper head and foot plates. The baby must be held flat with legs and neck extended by one person while another takes the measurement.
- Children over 2 years old are measured standing up in bare feet with the back against a vertical surface.
- The heels must be on the ground and the neck is gently extended by the examiner's fingers under the angle of the jaw.
- The child's bottom should touch the vertical measure.
- The height is measured by a head plate touching the top of the head and at right angles to the measure.
- The head is positioned with the occiput touching the vertical measure and eyes level with the external auditory meatus.
- Only specially designed apparatus (e.g. Minimeter) should be used. It must be carefully and permanently fixed to a vertical wall and the position checked periodically.
- Lengths and height must always be recorded and charted in the PHCR.
- Tape measures should never be used to measure length or height.
- The most important measure of growth is growth velocity, which requires a minimum of 2 measurements separated by at least 3 months. If this is reduced, as shown by a fall off a percentile line, the child should be referred for a secondary paediatric opinion.

Head circumference

- Measure only at the neonatal and 6-week check unless abnormality of head growth is suspected.
- The maximum measurement is recorded (occipito-frontal circumference).
- Use disposable paper or non-stretchable metal, plastic or fibreglass tape.

COVERAGE OF HEALTH SURVEILLANCE

Controversy surrounds the need for universal as opposed to targeted coverage. Should a particular screening test be aimed at all children in the appropriate age range (with likely high cost and low yield), or should there be targeting only to the population most *at risk* of developing the condition? There is no agreement as to how the coverage rate of a total population should be calculated nor how significant a low coverage rate might be.

Targeting

Targeting is an intuitively attractive concept which allows concentration of inevitably limited resources where they will be most useful. An associated concept is that children identified as being 'at risk' of developmental problems should be kept under surveillance until their development is seen to be progressing entirely normally, with the assumption that, among a cohort of children developing a particular disorder or handicap, a very high proportion would have had the risk factor(s) selected as being the precursor(s). There have been recommendations, supported by mathematical models, that health providers keep 'at risk' registers of *vulnerable* children for health surveillance purposes. Such a selective approach to screening was thought to be particularly beneficial in situations of resource constraint.

Unfortunately, this 'at risk' register concept, which generated much enthusiasm and confidence, was introduced without pilot studies and the registers were not designed to permit easy continuing evaluation. Experience soon revealed discrepancies and shortcomings, including problems with definitions and lack of uniform implementation of criteria. Such criticisms of 'at risk' registers led the (Court) Committee on Child Health Services in 1976 to reiterate an approach to surveillance in which health care staff should be alert to *any* child displaying evidence of a greater than average risk of ill health, developmental disorders or handicaps. Health workers were advised to 'avoid a categorisation of children "at risk" on account of selected social factors', and that 'at risk' registers 'should not be used to restrict the coverage of the basic surveillance programme'. The main argument against 'at risk' registers was that they 'have in the past proved unsuccessful in accurately identifying children at risk of developing handicaps'.

Another selective screening approach proposed is that children should be selected not on the basis of predefined risk factors but on the basis of a health visitor's concern about some aspects of the child's health and development, i.e. a child would be examined only if the health visitor was worried about his or her health and/or development. This 'pre-screening' approach by a health visitor has been seen as a highly efficient way of using the time of a screening doctor, although the study on whose basis this approach was recommended has not yet been reproduced. The debate on these key issues of health surveillance of pre-school children (i.e. 'at risk', targeting and objectives) is far from over.

Coverage

The coverage rate is the proportion of the target population that is *actually* screened within the relevant time. If the aim of surveillance is to reach all children within the relevant age ranges for each individual screening test, the coverage rate is one indicator of the effectiveness of a screening programme, but by no means the only one: firstly, if a high coverage is obtained, the yield of positive cases may be too low to justify the cost of screening for them; secondly, the proportion of false positive or false negative results may be unacceptably high; thirdly, even if these

indicators are within tolerable limits, screening programmes may not confer any distinctive or worthwhile advantages upon the children undergoing them.

The calculation of coverage rate per se may be misleading, with deficiencies in both the numerator and denominator. Numerators must include all children in a given community who receive the component or components of the surveillance programme being assessed for coverage; since children may be screened either in general practice or in community child health clinics, the records from both sources must be merged to obtain a reliable numerator and build up an overall picture. Denominators can also be problematic, as they must reflect a defined 'true' population. General practice age/sex registers have been widely used as true population denominators, but major doubts have been raised about their reliability and validity: comparisons of health visitors' records, age/sex registers and the immunisation and vaccination computer appointment files have demonstrated that practice age/sex registers were the least accurate of the three. In one study about 15% of children aged between birth and 4 years no longer resided at the address given for them in any of the three registers, and a further 8–12% of children in the age group were not on the age/sex register.

Benefits and some limitations of child health computer systems for surveillance

The introduction of computers into child health programmes—initially on a local and then on a national scale—ought to have alleviated such problems: the registration/pre-school module of a computerised child health system allows the creation of a centralised record for each child in a defined local population, into which details of all developmental and other examinations can be fed, whether conducted in community child health clinics or general practitioners' surgeries. The need for administrative/geographic boundaries, however, means that many general practice populations include children from adjacent child health populations, and links between child health computing systems remain infrequent and unsophisticated as do the links between health authority, GP and child health systems, with little ability automatically to update or rationalise the population databases.

Coverage rate

There are difficulties in interpreting the coverage rate. Unlike immunisation uptake, for which concrete targets have been set (e.g. '95% in 1995'), there are no hard-and-fast rules for determining the cut-off point below which the coverage rate of surveillance is evidence of the failure or unacceptability of a screening programme. A fundamental concern when evaluating something like a screening programme is the possibility of bias. The relevance and importance of a coverage rate will depend upon the extent to which the attenders of a screening programme contain the children in the target population who are *truly* affected by the condition that the test is seeking. Thus if the attenders were such a biased group as to contain *all* the children in the target population who were *truly* affected the yield would be high, however low the coverage rate might be. At the other extreme if the attenders were so biased as to contain *none* of the children in the target population who were *truly* affected the yield would be zero, however *high* the coverage rate might be. The real situation is that the attenders for screening generally contain a proportion of truly affected cases somewhere between these two extremes. In this circumstance, a higher coverage rate and a larger proportion of truly affected cases would normally generate a higher yield of a screening test.

In practice, however, the situation has been far from satisfactory with large biases existing in the selection of attenders. One study of high and low risk groups, totalling 1878 children, concluded that 'a larger proportion of children not brought to child health clinics, and thus not using available services, were in a group with a higher risk of developmental problems than in the study population as a whole', and 'even high clinic attendance rates are not grounds for complacency. More of the children who do *not* attend were those in *greatest* need' (inverse care law).

A review of 25 papers on coverage rate, mainly from general practice, found no evidence of any trend towards higher coverage rates over the 10 years 1974–84; there were marked variations in coverage rates ranging from under 60% up to over 90%; there was great variability in rates at individual screening ages (median coverage ranging from about 60% for the 48--54-month screening to 80% for the 6-week check). No national figures of coverage rate are available.

CHILD HEALTH SURVEILLANCE: CHANGING PRACTICE

Until the late 1980s pre-school surveillance in the UK was mainly undertaken by clinical medical officers. With the development of consultant-led community child health services orientated towards disability care and other special needs and the continuing development of primary care, most surveillance is now carried out by members of the primary health care team—often the health visitor. The PCHR and developments in information systems and recording have led to greater uniformity in practice. Many areas remain, some of which are outlined in Box 2.4, where improvements could and should be made. There has been an appropriate trend towards opportunistic surveillance rather than subjecting a child to a routine battery of tests at a fixed age; health professionals are encouraged to consider the child's developmental progress whenever he or she is seen. Is the child doing what he or she ought for the age and circumstances? Has the care-giver any concerns about behaviour or the child's progress?

The health professional, working in partnership with the parent/s, should follow the four Rs of surveillance:

Reassure—the bulk of contacts. Reassurance based on the professional's experience and judgement and where there are no parent/care-giver's concerns. Any such concern should be taken seriously.

Review if the professional is uncertain but feels there is no problem or if the child is perhaps under par with an intercurrent infection and not performing on the day.

Box 2.4 Areas of surveillance practice needing modification and/or development

Screening
- Universal neonatal hearing screening to replace the 8-month distraction test
- Neonatal screening for haemoglobinopathies, cystic fibrosis, biliary atresia
- Early infancy screening for maternal postnatal depression
- Toddler screening for iron deficiency anaemia, autism

Preventive activities
- Cot death
- Accidents
- Support to stressed parents

Informatics and audit
- Better standardisation of terms and tests
- Method to record outcome of referral following identification of possible problem
- Quality assurance and accreditation of local systems
- Use of local and regional data, to identify information and practice shortcomings (so leading to improvements in present activity), and to the development/testing of innovations.
- Clear programme guidelines and quality requirements from the Department of Health
- Central co-ordination of programme with involvement of professional bodies

Refer to a second-tier service, usually run by the local community child health department, if the parent or professional feels there may be a significant developmental problem. Such referral services may include audiology, single specialty assessment such as paediatric occupational therapy or multidisciplinary assessment in a child development centre depending on the problem.

Record. The findings of any surveillance contact should be recorded in the clinical record and at the appropriate ages in the PCHR with a copy sent to the local child health computing department. It is important to record details of any referral made and the result of such a referral. Was a problem confirmed? Have any arrangements been made for further tests or assessments?

CONCLUSIONS

Pre-school surveillance is an imprecise science with many unresolved questions regarding its aims, practice and outcome. That there is such a lack of definition is surprising in the light of the magnitude of the resources involved in the process. The topic is at present under intense scrutiny. Even though many current procedures may not be confirmed as useful and there is a need to provide an evidence base for practice, the systems in place provide an invaluable resource to promote child health.

FURTHER READING

Butler J 1989 Child health surveillance in primary care: a critical review. HMSO, London
Committee on Child Health Services 1976 Fit for the future. (The Court Report). HMSO, London
Department of Health 1996 Immunisation against infectious disease. HMSO, London

Hall DMB (ed) 1996 Health for all children: report of the Joint Working Party on Child Health Surveillance, 3rd edn. Oxford University Press, Oxford
NHS Management Executive health service guidelines 1992 Child health surveillance—a recommended "core" programme. HSG(92)19

Internet address

Child Health Informatics Consortium
http://www.capita-ec.com/childinf

3

The newborn infant

Michael Williams

ROUTINE CARE AT DELIVERY

Temperature

The newborn baby is well adapted to survive—the most important factor is maintaining body temperature. A wet 2 kg baby left exposed in a room at 21°C can lose as much as 1°C of body temperature every three minutes, significantly increasing the risk of morbidity as the temperature falls. The room used for the delivery should be warm and draught free; the baby should be dried off as soon as possible after birth and wrapped in a warm towel which should also cover the head. When the mother wishes the baby to be delivered onto her abdomen and put directly to the breast, the baby is partly warmed by maternal contact and the temperature can be maintained by covering mother and baby together with the towel. Later, the wrapping towel can be used to dry and clean the baby. Bathing babies with warm water soon after birth removes maternal blood from the skin, thus lessening the risk of human immunodeficiency virus (HIV) transmission. It should be noted if the baby passes urine or stool.

Vitamin K

Vitamin K_1 should be administered to babies following delivery to avoid later haemorrhagic disease of the newborn which results from a deficiency of vitamin K dependent clotting factors. The intramuscular dose is 1 mg for babies of 36 or more weeks' gestation and 0.4 mg/kg for babies of less than 36 weeks' gestation. An alternative oral regimen for term babies is to give 2 mg at birth and again at 4–7 days. For breast fed babies, the manufacturers recommend a further dose of 2 mg at one month.

RESUSCITATION AND BIRTH ASPHYXIA

Wherever possible, the risks of birth asphyxia should be anticipated by monitoring maternal and fetal health during pregnancy. The risk is highest when the fetus is growing poorly as a result of failure of the placenta, but even an apparently healthy placenta can start to separate unexpectedly from the uterine wall and result in asphyxia. Monitoring the fetal heart rate during delivery and measuring the fetal pH may help to identify intrapartum asphyxia, as may the presence of meconium in draining liquor. Fetal tachycardia and the presence of late decelerations in fetal heart rate following uterine contraction are indicators of utero-placental insufficiency. Early decelerations in fetal heart rate are thought to be caused by compression of the fetal head. Wherever possible, high risk deliveries should take place in an obstetric unit which has full paediatric support.

A hospital labour ward should have all the equipment needed for advanced resuscitation, supported by trained paediatric staff. In a low risk department or in a home delivery advanced resuscitation may require a paramedic ambulance or immediate transfer to a specialist setting, but basic resuscitation should be started immediately. A midwife or general practitioner attending low risk deliveries should have the minimum equipment required for simple resuscitation (Box

---

Box 3.1   Resuscitation equipment
Basic
• Simple oro-pharyngeal suction device (mucus extractor)
• 'Bag and mask' set with range of soft masks of different sizes
• Portable oxygen cylinder
Specialist
• Neonatal laryngoscope
• Range of sterile endotracheal tubes
• Adapter for inflation bag
• Naloxone

3.1). All the items need to be checked regularly and kept clean; sterile items must be replaced by the expiry date. Spare batteries and bulbs are needed for a laryngoscope.

The Apgar score is a universal method of assessing the well-being of a newborn baby (Table 3.1). The score is estimated at one minute and five minutes after delivery and should be repeated every five minutes during resuscitation. Following normal delivery, it would be unusual for a baby with an Apgar score of more than 6 at one minute to require resuscitation. When the Apgar score is between 4 and 6, the baby may respond to physical stimulation such as drying with a towel or pinching a foot, or it may require basic resuscitation with a bag and mask. The baby with an Apgar score of less than 4 will usually require immediate resuscitation. If the doctor responsible for this does not have the equipment or experience for specialist resuscitation, it is essential to summon help as soon as possible while simple resuscitation (Box 3.2) is carried out. For a home delivery this means sending a helper to telephone for an emergency paramedic ambulance.

Table 3.1   The Apgar score

Observation	Score 0	Score 1	Score 2
Heart rate	Absent	< 100/min	> 100/min
Respiratory effort	Absent	Weak cry	Strong cry
Muscle tone	Absent	Some flexion	Good flexion
Response to pharyngeal suction	None	Some movement	Cry
Colour	Pale or central cyanosis	Peripheral cyanosis	Pink

Box 3.2 Basic resuscitation follows the usual principles used for any age group

- The mouth, nostrils and pharynx should be cleared of mucus, blood, amniotic fluid or meconium by gentle aspiration with a mucus extractor.
- When there is meconium in the upper airway, the ideal practice is to check for its presence below the vocal cords if the examiner has sufficient experience and equipment.
- If respiration is not established then artificial ventilation should be given with the bag and mask. The mask should fit closely around both the chin and the nose without leaking or causing nasal obstruction. The jaw is held closed and slightly forward with one hand, which also holds the mask on the face. The other hand squeezes the bag at a rate of about 35 breaths per minute. Inadequate bag pressure will fail to inflate the chest but excessive pressure can increase the risk of pneumothorax. A pharyngeal airway can be used if inflation appears poor.
- The baby's colour and heart rate should be monitored; if the condition is not improving, cardiac massage may be needed while advanced resuscitation help is awaited.
- Keep the baby as warm as possible during resuscitation.

Box 3.3 Advanced resuscitation

- The baby's airway must be cleared under direct vision using a laryngoscope; when meconium is present in the mouth or pharynx, this should also be suctioned from below the vocal cords.
- A term baby should be intubated with a size 3.0 endotracheal resuscitation tube so that the tapered end is just above the vocal cords. This is then held in place close to the mouth by one hand while the other is used to attach the resuscitation bag or the pressure limited oxygen supply from a resuscitaire.
- If the heart rate is not above 50 per minute and rising, cardiac massage is also required. This is given by a second operator who places both hands around the baby's thorax such that the thumbs are over the lower part of the sternum. Compression with the thumbs should be at a rate of about 80–100 per minute and there should be three compressions followed by a pause to allow for a breath.
- When narcotics administered to the mother may be depressing spontaneous breathing, high dose naloxone (0.1 mg/kg) may be given intravenously or intramuscularly. When the heart rate is absent, 1 ml adrenaline (1:10 000) can be administered down the endotracheal tube. Sodium bicarbonate (8.4%) diluted 1:1 with water for injection may be required in a dose of 2–5 mmol/kg by slow intravenous injection when assisted ventilation is adequate and there is no response. The possibility of hypoglycaemia should also be borne in mind.

Advanced resuscitation (Box 3.3) is required for any baby who does not respond rapidly to simple measures.

It is generally accepted that if resuscitation has not been successful in maintaining an adequate heart rate it should be stopped at about 20 minutes. This decision should be taken by a senior member of the resuscitation team and sensitively communicated to the family.

Hypoxic-ischaemic encephalopathy (HIE)

Asphyxia during birth may affect a baby to varying degrees according to the duration and severity of hypoxia. The worst effects are usually seen when an acute anoxic event has been added to a longer period of hypoxia or when there is sudden and severe hypoxia and delay in delivery. The complex of central nervous system signs and symptoms seen in the asphyxiated infant is termed hypoxic-ischaemic encephalopathy; a classification for the condition is shown in Table 3.2. Acidosis and hypoxia within the brain cause cerebral oedema, the severity of which is related to the degree of insult suffered:

- The most mildly asphyxiated baby will recover with no symptoms or only mild irritability which resolves within a few hours.
- The moderately affected baby may be floppy and rather unresponsive at first, although normal spontaneous respiration will be established. This gives way to excessive muscle tone and irritability which may last for several days before resolution and may interfere with normal feeding. There may be seizures but these are usually fairly easy to control.
- More severely affected babies may require assisted ventilation and drugs to support cardiac output. Seizures in these infants can be severe and prolonged, adding further to the cerebral insult. The management of cerebral oedema in such infants is a complicated matter requiring the services of an experienced neonatal intensive care unit.

Table 3.2 Outcome for hypoxic-ischaemic encephalopathy

Grade	Features	Prognosis
Mild—Grade I	Irritability Hyper-alert Mild hypotonia Poor sucking	Prognosis excellent Normal later development
Moderate—Grade II	Lethargy Seizures Marked abnormalities of tone Requirement for tube feeding	Guarded prognosis About half the infants will have normal later development
Severe—Grade III	Coma Prolonged seizures Severe hypotonia Failure to maintain spontaneous respiration	Poor prognosis About 25% die All survivors will show degree of neurological disability

Other complications of asphyxia

- Asphyxiated babies may have uncorrected metabolic acidosis after successful resuscitation. This may correct spontaneously as the pH is temporarily balanced by hyperventilation and respiratory alkalosis. More severe acidosis may require the administration of buffer.
- Inhalation of meconium or amniotic fluid can lead to respiratory distress.
- Myocardial ischaemia can cause dilatation of the heart with functional tricuspid incompetence and congestive cardiac failure.
- The pulmonary blood pressure can remain high, preventing adequate oxygenation even with normal ventilation—this is known as persistent fetal circulation.
- There may be renal failure associated with renal venous thrombosis, acute tubular necrosis or acute cortical necrosis.
- In the most severe cases there may be adrenal or pulmonary haemorrhage.

Parent counselling

The two major concerns for the families of asphyxiated babies are survival and possible brain damage. When only minimal measures have been required, the doctor should be very reassuring and optimistic. When the baby has needed more intensive resuscitation, the detailed exploration of these issues is the task of the consultant paediatrician or neonatologist who is caring for the baby. There is usually a degree of uncertainty about the future and the parents find this difficult to manage, often moving between extremes of optimism and pessimism as events unfold. Even at discharge from the hospital, the final outcome can only be a matter of informed opinion and the parents will face months of uncertainty before the situation becomes clearer. General practitioners and other health professionals may be contacted by family members for support or information and it is important that the hospital keeps the GP up to date. The GP should listen to the family's concerns and give support, but should not be tempted to give information which is beyond his or her expertise. Families should be encouraged to write down a list of questions to take with them for meetings with the consultant.

EXAMINATION OF THE NEWBORN INFANT

General principles

The newborn examination is essentially a screening examination which only detects the abnormalities and problems apparent at that time. It is best to discuss this limitation with family members. An example is the heart murmur of a small ventricular septal defect (VSD) which may not be heard at birth but should be found at the 6-week check.

Immediately after birth, the baby should be checked for obvious problems; this is usually the responsibility of the midwife. In some districts midwives have been trained to take total responsibility for newborn examination.

The best time for a more detailed examination is the day after delivery when the infant should have settled and enough time has passed to assess feeding and record the passage of first urine and stool. A later examination would then be required only if the family, midwife or health visitor were concerned about the baby.

Ideally babies are best examined about one hour after the last feed, but such a counsel of perfection is rarely achievable. The way in which a baby behaves and reacts is determined by its sleep/wake states, as described by Brazelton (Box 3.4).

The mother should be asked if she has any particular concerns about her baby so that these may be specifically addressed.

Before the baby is undressed, the covers should be removed to observe the general appearance and posture. The examiner should always undress the baby and not allow parents or staff to do this. Much can be learnt from handling the baby, and techniques can be developed which allow the baby to wake up gently without becoming distressed. The ideal is for the baby to be in Brazelton state 4, when most functions and activities can be checked.

Many different methods are used for conducting the examination but it is preferable to work in a way that minimises disturbance and distress until the end. The exact routine can be varied according to the individual baby's response to handling: in more unsettled babies auscultation of the heart may need to be performed early in the process.

It is useful to learn some methods of quieting restless babies. These include talking in a soft, firm voice, holding the baby's arms gently across the front of its chest, and placing the baby's own fingers in its mouth to encourage sucking.

Families like to hear a doctor talking to their baby; for a first-time mother it can give clues as to how babies can be handled and stimulated. Within a week of birth, a baby will be able to distinguish its mother from other people by sound, vision and smell. Vision is best about 8–12 inches from the face, the distance between the mother's and baby's face when breast feeding. It is surely no coincidence that babies have their eyes open when starting a feed.

Babies should normally pass stool and urine within the first 24 hours after delivery. Occasionally urine passage may be delayed another day and it can be difficult to know whether urine was passed during delivery. If babies fail to achieve either of these goals they should be referred immediately for paediatric advice.

Birth trauma

Caput

The presenting part of the fetus is subject to pressure injury during delivery, and there will usually be associated swelling after delivery. When this occurs over the scalp it is known as the *caput succedaneum*. Where the caput has been haemorrhagic, it may resolve to leave a disc of bruising which takes longer to settle. This appearance can be particularly prominent following ventouse extraction, when the swelling is referred to as a *chignon*. Extensive bruising may

Box 3.4	Wake/sleep states
State 1	Deep, quiet sleep. The eyes are closed. There is regular breathing and no spontaneous movement apart from respiration.
State 2	Light, active sleep. The eyes are closed. There is rapid eye movement (REM). Breathing is irregular and there is some spontaneous movement which is often twitchy.
State 3	The baby is semi-wakeful and the eyes could be open or closed. Muscle activity is variable and the movements tend to be smooth rather than twitchy.
State 4	The baby is awake and alert. The eyes are open and the baby is interested and 'co-operative'. Little muscular activity is present.
State 5	The baby is awake and very active. The eyes are open but there is less interest and 'co-operation'. There is considerable muscular activity but no crying.
State 6	The baby is crying. With a newborn baby the eyes will be closed and muscular activity is considerable.

occur when the presenting part is the breech or the brow, and subsequent jaundice is a potential problem.

Cephalhaematoma

It is quite common for the periosteum to separate from the outer surface of one or both parietal bones, allowing blood to accumulate gradually below the periosteum and resulting in a swelling termed a cephalhaematoma. This is limited by the edges of the parietal bone and requires no treatment. Most cephalhaematomas settle spontaneously, although jaundice is more common in affected babies. Calcification can occur around the edge of the lesion during resorption of the clot and give rise to a crater-like appearance. Rarely, the swelling calcifies completely and then only disappears very slowly with remodelling and growth of the skull over the first years of life.

Subaponeurotic haemorrhage

This is bleeding in the potential space just below the scalp. It is not limited by the skull bones and can cross the midline, moving to a dependent position wherever the head is turned. The potential cavity is limited only by the insertion of the scalp around the skull and can accommodate sufficient blood to endanger the baby.

Fat necrosis

This is caused by pressure over bony facial prominences during delivery and is most often seen over the angle of the lower jaw or over the zygomatic arch. A small area of redness and swelling develops over the first few days and may be quite tender. The lesion usually resolves entirely but can discharge from the skin.

Facial palsy

Facial palsy can result from pressure over the facial nerve during delivery. This may be associated with the use of forceps but is also seen in normal deliveries. Recovery is usually rapid and complete; rarely a more serious nerve injury can be present with delayed recovery which might be incomplete.

Brachial plexus injury – see page 212

Fractured clavicle is a possible complication of shoulder dystocia but can occasionally be seen after normal deliveries. It may present at delivery but is often only discovered later as a callus develops over the fracture site. No treatment is required but there is often considerable parental anxiety.

Sternomastoid tumour is thought to be caused by bleeding within the middle third of the sternomastoid muscle. It is not usually noted in the first days of life and will often be discovered later by the parents. It presents as a rounded, tender lump which causes shortening of the affected muscle and limiting rotation of the head towards the lesion. It is usually treated with physiotherapy and asking the family to approach the baby from the affected side to encourage movement in that direction.

Birthmarks

Capillary naevi are very common pink patches over the nape of the neck and in the central area of the face. Those on the neck vary in size and are virtually universal. They are of no importance and will later be largely covered by hair anyway. The facial marks are most common on the upper eyelids but can also involve the central area of the forehead. At their most extensive they are also seen on the upper lip and around the nares. They look more florid when the baby is active or crying; the family can be reassured that they will gradually fade over the first weeks and months of life.

Strawberry naevi are also common but are not present when the baby is born and gradually appear over the first weeks of life. The colour is usually bright red unless the naevus is very large and thickened, when stagnant cyanosis may make it more blue. The surface may become marked with tiny dimples, giving rise to the strawberry analogy. These naevi are often multiple and sometimes very extensive. Even though such a naevus can affect virtually the whole surface of an arm, eventually it will clear entirely. The naevus starts to resolve within weeks or months, with the development of paler areas in the centre which gradually become confluent. Occasionally the very large ones may leave slightly more obvious surface veins behind. Some have a much larger deep portion which is usually termed a *cavernous haemangioma*. These will also resolve with time but may require intervention if they interfere with vision or the airway; steroids and laser treatment have been used.

Port wine stains are present at the time of birth and do not change with age. They are a significant cosmetic problem and may later be treated with laser therapy. If they occur over the distribution of the trigeminal nerve they may be part of the Sturge–Weber syndrome and be associated with an intracranial haemangioma which may calcify and cause seizures.

Naevocellular naevi are dark pigmented lesions of varying shades, sometimes with tufts of hair within them. They are commonly small but may be much more extensive and surrounded by smaller lesions at the edges in an irregular fashion. If they occur over the base of the spine they may be associated with spina bifida at the same level. Excision and dermabrasion have both been used to treat these lesions; some naevocellular naevi are thought to have a risk of malignant change in adult life.

Café-au-lait patches can be present from birth and are usually quite small. A diagnosis of neurofibromatosis should be considered when there are more than five significant patches.

Mongolian blue spot is an area of bluish pigmentation seen over the base of the spine in babies with pigmented skin. It can be localised or so extensive that it covers much of the lower back. Occasionally it consists of discrete separate areas over the back which can look like bruises at first glance. It is most obvious in babies who have mildly pigmented skin, such as those from Mediterranean countries or China. These lesions fade as the child grows but can be present into the second year of life.

Fontanelles and sutures

The cranial sutures are spaces between the bones of the skull that allow for growth and also for flexibility of the skull during birth. They are usually not more than a few millimetres across, with the exception of the sagittal suture which can be slightly wider. The anterior fontanelle is roughly diamond shaped and can be too small to admit a finger tip at birth. It can also be several centimetres across and is often larger than average in black or Asian babies. The posterior fontanelle is usually not felt at birth but may persist in some infants. Occasionally there is a 'third fontanelle' within the posterior part of the sagittal suture; although this is a normal variant it is seen more commonly in Down's syndrome and with hydrocephalus. Hydrocephalus should be considered in any baby who has wide sutures and a large bulging fontanelle. Early referral should be made to a paediatrician for further assessment if this is suspected, and a cranial ultrasound scan will easily resolve the issue.

Eyes

The eyes are best examined in an infant who is awake and quiet. The eyelids are commonly initially oedematous and will settle over the first few days. Oedema is most prominent in the dependent eye after the baby has been asleep and results in that eye opening after the other one. Bleeding within the sclera around the iris is not uncommon after normal delivery and resolves spontaneously. Both eyes should show a normal red reflex when seen through an ophthalmoscope. If this is not present, the baby should be referred urgently to the local ophthalmic surgeon who has an interest in children. Most alert babies can be encouraged to follow a face through a wide horizontal arc.

Ears and hearing

The ears can be folded over during pregnancy to give rise to deformity at birth. There is now good evidence that in most cases the appearance can be corrected by taping the ears back in a normal position over the first months of life, thus avoiding the use of cosmetic surgery later. The presence of the meatus should be noted and the baby referred to a paediatric audiologist if this is absent. Accessory auricles are common just at the front edge of the ear and may be treated surgically. If they have a very narrow pedicle, it may be possible to tie the base with black silk thread and allow the accessory auricle to separate following infarction. Hearing can be tested at birth by measuring oto-acoustic emissions.

Mouth

Cleft lip and palate may be detected by good antenatal ultrasound scan but is most commonly first seen at birth. The condition can be unilateral or bilateral and cause major parental concern because of the disruption of the facial appearance. The cleft lip is usually repaired within a day or so of birth, greatly improving the facial appearance. The palatal lesion is usually repaired at a few months of age but there can be long-term problems with the dentition which require subsequent orthodontic help. The incidence of glue ear is higher in these babies and they need carefully co-ordinated care involving paediatric audiologists, ENT surgeons and speech therapists. Most paediatric units have 'before and after' photographs to reassure parents about the possible appearance after surgery.

Occasionally babies are born with a tooth present and will need referral to a paediatric dental surgeon. If the tooth is firmly in the gum it will probably be left there but if it is only loosely attached it will be removed.

Chest and cardiovascular system

Babies usually have a resting respiratory rate of about 40 breaths per minute after birth; a rate of more than 60 per minute should be considered abnormal. Parents often note the prominence of the xiphisternum in the first days of life and need reassurance that this is quite normal.

Cyanosis can be surprisingly difficult to see—the baby needs to be in good light. The resting heart rate is usually between 110 and 130 per minute but is occasionally lower in large babies or much higher with activity. The femoral pulses should be checked to exclude coarctation of the aorta. The presence of cyanosis or any heart murmur needs further investigation, including oximetry, chest X-ray and ECG. Further evaluation by ultrasound scan may be required in some babies.

Breasts

Breast enlargement is common in the first days of life in either sex. It may also be associated with milk secretion and will resolve spontaneously.

Abdomen

The abdomen should be examined for distension and visible peristalsis. A recent feed can cause considerable stomach enlargement in some babies and make examination difficult. There is commonly wide divarication of the rectus muscles which will resolve in the first years of life.

The umbilical cord usually contains two arteries and a single vein. A single artery is occasionally associated with other abnormalities: some consultant paediatricians favour ultrasound scanning of the urinary tract in such cases. The umbilical cord usually separates by about 10 days and most of the cord dries out. The base where separation takes place is often moist and can be smelly, as the process is one of 'wet' gangrene. Infection should be suspected if surrounding tissues become inflamed or discharge or blistering is present. Discharge of urine or meconium from the stump is due to the presence of a patent urachus (urine) or an omphalo-mesenteric duct (meconium) and requires intervention from a paediatric surgeon.

Exomphalos is protrusion of the bowel covered with peritoneum through the umbilicus. In *gastroschisis* the bowel emerges through the abdominal wall to the side of the umbilicus and has no covering. These lesions should be wrapped in clean 'cling' plastic film to keep them moist; no feeds should be given. Transfer to a neonatal paediatric surgeon is urgently required. Occasionally a small exomphalos may be mistaken for a large base to the umbilical cord with the risk that it is clamped at delivery, causing intestinal obstruction.

A pink granuloma may develop in the umbilicus following separation and lead to constant minor weeping of the area. This will resolve after one or more treatments with silver nitrate, which should be applied to the whole granuloma including the pedicle at the base.

Umbilical hernias are not uncommon in the first year of life and almost always resolve spontaneously. They are more common in black or premature babies. The larger ones may take many years to resolve and parents often request surgery if the hernia is prominent at school entry.

The liver is often palpable for up to about 1 cm below the right costal margin, possibly more if the diaphragm is pushed down. The liver often enlarges when haemolysis is present.

The spleen is palpable in about a quarter of newborn babies but may also be enlarged in haemolysis or infection.

The kidneys are often easily palpable when a baby is quiet or asleep. Kidney enlargement may cause them to be more easily felt: causes include hydronephrosis, juvenile polycystic kidneys or multicystic dysplastic kidneys. Further investigation usually commences with an ultrasound scan.

Genitalia

Unless a female baby is growth retarded during pregnancy, the labia majora are usually large enough to cover the labia minora. Mucosal tags are commonly seen attached to the hymen and need no intervention. There is usually a mucous discharge from the vagina and occasionally there may be 'withdrawal bleeding' a few days after birth. The clitoris is of variable size at birth, but if it appears very large then the adrenogenital syndrome should be considered.

The male baby should be examined closely for the presence of *hypospadias*, where the urethral meatus is displaced ventrally down the glans or shaft of the penis. This requires surgical treatment by a paediatric urologist; circumcision should not be carried out until it is known whether or not the tissue of the prepuce will be required for reconstruction. It is also advisable to carry out ultrasound scanning of the kidneys and bladder to exclude an obstructive lesion.

The testes are not fully descended in all term babies and are more commonly absent from the scrotum in babies who are premature. All babies with absent testes should be checked carefully again at the 6-week examination.

It is quite common for there to be hydrocoeles in the scrotum at birth. These can be confirmed by transillumination and do not require treatment at this stage as most resolve spontaneously during the first months of life.

Ambiguous genitalia

It is sometimes difficult to be certain of the sex of an infant from the appearance of the genitalia; this situation must be handled very sensitively. The baby must not be casually assigned a sex, and urgent consultation with a paediatric endocrinologist should be sought. The eventual gender assignment needs to take into account the future physical, emotional and sexual development of the child. The language used to describe the situation to the parents should be simple: technical words should not be used, especially when they may have emotive meanings to lay people.

The infant with ambiguous genitalia usually has a small phallus and an underdeveloped 'scrotum'. Examination takes into account the size of the phallus and the presence or absence of palpable gonads. Where gonads are present in the 'scrotum' or inguinal regions the baby is probably an undervirilised male. Further investigation may include a karyotype, ultrasound scans, a 'genitogram' and hormone studies. The assigned sex will not automatically be the sex determined from the karyotype.

Congenital adrenal hyperplasia (see also p. 246) is one important cause of ambiguous genitalia. It is an autosomal recessive condition that may be caused by a number of enzyme deficiencies in the production of cortisol by the adrenal glands. The low levels of cortisol cause an increase in ACTH production in the pituitary gland and resultant increase in adrenal size. Precursors in the production of cortisol accumulate and may result in excessive production of androgens. These can produce an enlarged penis in the male with excessive genital pigmentation. In the female, the clitoris may be enlarged and there can be labial fusion and increased genital pigmentation. While all the affected infants may lack adequate cortisol production, about half of all the babies also lack mineralocorticoid production and lose salt excessively in the urine. If this is not investigated and recognised at birth, the affected infants present during the first few weeks of life with hyponatraemia and possible circulatory collapse. Treatment involves oral replacement of the missing hormones.

Back

Spina bifida occulta may be associated with dark pigmentation, vascular birthmarks, lipoma or a tuft of hair over the spine. This requires further evaluation by X-ray and, if confirmed, a later MR scan to look for any tethering of the spinal cord which would require surgical release.

Hips

Examination of the hips is best accomplished with a quiet, awake baby. Most cases of congenital dislocation of the hip (CDH) are detectable at this stage, and the problem is more common with a family history or with breech presentation. The legs should be examined for unequal length or asymmetry of the leg creases around the buttocks and thighs. 'Limited abduc-

tion' may be one of the associated findings but this term has no accepted definition.

For Ortolani's test (Fig. 3.1) the baby should be placed supine on a firm surface and the hips and knees flexed to 90°. Each leg is examined in turn and is grasped with the examiner's middle finger over the greater trochanter. The thigh is lifted and gently abducted to allow a dislocated femoral head to return to the acetabulum with a notable 'clunk'. It will be noted that the femoral head moves forward if this occurs.

For Barlow's test the pelvis is fixed with one hand, placing the fingers at the back and the thumb over the symphysis pubis. The other hand is used to grip the opposite thigh and this is adducted with gentle downward pressure encouraging the femoral head to slip backwards over the lip of the acetabulum. Many paediatric departments have a 'doll' with specially made hips which can simulate the feeling of abnormal hip examinations.

When dislocation is suspected, the baby should be referred to an orthopaedic surgeon with paediatric interest. Treatment aims at keeping the femoral head within the acetabulum by immobilisation for the first few months of life using a splint or harness device. An open reduction may become necessary if the condition is missed or early treatment fails. Avascular necrosis of the femoral head is more likely with delayed treatment for the condition.

Screening tests for CDH are widely used but there is continuing controversy about their role and effectiveness. It is probable that some cases will go undetected, but the number can probably

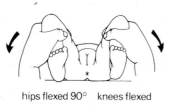

hips flexed 90°   knees flexed

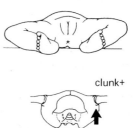

clunk+

Figure 3.1   Ortolani test for congenital dislocation of the hip.

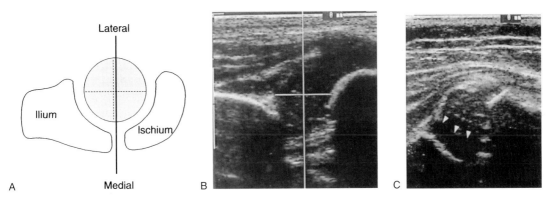

Figure 3.2 A: Transverse section through the infant hip showing the normal relationship of the ball of the femoral head to the acetabulum. B: Normal transverse section showing the axes indicated in A. C: Inferior subluxation with interposition of poorly echogenic limbic cartilage (arrowheads) between the moderately echogenic femoral head and the floor of the acetabulum.

be minimised by improved training for those who carry out examinations. Ultrasound examination of the hip (Fig. 3.2) has been used in some centres and is probably best considered as an aid to diagnosis in high risk or suspected cases, rather than as a primary screening test.

Limbs

It is not uncommon for there to be extra digits on the hands (polydactyly). These are most commonly small pedunculated structures attached to the ulnar side of the hand: they have a dominant inheritance. When the digit has a very narrow base it may be tied off firmly with a black silk suture and allowed to separate. If the base is thick or there is any bony structure present it will need surgical treatment, possibly after an X-ray. Extra toes may also be found and tend to be more substantial.

Webbing of adjacent digits (syndactyly) is not uncommon and is usually incomplete. Both hands may be similarly affected but this is not always the case. The webbing can be separated by a plastic surgeon. Webbing of the second and third toes is more common and does not need treatment.

After birth, all babies tend to hold their feet out of line with the leg when they are relaxed. This positional talipes is easily corrected with minimal effort by the examiner and is due to the way the baby's feet are folded together in the uterus. True talipes or club foot is present when the deformity cannot be over-corrected by pressure; such a deformity will require the opinion of an orthopaedic surgeon with paediatric expertise. The foot may be treated by passive stretching, taping or plastering, depending on local practice and severity. The worst deformities will require surgical correction.

Many babies show adduction of the forefoot (metatarsus varus). This almost always corrects itself as the child grows and should not normally require intervention.

Skin rashes

Erythema toxicum (neonatal urticaria) is seen in many babies by about the third day of life. The rash consists of small pustules filled with eosinophils and surrounded by a larger area of erythema. They occur mainly over the trunk and proximal parts of the limbs, disappearing within a few days without treatment. (See also p. 356.)

Milia are tiny white sebaceous plugs within the skin. They are very common around the nose but can be more widespread. They will resolve without treatment.

Miliaria are small blisters under the skin, caused by sweat being trapped under the upper layers of the epidermis, and may be associated with areas of erythema. They are more common in hot climates and can be treated by rubbing the skin with a towel after bathing.

Candida may cause a pustular skin rash, often in the nappy area. It can also appear as white patches within the mouth, especially within the buccal pouches and along the gums. As it spreads it causes distress to the baby during feeds. Treatment is with nystatin 100 000 units dripped into the sides of the mouth after feeds until it is cleared. When the baby is breast fed, the infection can return after treatment has stopped, presumably by re-infection from the mother. This can usually be prevented by giving one dose of nystatin to the baby after the last feed while breast feeding continues. If the baby is bottle fed, special attention should be paid to sterilisation techniques and the teats should be replaced.

Primitive reflexes

A large number of reflexes have been described in the newborn infant, many of which are dependent on the wake/sleep state. A few of these are tested routinely as a part of the examination.

The rooting reflex is elicited by stroking the cheek just to one side of the mouth with a finger. The alert infant will move the head towards the stimulus and the baby's mouth will seek to suck the finger.

The sucking reflex is elicited by gently placing the little finger into the corner of the baby's mouth. The alert infant will move around to accommodate the finger within the mouth and start to suck it.

The grasp reflex is elicited by placing the examiner's thumbs into the palms of the baby's hands with the arms outstretched. In an alert baby the resulting grasp will support some of the weight of the trunk as the examiner lifts his/her thumbs upwards.

The Moro reflex is elicited by holding the trunk of the baby carefully in one hand and the head in the other. The head must be in the midline or the tonic neck reflexes will cause asymmetry. The hand holding the head is suddenly moved down through a few centimetres, allowing the baby's neck to extend partially. The baby's arms should move away from the trunk and then extend fully at right angles to it. Following this the arms will begin to flex again at the shoulders, elbows and wrists, so that the outstretched fingers come back towards the midline. The response should be symmetrical but can vary with gestational maturity and wake/sleep state.

The placing reflex is best demonstrated in a baby in a high state of alertness and activity. The baby is held by the examiner with a hand around either side of the trunk. If the dorsum of one foot is placed against the undersurface of a flat edge such as a table, the leg and foot will be lifted up and the sole of the foot placed down on the upper surface.

The walking reflex requires the baby to be in a similar state as the placing reflex. The baby is held in the same way with the feet touching the top of a firm surface. The baby will place alternate feet on the surface and lift the other leg in a 'walking' movement.

INFANT FEEDING

Breast feeding

Breast feeding offers an infant many advantages over artificial feeding and these are generally well publicised to mothers during pregnancy (Box 3.5). Not all mothers will wish to breast feed; some will not succeed and they must not be allowed to feel guilty as a result. Mothers may doubt the adequacy of feeds as they are not measured, however successful feeding will be demonstrated by adequate weight gain; 'test

---

Box 3.5 Advantages of breast feeding

- Appropriate protein, carbohydrate and fat content
- Inexpensive
- Ready prepared
- Clean
- Antibodies and white blood cells transmitted which protect against infection
- Iron in breast milk is protein bound and available to infant but not bacteria
- Infant's bowel becomes colonised with lactobacilli, and the number of coliform organisms is low
- Mother/infant feeding relationship more intense than for bottle feeds
- Supply/demand feedback ensures that the infant consumes the correct amount of milk to give adequate fluid and nutrition intake

weighing' a baby before and after a feed is not accurate enough to be a valid exercise.

Breast feeding babies can lose up to 15% of their body weight in the first three days of life but most will have regained their birth weight by the end of the first week. Stools tend to be explosive with a mixture of liquid and small 'seedy' particles. The colour can vary from orange through yellow to green. The frequency can be anything from 12 or more per day to only one stool in a week. The extremes of this range often cause anxiety to families and professionals alike, but if the stool is of a typical consistency and the baby is thriving and well, the family should be reassured.

Bottle feeding

Bottle feeding requires good maternal education about the risks of contamination of feeds. The infant will take the feed more slowly and may not limit intake as successfully as the breast fed baby. All infant formulae have to conform to the same regulations concerning their composition and preparation, so the choice is largely a matter for the family. Frequent changes of milks should not be encouraged. Most bottle fed infants will take about 150 ml/kg of milk in each 24 hours but there is considerable variation. A bottle fed baby typically loses 5–10% of body weight in the first five days of life and only regains its birth weight in the second week of life. The stools tend to be fairly solid or clay like, and the modern milks produce colours ranging from pale yellow to pale green. Stool frequency is not as varied as that seen for breast feeding.

Vomiting

Most babies tend to bring up some of the milk that they take: this is usually effortless or associated with 'burping'. This is known as posseting, and parents may need confident reassurance to view it as normal. True vomiting can be caused by overfeeding, crying, swallowing air and excessive parental handling. An anxious parent with a crying baby may even give more milk to replace that lost by vomiting.

Vomiting is less commonly caused by prob-lems such as infection, gastro-oesophageal reflux, cow's milk protein sensitivity, metabolic prob-lems or bowel obstruction. The baby should be examined carefully for lethargy, failure to gain weight, abdominal distension and visible peri-stalsis. The presence of any of these features indicates the need for further investigation.

CRYING BABIES

One of the common concerns for a new mother is that her baby appears to cry excessively. Before birth, mothers usually report that their baby is quiet by day and active when they are trying to sleep. Many babies seem to carry on this diurnal rhythm after they are born and are more awake during the night when the mother wishes to rest. Over the first days of life, babies begin to wake regularly for feeds and it is usual for them to cry to alert their mothers. After feeds, most new babies return to sleep, but as they get older they will be more alert after feeds.

Babies who have suffered minor birth trauma or asphyxia are often irritable during the first few days and may cry more than average. Babies who are withdrawing from maternal drug use may also be irritable but the behaviour is more prolonged and may be severe enough to require sedation. Some babies who are sensitive to cow's milk protein may cry excessively during or just after feeds and this behaviour may worsen steadily with the baby becoming reluctant to feed. The problem is not confined to bottle fed infants: it can occur in infants whose mothers secrete unchanged cow's milk proteins in breast milk. The bottle fed infant will improve dramati-cally on a cow's milk protein free formula such as Prejomin, Nutramigen or Pregestimil. Soy milk has also been used but a significant propor-tion of babies treated with it will develop soy protein sensitivity. If the baby has a period of several months free of cow's milk protein, the problem often resolves spontaneously. Some doctors prefer a later cow's milk challenge to be carried out in hospital in case there is a severe allergic reaction. The breast fed baby can be simi-larly treated by asking the dietician to arrange a cow's milk protein free diet for the mother.

Some crying babies have no medical cause for their problem but have parents who find the situation difficult to handle. They may find it impossible to put a crying baby to sleep, even though that is how many babies indicate they are tired. As a result, the baby is picked up, offered more feeds and carried around. The baby gets used to this attention and becomes even more reluctant to sleep. Friends and relatives confirm the parents' worries that the baby 'must have something wrong' and professionals often compound the problem by referring to the baby as having 'colic', for which medication is prescribed. The baby usually does not respond and the situation becomes more fraught as the parents get little sleep and begin to argue. Crying behaviour of this type is more common where the baby is seen as 'precious', especially after infertility, threatened miscarriage, previous fetal loss, previous infant death or a difficult labour. When faced with the problem of a crying baby like this, it is important to spend time exploring the background and the parents' feelings as well as considering medical problems. On many occasions, the parents begin to understand their own difficulties as the history unfolds and they can be given help to allow the baby to cry itself to sleep without intervening.

NEONATAL JAUNDICE
Physiological jaundice

Jaundice is a very common finding in the first week of life—possible causes are listed in Box 3.6. It usually reaches a peak by 4–5 days of age and then settles rapidly. Physiological jaundice is caused by a combination of circumstances which allow the accumulation of bilirubin within the tissues. Haemoglobin levels are high at birth (15–23 g/dl) and red cells containing fetal haemoglobin are gradually replaced by new ones with adult haemoglobin. The baby will have a higher red cell mass if the cord is clamped late or the infant held low down during delivery: these factors contribute to higher rates of haemolysis in the first days. Bilirubin is one of the breakdown products of haemoglobin and is fat- rather than water-soluble, being transported in the blood

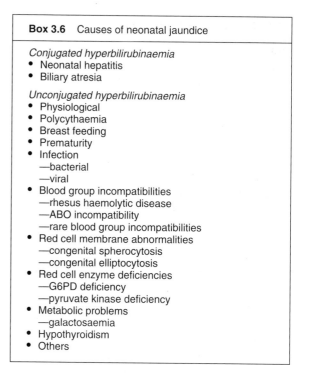

Box 3.6 Causes of neonatal jaundice

Conjugated hyperbilirubinaemia
- Neonatal hepatitis
- Biliary atresia

Unconjugated hyperbilirubinaemia
- Physiological
- Polycythaemia
- Breast feeding
- Prematurity
- Infection
  —bacterial
  —viral
- Blood group incompatibilities
  —rhesus haemolytic disease
  —ABO incompatibility
  —rare blood group incompatibilities
- Red cell membrane abnormalities
  —congenital spherocytosis
  —congenital elliptocytosis
- Red cell enzyme deficiencies
  —G6PD deficiency
  —pyruvate kinase deficiency
- Metabolic problems
  —galactosaemia
- Hypothyroidism
- Others

stream attached to albumin. This unconjugated bilirubin is normally conjugated within the liver by the enzyme glucuronyl transferase, producing the water-soluble form of bilirubin which can be excreted in bile. The enzyme levels are initially low, allowing accumulation of the pigment in body tissues, including the skin.

Jaundice is first apparent in areas with the best blood supply and is thus observed as spreading from the face to the trunk and thence down the limbs. If it is limited to the face and trunk, the blood level is probably less than 200 µmol/l. If the limbs are involved, especially the hands and feet, then the level is probably higher. The skin must be pressed briefly to blanch it so that the underlying colour can be seen. Care must be taken with babies who have pigmented skin as jaundice can easily be underestimated. Jaundice within the first 24 hours of life should always be investigated immediately. Jaundice of later onset thought to be greater than 200 µmol/l should be checked by blood test and investigated if the level is confirmed. Jaundice persisting for more than 2 weeks after birth also needs investigation.

The complications of jaundice

High levels of jaundice, especially in ill infants, can be a cause of high tone deafness. Bilirubin may also be deposited within the basal ganglia of the brain—kernicterus. There is no defined bilirubin level which constitutes a risk: in the first three days of life the rate of rise is as important as the absolute value. After the third day, photo-therapy would be started in a normal birth weight term infant at about 250 µmol/l, and exchange transfusion considered at about 350 µmol/l. Hospital paediatric departments keep charts on which it is easy to plot bilirubin values allowing for size, gestation and age, giving guidance about suitable treatment. Kernicterus was most commonly seen in the past in babies affected by rhesus haemolytic disease and is fortunately now very rare. Kernicterus causes increased lethargy, progressing to irritability, opisthotonos and convulsions. The mortality used to be about 50% and survivors could develop choreo-athetoid cerebral palsy and learning difficulties.

The treatment of jaundice

Phototherapy is an extremely effective treatment for jaundice and uses the visible blue spectrum of light. The bilirubin in skin undergoes photo-isomerisation to a form that is water-soluble and readily excreted in bile without conjugation. The baby develops loose stools and there is thus a need to watch fluid balance carefully as the baby is undressed and has high evaporative losses. It is usual to shield the eyes to prevent damage to the retina, although the risk is unproved.

Exchange transfusion has become quite rare now that phototherapy is so effective and rhesus haemolytic disease is less widespread. The ex-change is carried out through a centrally placed catheter inserted into the umbilical vein or using the umbilical or radial artery and a peripheral vein. Using small aliquots of around 10 ml at a time, the baby is exchange transfused with about twice its blood volume of fresh, cross matched, anticoagulated blood. This process removes not only bilirubin but also any maternal antibodies or antibody coated red blood cells. It replaces red blood cells lost through haemolysis and provides albumin which can bind bilirubin and help prevent kernicterus.

Conjugated hyperbilirubinaemia
(see also p. 151)

One of the most important investigations for jaundice, especially prolonged jaundice, is to check whether the bilirubin is conjugated or un-conjugated. The rare finding of high levels of conjugated bilirubin indicates that the jaundice is obstructive and the prognosis is usually more serious. As the condition progresses it may be associated with pale stools, dark urine and a greenish tinge to the skin colour. The most common causes are biliary atresia and neonatal hepatitis. In biliary atresia there is a failure of development of some or all of the bile ducts; this can often be treated surgically by porto-enterostomy (Kasai procedure). The procedure needs to be carried out before the baby is more than about 8 weeks of age, and early referral to a paediatric liver specialist is imperative.

Neonatal hepatitis can be caused by congenital infection and some inborn errors of metabolism, including α_1-antitrypsin deficiency, fructosaemia and tyrosinaemia. These conditions also neces-sitate early specialist referral.

Unconjugated hyperbilirubinaemia

Unconjugated hyperbilirubinaemia has many possible causes apart from physiological jaun-dice. Any form of infection can be responsible: the baby should be examined carefully with appropriate attention to feeding and the way in which the baby is behaving. If there is any doubt, the baby will need to be reviewed in hospital with bacterial cultures, blood tests and possible antibiotic treatment.

Breast milk jaundice

Breast feeding is a common cause of jaundice; the jaundice may be prolonged, lasting for up to three months. A steroid excreted in breast milk inhibits liver conjugation. This is a diagnosis of exclusion and breast feeding should not be stopped. Phototherapy is occasionally required for a time but the baby will remain healthy.

Rhesus haemolytic disease

Rhesus haemolytic disease is caused by the passive transfer of rhesus D IgG antibodies across the placenta from a rhesus negative mother to a rhesus positive fetus. The problem does not usually occur in a first pregnancy but only in subsequent pregnancies, perhaps becoming more severe with each new baby. It is caused by significant leaks of fetal red blood cells into the maternal circulation, especially during delivery and manoeuvres such as external cephalic version of a breech presentation. Leaks of fetal cells can occur spontaneously and this is the rationale for the regular administration of anti-D gamma globulin injections to rhesus negative mothers to prevent sensitisation. Transfusion of rhesus positive blood to a rhesus negative mother may also cause sensitisation.

In severe cases of rhesus haemolytic disease, fetal red cell haemolysis may occur with fetal anaemia and enlargement of liver and spleen to cope with increased erythropoiesis. The liver fails to make adequate amounts of albumin, and fetal oedema or hydrops occurs. Intrauterine transfusions may be used to suppress these problems and allow sufficient maturity for delivery. The accumulation of bilirubin and related pigments in the liquor is also monitored and will give an indication for the timing of induced delivery. Haemoglobin and bilirubin in the cord blood should be measured at delivery and appropriate treatment given according to the severity of the problem. This might include phototherapy, exchange transfusion or top-up transfusion for anaemia. All babies of rhesus negative mothers should have cord blood sent for a Coombs' test as well as bilirubin and haemoglobin estimation.

Other blood group incompatibilities

ABO incompatibility is now probably a more common cause of jaundice than rhesus haemolytic disease. In this situation, the baby has a group A or B red cell antigen that is not possessed by the mother. This does not require a sensitising pregnancy and does not necessarily recur even when the blood group of a subsequent baby presents the same risk. Antibodies to the A and B blood antigens are normally of the IgM type and therefore too large to cross the placenta. Following a leak of fetal red cells into the maternal circulation the mother can make antibodies of the IgG type, and it is these which can cross the placenta and cause haemolysis. The pregnancy is usually normal and the problem is only identified when it causes neonatal jaundice. The direct Coombs' test may be weakly positive at delivery but is often negative later, though the indirect Coombs' test may be positive. The problem can be positively diagnosed by the identification of appropriate haemolysins in maternal blood.

Other rare blood group incompatibilities may cause haemolysis of varying severity: these include C, E, Duffy, Kidd and Kell antibodies.

Red blood cell enzyme deficiencies

Glucose-6-phosphate dehydrogenase deficiency (G6PD) is an X-linked recessively inherited disease causing jaundice. Male infants are usually affected but the heterozygote female may also have problems. The groups mainly affected are those of Chinese, Mediterranean, black African and black American origin. Some infants with this condition develop spontaneous haemolysis in the first days of life, while others may have the problem triggered by drugs transferred in breast milk. A list of conditions and agents which may cause haemolysis in affected individuals is given in Box 3.7. Affected infants develop not only jaundice but anaemia: a blood film may show spherocytes, Heinz bodies and crenated red blood cells as well as a reticulocytosis. A screening test is available for this condition and the enzyme can also be estimated when the screen is positive. Advice to families is directed at understanding the condition and avoiding the trigger factors.

Pyruvate kinase enzyme deficiency is another cause of neonatal haemolysis and jaundice.

Box 3.7 Possible causes for haemolysis in individuals with G6PD deficiency

- Antibiotics:
  —nitrofurantoin
  —sulphonamides
  —nalidixic acid
  —chloramphenicol
- Anti-inflammatory drugs:
  —acetylsalicylic acid
  —phenacetin
- Antimalarials:
  —quinine
  —primaquine
- Naphthalene
- Methylene Blue
- Vitamin K (only in large doses)
- Fava beans
- Respiratory viruses
- Viral hepatitis

The inheritance is autosomal recessive and the enzyme can be assayed.

Hereditary spherocytosis (see also p. 281)

This is an autosomal dominant condition but there is also a high level of new mutation. The blood film may show spherocytes but this is also true of other conditions. There is increased fragility of the red blood cells when exposed to an osmotic gradient, however this test is unreliable until the infant is several months old. Some affected children suffer with hypersplenism as they get older and require splenectomy; others suffer only mild haemolysis which causes them no long-term problems. Other family members should be screened if there is no family history of the condition.

Polycythaemia

Polycythaemia is defined as a haematocrit of more than 65% during the first days of life. It is more common when there has been intrauterine growth retardation, maternal diabetes, twin to twin transfusion or materno-fetal transfusion, or in Down's syndrome. Polycythaemia is a cause of jaundice but it can also contribute to hyperviscosity of the blood which may cause other problems including pulmonary hypertension, heart failure, jitteriness and necrotising enterocolitis. Treatment is by dilutional exchange transfusion with plasma when the infant is symptomatic with a haematocrit over 75%.

RESPIRATORY DISTRESS

Babies are defined as having respiratory distress if the resting respiration rate is consistently above 60 per minute. Respiratory distress may also be associated with flaring of the nostrils, marked head movement in time with respiration, intercostal recession, subcostal recession and grunting. Very often it is the grunting which draws attention to the condition, and when grunting is marked it may significantly depress the respiratory rate. The problem for the clinician is that there is a very wide range of causes, involving many body systems. Cyanosis may be an additional feature and indicates a degree of urgency in resolving the cause. Hypothermia is a significant cause of grunting—babies should not be allowed to become cold after delivery.

Causes of respiratory distress

Upper airways obstruction. Obstruction of the upper airways should be excluded; there may be choanal atresia or stenosis, when a membrane completely or partially occludes the nasopharyngeal airway posteriorly. An airway placed in the mouth and fastened with adhesive tape allows the baby to breathe normally while specialist surgical care is arranged.

Metabolic acidosis. Metabolic acidosis resulting from birth asphyxia may cause respiratory distress as the baby attempts a respiratory compensation by hyperventilation. Measurement of arterial blood gas is required to confirm diagnosis. Metabolic acidosis may also be present in infection, metabolic problems and cyanotic heart disease. Provided there is no continuing cause for the acidosis and the problem is mild, the baby will correct the situation without help. More severe problems require slow correction with a buffer such as sodium bicarbonate. This is administered as an 8.4% solution, diluted to half that strength with water for injection and infused slowly. The volume of 8.4% bicarbonate is calculated from the base deficit, the baby's weight and a factor representing the proportion of extracellular fluid as 30% of body weight:

$$\text{Volume of 8.4\% NaHCO}_3 \text{ (ml)} = \text{base deficit} \times \text{body weight (kg)} \times 0.3$$

This formula will not result in excessive correction and the blood gases need to be reviewed after the infusion has been completed. The cause of the acidosis must also be treated effectively or the problem will recur.

Pneumonia. Congenital pneumonia is a serious cause of respiratory distress and requires urgent treatment. One of the most common causes is the group B haemolytic streptococcus (GBS) which can be acquired from the mother during delivery, but other organisms can also infect the lung. Treatment is with appropriate antibiotics and respiratory support with oxygen and artificial ventilation where required.

Pneumothorax. Term babies can develop a spontaneous pneumothorax at birth; the condition may also follow resuscitation with artificial ventilation. It can usually be demonstrated in a darkened environment by transillumination of the chest with a cold light source, when the affected side will be notably brighter. It can be confirmed with a chest X-ray (Figure 3.3) and may require needle aspiration or the placement of a chest drain with a one-way valve. Pneumothorax is seen more commonly after prolonged ventilation for respiratory pathology.

Transient tachypnoea of the newborn (TTN). TTN is caused by failure to clear the lungs of fetal lung fluid during the process of delivery. The usual mechanism for clearance is the squeezing of the fetal chest by the contractions of normal labour. TTN is more frequently seen following elective Caesarean section or precipitate labour and in babies of 34–36 weeks' gestation. An X-ray shows fluid in the lung fissures and streaky shadowing caused by interstitial fluid. Treatment is supportive and the condition usually resolves within 48 hours.

Heart disease. Congenital heart disease can cause respiratory distress through the mechanisms of pulmonary oedema, increased pulmo-

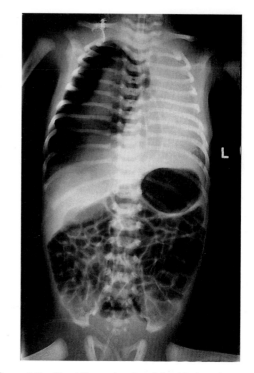

Figure 3.3 Chest X-ray showing right-sided tension pneumothorax.

nary blood flow or metabolic acidosis. Evaluation of cardiac function is an important part of investigation of respiratory symptoms.

Meconium aspiration. Meconium aspiration can be a very serious neonatal illness and is mainly preventable by careful management of the baby at the time of delivery. The passage of meconium during delivery may be seen in babies who are suffering a degree of intrapartum asphyxia and also in larger babies without obvious asphyxia. Meconium can block airways with resultant collapse or hyperinflation due to a 'ball valve' effect. It is also irritant to the airway and causes widespread inflammation with a risk of secondary bacterial infection.

When meconium is present in the liquor at delivery, the baby should have the mouth and nose aspirated following crowning of the head. After delivery the baby's pharynx must be aspirated without delay using a laryngoscope under direct vision. If meconium is seen at or below the vocal cords, the baby should be intubated and meconium aspirated from the trachea. The stomach should also be aspirated and can be lavaged with normal saline if any meconium is present in the initial aspirate.

Respiratory support and antibiotics are the routine treatment for meconium aspiration. In some babies the condition can be associated with persistent fetal circulation, and in the worst cases treatment with an extracorporeal membrane oxygenator (ECMO) may be extremely effective.

Congenital anomalies. Diaphragmatic hernia and oesophageal atresia are dealt with in Chapter 15, pages 309 and 310.

CONGENITAL HEART DISEASE (CHD)

Congenital heart disease is the most common major congenital abnormality: its incidence in the first week of life is approximately 2 per 1000 deliveries. Throughout childhood the prevalence of congenital heart lesions is greater than 1 in 100 children. Defects are more frequent in premature babies and those with Down's syndrome or other chromosomal abnormalities. Some maternal conditions (Box 3.8) can also increase the risk.

Infants with heart lesions may present with respiratory distress, cyanosis or even sudden collapse, but CHD may also be diagnosed on routine examination of a well baby.

Cyanotic heart disease

Peripheral or stagnant cyanosis of the hands and feet is very common in babies during the first hours of life while the baby adapts to an independent life. It is more noticeable while the baby is quiet and clears when there is crying. Central cyanosis is diagnosed by seeing it in tongue and lips as well as the peripheries. It can be surprisingly difficult to recognise in an otherwise well baby unless examination is carried out in a good level of natural lighting. When there is also respiratory distress it can be difficult to decide whether the cause is chest disease or heart disease. To help resolve this the baby can be placed in 100% oxygen for 10 minutes and the effect on pO_2 noted. If there is little or no rise, the problem is one of right to left shunting due to cardiac disease. Further information may be gained from cardiac examination, ECG, chest X-ray and cardiac ultrasound scan. Cyanotic heart disease usually requires surgical intervention: this may initially involve a palliative shunt to allow sufficient oxygenation. Box 3.9 lists conditions which may present with cyanosis.

Congestive cardiac failure

Most babies with congestive cardiac failure (CCF) have structural lesions of the heart (Box 3.10) but some may have other diseases which adversely affect cardiac function.

Box 3.9 Cyanotic congenital heart lesions

- Tetralogy of Fallot when the pulmonary stenosis is severe
- Pulmonary atresia
- Severe pulmonary stenosis
- Tricuspid atresia
- Transposition of the great arteries
- Total anomalous pulmonary venous drainage
- Hypoplastic right heart syndrome

Box 3.8 Maternal conditions which predispose to CHD

- Diabetes mellitus
- Alcohol abuse
- Drug therapy, e.g. anti-epileptics
- Drug abuse
- Infections in pregnancy, e.g. rubella

Box 3.10 Structural cardiac lesions causing congestive cardiac failure

- Patent ductus arteriosus
- Ventricular septal defect
- Coarctation of the aorta
- Hypoplastic left heart syndrome
- Persistent truncus arteriosus
- Defects of the endocardial cushions (e.g. atrio-ventricular septal defect)
- Severe aortic stenosis

Clinical features

Cardiac failure is recognised by the presence of respiratory distress associated with an enlarged liver. There may also be oedema but this is not always obvious and may be represented by excessive weight gain. The baby may also show sweating, heart murmurs, gallop rhythm and crepitations on chest auscultation.

Management

Apart from the clinical signs, further information may be gained from ECG, chest X-ray or cardiac ultrasound scan. Immediate treatment involves diuretics, and cardiac surgery may also be required. Most cases involve a left to right shunt or an obstruction to blood flow.

Other conditions which can present with cardiac failure are listed in Box 3.11. These are diagnosed by exclusion of structural defects and by specific tests or circumstances.

Heart murmurs

Routine examination may reveal the presence of a heart murmur in an otherwise healthy infant. The whole cardiovascular system should be carefully examined for any other signs which might be helpful; the baby also requires blood pressure measurement in upper and lower limbs, an ECG and a chest X-ray. If these investigations are normal, a routine referral to a paediatrician or paediatric cardiologist can be made but, if there is concern that the tests are abnormal, the child may need a more urgent cardiac ultrasound scan.

Box 3.11 Other causes of congestive cardiac failure
• Myocardial ischaemia caused by birth asphyxia   • Viral myocarditis   • Hydrops fetalis   • Polycythaemia   • Endocardial fibroelastosis   • Fluid overload   • Arrhythmias

INFECTIONS

Neonatal immunology

The newborn infant has a less efficient immune system than an older child or adult. The physical barriers of the skin and mucous membranes are more easily breached and antibody levels are generally low. IgG antibody crosses the placenta during the last trimester of pregnancy and helps to protect the infant against organisms that the mother has been exposed to and which may colonise the baby following delivery. The infant's polymorphonuclear leukocytes are also inefficient, allowing bacterial infections to spread easily to the blood stream rather than remain localised. All this means that the infant is particularly vulnerable to bacterial infections. The baby may have very few clinical signs of infection and may not be febrile. Symptoms like irritability, lethargy, floppiness, jaundice, poor feeding and vomiting should all be taken very seriously in the first weeks of life, and treatment will often be required before the diagnosis is certain.

When a baby is unwell and sepsis may be the cause, the baby should be examined carefully for any signs of localised infection. The temperature, heart rate and respiratory rate should be monitored. Swabs should be taken from the nose, throat, umbilicus and any obvious site of superficial infection. Without evidence of localised infection, the baby will also require a chest X-ray, blood cultures, a suprapubic urine aspirate and probably a lumbar puncture. Antibiotic therapy is usually given intravenously; the drugs used depend on the likely cause of infection and the age of the baby.

Bacterial infections

Septicaemia, meningitis and pneumonia

The group B haemolytic streptococcus (GBS) represents one of the most serious potential pathogens for the newborn infant. It is carried in the bowel or throat of up to about one third of the population but causes relatively little adult infection. During pregnancy it may also be carried within the vagina and can gain access to the fetus. Usually, but not always, this happens after rupture of the membranes; the organism may infect the lungs and rapidly spread to cause septicaemia and occasionally meningitis. Considering the carriage rate for the organism, the infection rate is very low (about 1 in 3000 deliveries) but the severity of the illness makes it important that GBS is suspected in any baby falling ill in the first few days after birth. The organism is sensitive to a combination of penicillin and gentamicin; recently the modern cephalosporins have also been successfully used.

Listeria monocytogenes is another organism that can be acquired from the mother during pregnancy. It is found in soft cheeses and it is usually recommended that these are not eaten by pregnant women. Listeriosis often causes premature onset of labour in a mother who is herself unwell. The pre-term infant often passes meconium during delivery: this is a useful clue since meconium is otherwise rarely passed in this way by pre-term infants. The organism causes septicaemia and pneumonia. Diagnosis is by blood culture.

Gram-negative organisms from the bowel such as *E. coli* can also be responsible for septicaemia. In many cases this follows a urinary tract infection which in turn may be caused by a urinary tract anomaly. Gram-negative septicaemia may progress rapidly to meningitis; when this occurs the prognosis may be poor. Intensive support and broad spectrum antibiotic cover are required. Survivors require a hearing test and developmental surveillance.

Skin infections

Staphylococcus aureus may be acquired from the family but professionals also represent a risk, as does cross infection from other babies in a nursery. Careful hand washing is important in the prevention of cross infection. Staphylococcal infections commonly present as blisters or pustules on the skin but may also cause paronychia. Any such area of skin should be cultured and the baby started immediately on flucloxacillin as the organism can easily spread systemically. Hexachlorophene skin preparations may also be used. If there is extensive erythema with the formation of bullae, the condition is known as *toxic epidermal necrolysis*. The baby must be treated with intravenous antibiotics and the affected skin managed like a burn.

Infections around the umbilicus are commonly caused by *Staphylococcus aureus* or Gram-negative organisms. Prompt culture and treatment are required because this site allows easy access to the portal system.

Conjunctivitis

Sticky eyes are very common in the first week of life and do not usually represent infection; it is more common for the nasolacrimal duct to be blocked. The stickiness can be cleared during routine washing of the face. This usually settles over the first weeks or months of life and only requires ophthalmological referral if it persists beyond six months.

Conjunctivitis is recognised by erythema of the conjunctiva and purulent discharge. A swab is sent for culture and appropriate treatment is given for the likely organism. Gonococcal infection usually presents with fulminant conjunctivitis occurring within the first three days of life. The conjunctival oedema can prevent the eye being opened easily and pus may squirt out under pressure as the eyelids are prised apart. Treatment is with systemic penicillin and penicillin irrigation of the eyes. It must be remembered that the parents also should be referred to a genitourinary medicine specialist.

Staphylococcal eye infection usually occurs about 3–5 days after birth and is milder. Topical treatment with gentamicin or neomycin eye drops may be given.

Chlamydia trachomatis is a cause of persistent conjunctivitis in the first week but can also present at about 7–10 days with more fulminant signs. Topical tetracycline is used as well as systemic erythromycin. This condition also necessitates referral of the parents for a genitourinary medicine opinion.

Congenital infections (see p. 327)

Toxoplasmosis

Rubella
Cytomegalovirus
Varicella.

Syphilis

Syphilis infection is now rare and only occurs in the fetus who is exposed after about four months of pregnancy. Treatment of the mother with penicillin also treats the fetus effectively.

Hepatitis B

All mothers should be tested in pregnancy for hepatitis B surface antigen (HBsAg); those who are positive should be further tested for the presence of the HBe antigen (HBeAg) and antibody to HBeAg (antiHBe). The greatest risk occurs when the mother is HBeAg positive but antiHBe negative, with a lesser risk when antiHBe is found. At risk babies are immunised with hepatitis B vaccine shortly after birth as well as being treated with hepatitis B immune globulin injections, repeated at monthly intervals for the first six months of life.

Human immunodeficiency virus

Human immunodeficiency virus (HIV) can be acquired by the fetus during gestation or at the time of delivery. The risk of fetal infection is probably greater if the mother has acquired immune deficiency syndrome (AIDS); the absence of any dysmorphic syndrome in the affected infants suggests that transmission rarely occurs early in the pregnancy. There is evidence to show that giving zidovudine therapy to the mother during pregnancy reduces the risk of transmission, as may Caesarean section.

Studies have suggested that vertical transmission of the virus occurs in 15–39% of pregnancies, but the risk is lower in Europe than in Africa and breast feeding may be an important factor in this. It appears that the risk of transmission from mother to baby is approximately doubled if the infant is breast fed, and breast feeding is usually contraindicated in developed countries. For a child living in a country where it would

run a high risk of malnutrition if not breast fed, the risk of breast feeding may be preferable.

The infant should be treated with zidovudine from birth until its HIV status is proved negative. Cotrimoxazole prophylaxis against *Pneumocystis carinii* is started once the risk of jaundice has subsided as there is a very significant risk of this organism causing severe pneumonia in an infected infant. Some authorities favour early BCG immunisation in all infants at risk.

HAEMORRHAGIC DISEASE OF THE NEWBORN (see also p. 43)

Haemorrhagic disease of the newborn is due to a deficiency of clotting factors that are dependent on vitamin K. Vitamin K is normally produced by bacteria within the bowel but the newborn infant has no organisms present. If vitamin K is not administered after birth, some babies will develop spontaneous haemorrhage from any site, most commonly from within the bowel but also possibly intracranial.

The condition is confirmed by a clotting screen which shows prolongation of the prothrombin time and a normal partial thromboplastin time. Treatment is replacement of blood loss through transfusion, where indicated, and the administration of vitamin K_1 in a dose of 1 mg i.v., repeated if necessary.

HYPOGLYCAEMIA

Hypoglycaemia is defined as a blood glucose of less than 2.6 mmol/l but the definition is empirical and has varied in the past; there has been considerable recent debate. The current acceptance of this value is based on the risks of brain injury with lower values and it is used for all infants regardless of their gestational age or state of intrauterine nutrition. There is every prospect of the value changing again or different values being used for different groups of babies in the future. Neurological symptoms are very likely if the level falls below 1.1 mmol/l.

Before birth, the fetal blood glucose level is about three quarters of the maternal level. After delivery, the baby uses glycogen in liver and

---

Box 3.12   Symptoms of hypoglycaemia

- Drowsiness
- Irritability
- High pitched cry
- Apnoeic attacks
- Cyanotic attacks
- Feeding difficulty
- Vomiting
- Jitteriness
- Seizures

---

muscle as an immediate source of glucose. Glucose can also be made from endogenous amino acids and fat but the process is slower. All these processes are eventually dependent on successfully establishing milk feeds. Hypoglycaemia may cause a variety of symptoms and needs a high level of suspicion (Box 3.12).

Untreated hypoglycaemia carries a 50% risk of irreversible brain injury if there are symptoms but only 5% if it is asymptomatic. The blood glucose level can be estimated by the use of a heel prick blood sample and a stick test (Dextrostix), the level being confirmed by a laboratory value if the stick test is low.

When the fetus has been malnourished during pregnancy because of poor placental function, there will be little stored liver glycogen or adipose tissue and poor muscle bulk. Such a growth retarded infant will often be small, but bigger babies can have the same problems if placental failure occurs late in pregnancy. These infants have a 20% risk of hypoglycaemia shortly after delivery because of the lack of glycogen; the risk remains for several days until feeding is well established. The blood glucose should be checked with a stick test shortly after delivery and before each feed on the first day. Less frequent checks are needed over the next two days if all is well. These babies should be fed soon after delivery and will usually tolerate more feeds than usual in the first days of life. Feeds may need to be more frequent and possibly supplemented with intravenous glucose infusion if hypoglycaemia is established.

Birth asphyxia is also associated with hypoglycaemia but the problem is usually short lived if the baby is well grown. Infants of diabetic mothers can develop hyperinsulinism when maternal glucose control is poor; this causes hypoglycaemia immediately following delivery, often without symptoms. Premature babies may also develop hypoglycaemia in the first hours of life.

HYPOCALCAEMIA

Hypocalcaemia is defined as a serum calcium level of less than 1.8 mmol/l but it is actually the amount of ionised calcium that is the critical factor. Symptoms may include irritability, tremors, apnoea and seizures, all of which may be indistinguishable clinically from hypoglycaemia. Causes include prematurity, birth asphyxia, maternal diabetes and disturbances of maternal calcium metabolism. Correction of the calcium is achieved with a slow intravenous infusion followed by supplements given orally or intravenously depending on the severity of the situation. Occasionally there is also a low serum magnesium level, and the calcium level cannot be corrected without first correcting the hypomagnesaemia.

CONGENITAL ABNORMALITIES OF THE CENTRAL NERVOUS SYSTEM

Anencephaly

Anencephaly has an incidence of about 1 in 1000 deliveries in the UK; it carries an increased risk of neural tube defects in subsequent pregnancies. It is usually diagnosed by routine antenatal ultrasound and is not compatible with life. Some parents may wish to consider the possibility of the baby's organs being used for transplantation.

Encephalocoele

This defect is caused by failure of closure of the skull in the midline posteriorly and results in an occipital herniation of the brain of varying size. When the defect is small, neurosurgical intervention is required. Very large lesions may be associated with microcephaly and have a poor prognosis.

Hydrocephalus (Figure 3.4)

Hydrocephalus is often diagnosed before birth by routine ultrasound scan but can present for the first time following delivery. The baby is likely to have an increased head circumference, wide sutures and increased pressure in the fontanelles. The rate of head growth will usually be excessive, and if hydrocephalus is left untreated there is a risk of irreversible neurological injury. The diagnosis is confirmed by an urgent ultrasound scan of the brain. Treatment is through the placement of a ventriculo-peritoneal or ventriculo-atrial shunt by a paediatric neurosurgeon. Shunts are prone to blockage and may become infected, so parents should be advised to be concerned about episodes of vomiting, drowsiness or unexplained fever. Families should be referred for genetic counselling to determine the risks for future pregnancies.

Spina bifida

This condition results from the failure of fusion of the posterior vertebral arches in a section of the spine and may be associated with herniation of meninges and spinal cord, with resulting neurological problems. The lumbar and sacral regions are the most frequently affected areas. A single vertebral arch is often found to be deficient on abdominal X-ray without other signs: this has no genetic significance. More severe defects carry an increased risk of neural tube defects in future pregnancies. The incidence may be lowered by encouraging mothers to take folate supplements before conception and during the first 12 weeks of pregnancy.

Spina bifida occulta is where the affected vertebrae are covered with skin.

Spina bifida cystica is where there is a swelling over the affected vertebrae.

A **meningocoele** is a skin or dura covered swelling containing cerebrospinal fluid and is found overlying an area of spina bifida.

In a **meningomyelocoele** (Figure 3.5) the spinal cord tissue is also involved and displaced superficially. Sometimes the swelling may be deflated because of leakage of the fluid.

All forms of spina bifida may have associated lesions in the same region, including pigmented naevus, lipoma, coarse hair or capillary naevus.

When spina bifida involves tissue of the spinal cord or spinal nerves, there can be associated problems. These include sensory and motor neurone deficiencies which result in paralysis and atrophic skin which is easily injured. The extent of the problem depends on the site and severity of spina bifida. Many children have a neurogenic bladder and may also have poor control of the bowels. The loss of mobility in the lower limbs in utero often causes deformities, including contractures, club foot and hip dislocation. The spinal problems may lead to scoliosis and kyphosis which compromise pulmonary and cardiac function. Many infants with meningo-

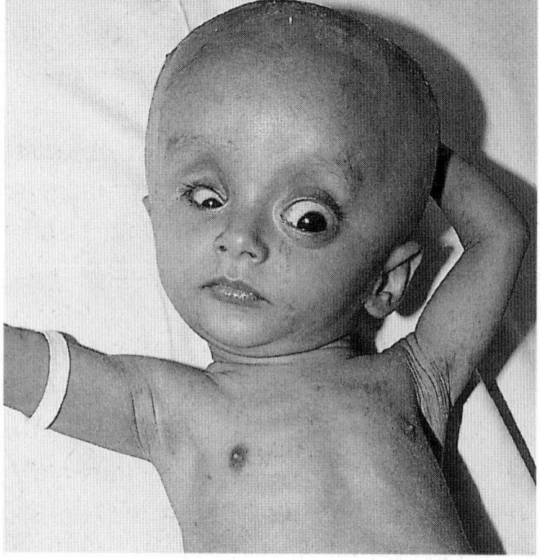

Figure 3.4 Hydrocephalus showing the setting sun sign.

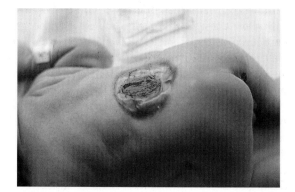

Figure 3.5 Open lumbar meningomyelocoele.

myelocoele will also develop hydrocephalus, as a result of the Arnold–Chiari malformation, although this may not be progressive in all cases. Some infants, despite multiple surgical procedures, may have severe physical and learning disabilities; others may die despite all the care given to them.

Antenatal diagnosis has lessened the impact of what can be a severely handicapping condition. The test used is based on determination of alpha-fetoprotein (AFP) levels in maternal blood and comparing them with normal ranges. Most high values are caused by conditions other than spina bifida, including multiple pregnancy, severe growth retardation and exomphalos. An abnormal value is followed by a repeat test; if this is also high, the baby can be further assessed by ultrasound and amniocentesis to determine the AFP and acteylcholinesterase level in the liquor. Termination is offered where appropriate. It should be remembered that the tests are based on leakage of CSF into the liquor through an open lesion; in closed lesions AFP levels will be normal. Screening by AFP levels has not been universal in the UK: in some places it is offered as part of the screening programme for Down's syndrome, which tends to cause low maternal AFP levels in pregnancy.

NEONATAL SEIZURES

Neonatal seizures are common and affect more than 1 in 200 of newborn infants. Seizures need to be distinguished from jittery movements—one of the best tests is to hold the limb that is shaking. If the movement is a seizure, the limb will continue to move rhythmically but jitteriness will stop. Seizures can be tonic or clonic but may also be more subtle, consisting of eye deviation, 'bicycling', lip or mouth movements and apnoea with no other signs of a fit.

Possible causes of fits are listed in Box 3.13. Asphyxia is the most common cause of neonatal seizures, and the timing of onset relates to the timing of the hypoxic insult to the brain. Intracranial haemorrhage can result from trauma during delivery but may also occur with deficiencies of platelets or clotting factors and in very

---

Box 3.13 Causes of neonatal seizures

- Perinatal asphyxia
- Hypoglycaemia
- Hypocalcaemia
- Hypomagnesaemia
- Meningitis
- Other infections
- Withdrawal from maternal drugs, especially narcotics and cocaine
- Structural anomalies of the brain
- Intracranial haemorrhage
- Inborn errors of metabolism
- Pyridoxine dependency
- 'Fifth day fits'
- Others

---

pre-term babies with no obvious cause. Serious infections can cause seizures, usually when associated with meningitis.

Seizures may be the first sign of a metabolic problem, including rare inborn errors of metabolism such as maple syrup urine disease, galactosaemia, urea cycle defects and organic acidaemias.

Some babies have seizures because of pyridoxine deficiency and require subsequent daily supplementation. 'Fifth day fits' are a self limiting condition with no known cause and are usually seen on the fourth and fifth days of life in an otherwise normal infant. The diagnosis can only be presumed after other causes have been excluded.

Diagnosis requires a careful history and examination to elicit possible causes. Blood should be obtained to exclude sepsis, clotting problems and metabolic problems. A lumbar puncture must be considered and an ultrasound scan of the brain is required.

Treatment is first directed at any preventable cause of the seizures, particularly metabolic or infective. Intravenous pyridoxine should be given under EEG control to infants who have no other obvious cause for the seizures. When seizures continue without a correctable cause, anticonvulsant treatment should be given. There are several first line drugs (Box 3.14) and benzodiazepines are also used when seizures are difficult to control. Treatment is usually stopped before discharge from hospital in a well infant with no long-term risk of recurrence.

Box 3.14 Treatment of neonatal seizures

Phenobarbitone
- Loading dose 20 mg/kg i.v.
- Maintenance 6 mg/kg orally as 2 divided daily doses

Paraldehyde 0.15 ml/kg i.m., repeated 4–6-hourly
Phenytoin
- Loading dose 20 mg/kg
- Maintenance 5 mg/kg orally as 2 divided daily doses

The long-term prognosis for neonatal seizures depends mainly on the underlying cause. The worst prognosis is seen with birth asphyxia, intracranial haemorrhage, hypoglycaemia and meningitis. About half of the infants with the first three conditions will develop normally but the figures for meningitis are less optimistic. Most infants suffering seizures from other causes will have no long-term problems.

LOW BIRTH WEIGHT

Definitions

A baby is termed 'low birth weight' (LBW) when the birth weight is less than 2.5 kg, regardless of gestational age. If the baby is less than 1.5 kg at birth then it is termed 'very low birth weight' (VLBW). Such small size can occur because of premature birth (defined as birth before 37 completed weeks of pregnancy). Babies may also be small at birth compared with other babies of the same gestation: one who is below the third centile for weight at that gestation is termed 'small for gestational age' (SGA). These terms are not mutually exclusive—a baby may be LBW, SGA and premature.

Problems

Temperature control

This is one of the biggest problems for LBW babies as the ratio of skin surface area to body mass is higher at lower birth weights and this exacerbates the problem of heat loss. Both premature and SGA babies may have little subcutaneous fat, decreasing their insulation. The smallest babies need an incubator to conserve body heat, the support required depending on factors such as weight, gestational age, age since birth, and state of health. Babies gradually become better at managing temperature control and the degree of support can be reduced.

Prematurity

Very often there is at least a short warning of premature delivery, although the reasons for most premature labours remain uncertain. Where possible, steps should be taken to ensure that delivery takes place in a maternity unit which has facilities for neonatal intensive care. Transfer before delivery is always preferable to transfer of the ill baby after delivery. Whenever possible the parents should visit the special care baby unit before delivery and see the equipment that may be used to support their baby; this reduces parental shock if the baby requires intensive care. If possible, steroids are given to the mother for up to 48 hours before delivery to decrease the risk of respiratory distress syndrome.

Respiratory distress syndrome (RDS). Premature babies are prone to development of RDS due to inadequate surfactant production. Surfactants are phospholipids with detergent like properties: they reduce surface tension within the alveoli. Without surfactant, the alveoli tend to collapse completely after each breath and the baby has to make a much greater effort to inflate them again. Exudate forms within the alveoli; at post mortem this appears as a hyaline membrane, hence the term hyaline membrane disease. Surfactant can be replaced by instillation down an endotracheal tube, usually in two doses a number of hours apart. It is usually given to babies who have an increasing oxygen requirement above an FiO_2 of about 0.4.

Babies with RDS may require an increased FiO_2 but may also benefit from the use of constant positive airways pressure (CPAP) via a nasal tube device. This helps to prevent the collapse of alveoli after each breath. Those babies who are most ill require artificial ventilation with the use of positive end expiratory pressure (PEEP) which has the same beneficial effect as CPAP. Larger babies may require paralysis and sedation with opiates to achieve this, as they tend to struggle against the respirator. There is a risk of pneumothorax with CPAP or artificial ventilation and the pressures used are kept to a minimum as this complication is a cause of serious anoxia and increases the risk of intracranial haemorrhage.

In most cases RDS recovers naturally after the first five days when the baby manufactures enough endogenous surfactant but the recovery may be faster with the use of artificial surfactant. Provided there have been no major complications, the recovery of the lung problem is complete and without long-term sequelae.

Longer-term oxygen dependency may develop in some of the smaller babies who have required high oxygen concentrations or high ventilator pressures. Usually this can be managed with low flow oxygen via nasal cannulae: this may be given at home if the baby is otherwise ready for discharge. This complication increases the risk to the baby from illnesses such as respiratory syncytial virus (RSV) bronchiolitis. Some babies affected by dependency on oxygen can be weaned off it using a short course of steroids.

Nutrition. Before about 36 weeks' gestation newborn babies may not be able to suck adequately to maintain their own nutritional needs. It is usual to supplement their own feeding efforts with tube feeds, which may be more frequent for smaller and more premature babies. Some babies will only tolerate hourly or continuous feeds without it affecting their respiration. Where a baby cannot tolerate nasogastric feeds it may be possible to use a weighted silicon tube to give nasojejeunal feeds. Sometimes parenteral nutrition is required; this is also used to maintain the nutritional intake of babies who remain ill on respirators but, apart from all the difficulties of the composition of the fluids used, there are potential risks of sepsis and mild disturbance of liver function.

Premature babies require higher protein and salt concentrations than term babies and there are special milks which allow for the extra requirements without increasing the fluid load. Premature babies are also given supplements of folic acid, iron and multi-vitamins for the first six months of life.

Breast milk is not always considered the best form of nutrition for more premature babies and may need to be supplemented to achieve adequate growth. Mothers who intend to breast feed should be encouraged to express their milk regularly; this can be stored refrigerated for a number of hours before being used for tube feeding. Breast milk can also be deep frozen for a few days, although some of the beneficial effects may be reduced by this process. The baby should be encouraged to the breast as early and as often as possible, with the mother staying in the special care nursery for a few days before discharge to establish feeding.

Apnoea. Before about 34 weeks of gestation, premature babies may have episodes of spontaneous apnoea which appear to be caused by immature respiratory reflexes. The milder episodes can be treated by physical stimulation but more persistent or frequent apnoeas usually benefit from the use of caffeine or aminophylline prophylaxis. The baby can usually be weaned off the stimulant medication by about 34 weeks of corrected gestational age.

Although apnoea is common with increasing prematurity, it is also a symptom of illness and should be investigated, common causes being sepsis, hypoglycaemia and hypocalcaemia. When there is suspicion of sepsis, immediate antibiotic therapy should be given pending the results of cultures.

Necrotising enterocolitis (see p. 147 and p. 315).

Periventricular haemorrhage. Very premature babies are prone to bleeding around the lateral ventricles and choroid plexus when they are unwell with other problems. The bleeding is often mild and clears up without long-term sequelae. When the bleeding spreads into the ventricles it can cause blockages within the ventricular system or prevent cerebrospinal fluid from being resorbed over the surface of the brain, with resulting hydrocephalus. This can often be treated with repeated ventricular taps while the problem resolves but may sometimes require the insertion of a shunt. Bleeding can also spread within the substance of the brain and this carries a greater risk of long-term neurological sequelae.

Periods of severely reduced brain perfusion

can lead to patchy infarction of the tissues around the ventricles. Serial ultrasound scans of the brain reveal bright areas which gradually develop into small cysts. This condition is known as periventricular leukomalacia and it is also very likely to be associated with long-term neurological sequelae.

Prognosis

Well premature babies carry little risk of long-term neurological problems and parents can be readily reassured. It is only babies with extreme prematurity or those with major illness who are likely to suffer with problems such as cerebral palsy and developmental delay. Those at greatest risk are likely to have been born prior to 28 weeks' gestation and to have had a stormy neonatal course with intracranial complications. Babies have survived from as early as 23 weeks' gestation but the morbidity is about 80%. For surviving babies born at 24–26 weeks' gestation, the incidence of cerebral palsy is between 10 and 20%. At 26 weeks' gestation, about 70% of the survivors will have a normal cognitive outcome, falling to 50% at 25 weeks and 30% at 24 weeks. Visual and hearing defects are also seen in about 40% of these early gestational survivors, but the defects are only likely to be severe in about 10%.

Parents are often quite gloomy when a baby is receiving the highest levels of intensive care, especially when ultrasound scans have shown intracranial pathology. They need strong support and must not be allowed to lose hope in this situation, as the outcome is often not as bad as they imagine. Parent support groups can be very helpful and the family should be encouraged to spend as much time with the infant as possible. Even at the worst of an illness the family should be encouraged to touch and, where possible, to hold their child.

COMMON SCREENING TESTS
Antenatal ultrasound scans

Most babies are now routinely scanned early in pregnancy to confirm the gestation and screen for common anomalies. When there is doubt about the findings, a more detailed anomaly scan with counselling should be arranged. When severe or life threatening conditions are diagnosed, a termination may be offered or an amniocentesis performed to exclude a chromosomal anomaly.

It is quite common for cysts to be found around the choroid plexus in the brain or within the abdomen. Most of these cysts resolve spontaneously during the pregnancy and may have disappeared by the time of birth. Parents become very worried about these and may need considerable reassurance.

It is also quite common for one or both of the renal pelvices to appear dilated, although there is no general agreement on what precise measurement should be considered abnormal. Most will resolve spontaneously but all babies should be investigated further after delivery (see Fig. 10.4): this may involve repeated ultrasound scans, possibly with a micturating cysto-urethrogram as well. Pelvi-ureteric junction obstruction may require surgical relief in a minority of cases.

The Guthrie test

This test is used to screen for phenylketonuria, a recessively inherited metabolic problem where the infant lacks the enzyme phenylalanine hydroxylase. The infant accumulates phenylalanine and its metabolites within the body, leading to epilepsy and developmental problems. The test requires the infant to have been on normal milk feeds for about 48 hours; the test is then carried out by collecting blood from a heel prick onto a piece of 'blotting paper' with printed information and a number of circles to mark where and how much blood should be collected. When the screening test is positive, a further blood sample is required for more detailed studies and the baby needs to be placed on a special milk, free of phenylalanine. Supplements of phenylalanine are then given according to blood estimations made at intervals. The condition should be followed by a specialist in paediatric metabolic disease.

Congenital thyroid deficiency

The Guthrie blood spots can also be used to estimate thyroid stimulating hormone (TSH) levels. These normally fall to very low levels within a few days of birth—a persistently raised level would suggest thyroid deficiency. A blood test is used to confirm the result and the baby started on replacement hormone, the dose determined by surface area or body weight. Untreated babies develop signs of cretinism, with prolonged jaundice, protruding tongue and coarse features. Umbilical hernia, abdominal protuberance and constipation can also be features. Untreated infants will suffer from a variable degree of learning disability.

Some babies only have a temporary problem with hypothyroidism and will not need life-long treatment with thyroxin. Sometimes this may be determined by the use of a thyroid uptake scan, but it may also be determined by gradually letting the infant outgrow the dose of thyroxin in the second six months of life while closely monitoring TSH levels.

Haemoglobinopathies

In some regions of the UK where the incidence of haemoglobinopathy is high, the Guthrie blood spot is also used to screen for conditions such as thalassaemia and sickle cell disease. This allows treatment to start early and may avoid serious illness in sickle cell disease, where pneumococcal meningitis may otherwise be the first sign. It is theoretically possible to screen only the infants of mothers who are noted to be carriers of haemoglobinopathies during pregnancy, but evidence suggests that this is not as effective because results are overlooked and the baby may not be brought back for testing after three months of age.

Cystic fibrosis

There is no uniform policy in the UK for screening for cystic fibrosis but there are some regional or local programmes. One of these involves screening Guthrie blood spots for the presence of known genetic markers and would probably miss about 15% of cases. The other looks for raised levels of immunoreactive trypsin, followed by a sweat test when the result is abnormal. It is argued that earlier diagnosis allows prompt instigation of treatment, as well as confirming the genetic risks for the family before further children are conceived.

TALKING TO PARENTS

Factors leading to parental anxiety

Parents usually have very high expectations of their unborn child and may even have quite vivid images of the baby's imagined appearance. Given the opportunity during pregnancy, many parents will also be able to express their fears that the baby might not be normal. Anxiety about the baby appears to be more common after infertility, previous fetal loss, threatened fetal loss or the previous death of a child. Self help groups and professional support programmes recognise this potential difficulty and offer various forms of help to families. A good example is CONI (Care Of the Next Infant), a programme aimed primarily at supporting parents who have suffered the loss of a previous baby through sudden infant death syndrome (SIDS). The programme is usually co-ordinated on a locality basis by a nominated health visitor using the support of a designated local consultant paediatrician and the family GP. The health visitor makes contact with the family during the pregnancy and the paediatrician may also help in agreeing the type of support needed after the baby is born. This can include the use of a breathing monitor or the use of scales and daily weight charts. The baby is examined after birth by the paediatrician and the family are given information about when they should contact their GP in the event of illness or significant weight change. Most families will begin to relax when the new baby passes the age at which the previous baby died.

Families often fail to express their anxiety directly and seek advice about symptoms that they perceive in the child. Common examples are feeding difficulties and crying but there may also be concern about colour changes, movements or apparent apnoeas. The doctor must always be sure that no medical issue does exist, but merely excluding this does not usually resolve the anxiety. A careful history of past events and exploration of issues that cause anxiety will help to resolve the problem but extended support will be required.

Breaking bad news (see also p. 82)

It is to be expected that giving bad news to a family will cause them distress but there is no need for this to be made worse by the manner in which the information is imparted. Sometimes, as with a cleft lip and palate, the problem is obvious to the family and they will already be upset. Down's syndrome in the baby may not have been recognised by the family, and the doctor may be the first to impart the diagnosis. The professional must recognise his or her own distress in having to give the information and the effect that this may have on his/her own behaviour. Training, observation of others and increasing personal experience are all factors which can improve this skill.

Whenever possible the information should be given to both parents together and in a situation of privacy. The doctor must not appear cold, detached or disinterested as the family will see this as uncaring. Equally the doctor must not appear light-hearted as this will have a similar effect. Handling the baby in a calm and confident manner and talking to the baby as for any other examination shows that the doctor cares about the situation. Explanations should be simple and brief initially, to allow the parents time to absorb them. Parents are usually very shocked and will almost always question a diagnosis that is not immediately obvious to them. The shock makes it difficult for them to take in information, and explanations need to progress at a pace appropriate to the family. Questions should be answered as simply as possible and the doctor must never be afraid to express ignorance, as this is always better than giving incorrect information. When a question cannot be answered, the parents should be given an indication that the answer will be available by referring to another source.

The family often need a further visit later the same day or the following day, when they have had time to talk and some of the shock has worn off. They should be encouraged to write down all their questions as they occur to them and to refer to the list while you are there. They will often need reassurance about guilty feelings that they have caused a problem by events such as drugs taken during pregnancy or previous termination of pregnancy. A plan for further referral will help the family to look forward and away from the paralysis that accompanies the initial shock.

The local community paediatric service should have details of suitable contact and support schemes for particular diagnoses or problems. Very often they are also able to offer advice from a social worker, who can be helpful not only through their professional role but because many families are pleased to talk to someone who is not a health professional.

FURTHER READING

Rennie J, Roberton N R C 1999 Textbook of neonatology, 3rd edn. Churchill Livingstone, Edinburgh

Internet address
http://silk.nih.gov/SILK/Cochrane/Cochrane.htm

4

Child development and disability

Martin Bellman

CHILD DEVELOPMENT

Nature

The brain grows in size and complexity from the sixth week of gestational age up to puberty. Developmental function may be damaged by insults (e.g. anatomical abnormalities, trauma, infection) at any time during this period: the most likely times are before, during and after birth. Many aspects of child development are directly related to the process of central nervous system maturation, the pattern of which is unstoppable, unalterable and consistent; thus, significant deviations from the recognised patterns indicate abnormality. The most important determining factor for the potential cognitive function of an individual is genetic endowment ('nature').

Nurture

The external experience of the child ('nurture') plays a major role, and the best way to promote optimal development is to offer consistent structured stimulation. Children learn from their environment by observation, copying and repeated trials and errors. The basic process is the 'stimulus–response' principle and children quickly learn to modify their own actions in order to achieve the best result. Conditioned and unconditioned reflexes are also important and are the basis for operant learning, which is used to deliver behaviour modification therapy in certain situations (see p. 180).

Personality

The process of personality development also depends on genetic and experiential factors. Sigmund Freud described several sexual stages (oral, anal, phallic) followed by a latent period leading to adolescent and adult sexuality. Abnormalities during these early stages may cause later psychological disorders.

Jean Piaget documented cognitive developmental progress in detail and formulated three major stages (sensorimotor, concrete operations, formal operations) through which children pass to discover their own abilities. These functions interact with the environment; children learn to modify their actions to adapt to circumstances and finally impose abstract thoughts to anticipate and plan strategies.

The importance of the mother–child relationship was described by Donald Winnicott. It is now clear that this is very much a two-way process and that the child is often the initiator and modifies the adult response. More recent work on attachment emphasises the infant's early social experience as an antecedent of later behaviour.

Fields of development

It is clear that all aspects of child development are interdependent. For example, the motivation to progress across the floor of a room comes from the wish to reach an object on the other side (e.g. person or toy) that has been seen and is wanted, and then social and play skills are developed by the resulting interaction. The complex cycle of factors which may interact and affect communication skills is shown in Figure 4.1.

Holistic development is difficult to analyse and record, and child development is therefore broken down into four major fields:

1. posture and large movements/gross motor skills
2. vision and fine movements/fine motor-adaptive skills
3. hearing and speech/language skills
4. social and play/personal–social skills.

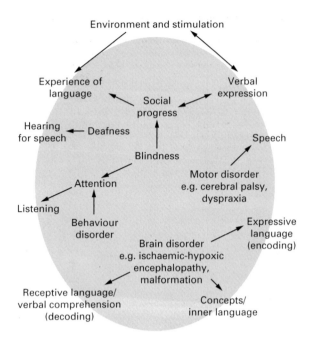

Figure 4.1 Verbal communication cycle showing interactions of various factors.

There are many methods for recording developmental status according to the above classification or a similar variant.

The tests listed in Box 4.1 produce results in terms of the age reached by the child in a particular developmental field relative to the performance of 'normal' children. Age equivalents can be converted to a quotient by the formula Performance age/Chronological age but this can give a false impression of accuracy and it is better to give the results as age ranges. These tests are very useful for screening purposes and for documenting developmental progress over time.

Box 4.1 Developmental tests commonly used by doctors

Screening tests
- STYCAR sequences
- Schedule of Growing Skills
- Denver Developmental Screening Test

Assessment tests
- Schedule of Growing Skills
- Griffiths scales

Table 4.1 Commonly used psychological tests of general cognitive ability

Test	Age range
Bayley scales	2 months–2½ years
Merrill–Palmer test	1½–5¼ years
McCarthy scales	2½–8½ years
British Ability Scales (BAS)	2½–17 years
Wechsler Pre-school and Primary Scale of Intelligence (WPPSI)	4–6½ years
Wechsler Intelligence Scale for Children (WISC)	6½–16 years

Most are fairly quick to perform (approximately 20 minutes), except the Griffiths test which takes around 1 hour. They can be used in an ordinary child clinic or surgery by a trained doctor or nurse.

When more detailed information is required, e.g. to analyse a global or specific developmental problem, a referral is made to a psychologist for psychometric assessment (Table 4.1).

Neurodevelopmental examination

Newborn infant

Gestational age can be estimated by the Dubowitz score which measures several different physical characteristics. Another well known method for neurological examination is the Brazelton assessment scale (see p. 47).

Later infancy and childhood

Primitive reflexes. Certain neonatal responses are programmed to appear or disappear at specific ages (Table 4.2); failure to follow this pattern indicates neurological abnormality.

Excessive muscle tone (especially extensor or adductor) or asymmetry of primitive reflexes is strongly suggestive of neurological abnormality, e.g. cerebral palsy.

Key developmental milestones

There are many good manuals of child development (see Further reading) which give detailed information. Some of the more important milestones for varying skills are outlined in Tables 4.3–4.13. A mean value for the normal population is given and, if available, a range which corresponds approximately to the 3rd to the 97th percentile. Failure to attain a skill by the latter age suggests abnormal development.

Table 4.2 Neonatal primitive reflexes

Reflex	Method to elicit	Response	Appears	Disappears
Moro	Suddenly extend head or arms	Symmetrical extension, abduction and then flexion of arms	Birth	6 months
Placing	Bring dorsum of foot up to edge of table	Foot is lifted and placed on surface	4 weeks	6 months
Stepping	Support in standing	Alternate legs flex at knees and hips and baby 'walks' forward	Birth	3 months
Grasp	Place finger in palm of baby's hand	Fingers close tightly round examiner's finger	Birth	4 months
Asymmetric tonic neck (ATNR)	Hold shoulders flat and turn head to either side	Limbs on face side extend and on occiput side flex	Birth	6 months
Head righting	In supine position turn head to either side	Pelvis and shoulders turn in same direction	4 months	2 years
Parachute	From ventral suspension suddenly lower the baby towards a surface	Arms and legs extend and abduct	6 months	Persists

Motor skills

Table 4.3 Prone position (adapted from Bellman et al 1996)

	Mean	Range
Lifts head momentarily	1 month	0.5–2 months
Lifts head about 45°	2 months	1–3 months
Head and upper chest up on forearms	3 months	2–5 months
Head and chest up on extended arms	6 months	4–8 months
Gets into crawling position	8 months	6–12 months

Table 4.4 Upright posture (adapted from Bellman et al 1996)

	Mean	Range
Bears some weight on feet	7 months	6–9 months
Takes full weight	8 months	6–12 months
Stands holding on	9 months	7–14 months
Pulls to stand	10 months	9–10 months
Stands alone	11 months	9–16 months

Table 4.5 Gross movements (adapted from Bellman et al 1996)

	Mean	Range
Rolls (or squirms) forwards or backwards	8½ months	6–11 months
Crawls	9½ months	7–13 months
Walks with support	10 months	8–12 months
Walks alone	13 months	11–18 months
Squats to pick up object	14½ months	12–19 months
Runs	16 months	15–20 months
Jumps	18 months	
Walks on tiptoe	20 months	
Runs on tiptoe	24 months	
Hops on one foot	3 years	

Table 4.6 Stairs (adapted from Bellman et al 1996)

	Mean	Range
Walks upstairs with hands held	16 months	12–24 months
Walks upstairs with two feet on each step	25 months	19–30 months
Walks upstairs, one foot per step and downstairs 2 feet per step	3 years	
Walks upstairs and downstairs, one foot per step	4 years	

Manipulative skills

Table 4.7 Building with bricks (1 inch) (adapted from Bellman et al 1996)

Number of bricks	Mean	Range
2	15 months	11–19 months
4	18 months	15–24 months
8	24 months	21–23 months
Bridge	3 years	27–39 months
3 steps	4 years	

Table 4.8 Drawing skills (adapted from Bellman et al 1996)

Drawing skill	Mean
Scribbles	15 months
Imitates vertical line	2 years
Imitates horizontal line	2½ years
Imitates circle	3 years
Imitates cross	4 years

Language skills

Table 4.9 Speech (adapted from Bellman et al 1996)

Speech sounds	Mean	Range
Grunts	4 weeks	1–6 weeks
Vocalises (coo)	6½ weeks	4–9 weeks
Laughs	3½ months	2–5 months
Babbles (monosyllabic)	6½ months	4–8 months
Imitates sounds	10 months	8–12 months
Jargon	12 months	10–15 months
One word	15 months	12–18 months
1–6 words	18 months	15–21 months
7–20 words	21 months	18–24 months
50 words	2 years	18–27 months
Joins 2 words	2 years	18–30 months
200 words	2½ years	24–36 months
Joins 3–4 words	2½ years	2¼–3 years
Questions 'why, what, where, who'	3 years	2½–3½ years
Pronouns ('I, you, he, she')	3½ years	3–4 years
Conjunctions (and, but)	4 years	3–4½ years
Sentences of 5+ words	4 years	3–4½ years
Complex explanations and sequences	4½ years	4–5½ years

Table 4.10 Comprehension (adapted from Bellman et al 1996)

	Mean	Range
Understands 'no'/'bye-bye'	7 months	6–9 months
Recognises own name	8 months	6–10 months
Recognises familiar names	12 months	10–15 months
Selects 3 out of 4 objects	15 months	12–18 months
Points to body parts on person	15 months	12–18 months
Points to body parts on doll	18 months	15–21 months
Follows a 2 step command	2 years	18–27 months
Understands prepositions ('in', 'on', 'under')	2½ years	2–3 years
Understands simple negatives	3 years	2½–3½ years
Follows a command with 2 instructions	3½ years	3–4 years
Understands complex negatives ('neither'/'nor')	4 years	3½–5 years
Follows a command with 3 instructions	4½ years	4–5½ years

Social skills

Table 4.11 Feeding (adapted from Bellman et al 1996)

	Mean
Holds spoon but does not feed	12 months
Holds spoon, brings it to mouth but cannot prevent it turning over	15 months
Holds spoon and gets food safely to mouth	18 months
Eats skilfully with spoon	2–2½ years
Eats with fork and spoon	3 years
Eats skilfully with little help	3½–4 years
Copes with entire meal unaided	5 years

Table 4.12 Toileting (adapted from Bellman et al 1996)

	Range
Reflex emptying of bladder	Up to 6 months
Empties bladder less frequently (CNS inhibition of reflex)	6–12 months
Indicates or vocalises toilet needs or wetness	1–2 years
Bowel control	2½–4 years
Dry during the day (occasional accident)	3–4 years
Dry at night (occasional accident)	3½–5 years
Able to control voiding, and micturate on command	4–5 years

Normal variation

Tables 4.3–4.13—milestones in different developmental fields—show that there is a wide age range of 'normal' development.

Table 4.13 Play

	Range
Shakes rattle	3–6 months
Transfers objects from hand to hand	6–9 months
Plays 'pat-a-cake' and 'peep-bo'	9–11 months
Casts	12–15 months
Imitates domestic activities	18 months–2 years
Isolated pretend play	2–3 years
Co-operative play with other children	3–4 years
Takes turns in play	4–5 years
Plays games to rules	4½–6 years

Most assessment or screening tools give a profile of results across the fields. Global developmental delay shows a consistent pattern throughout the fields: if there is mild discrepancy in only one field it is likely that this represents an insignificant variant or perhaps lack of co-operation in that area. In this situation the child should be reviewed after a period of 6–8 weeks. A severe delay in any field must, however, be taken seriously.

Developmental variation

- Racial—Negro children show more advanced motor skills than Caucasians.
- Familial—a tendency to late talking or walking may run in families.
- Bottom shufflers are invariably late walkers (this is familial).
- Twins may have their own unique system of communication with apparently delayed speech development.
- Sex—males tend to have slower language development than females.
- Nutrition—mild undernourishment and iron deficiency anaemia may cause slow development which improves after nutritional correction. Prolonged or severe undernutrition or anaemia can cause persistent developmental delay.
- Bilingual family—if the first language is not English, language skills may appear delayed. Most children cope well with two languages but the examiner must be aware of the mother tongue when testing.
- Understimulation—poor child rearing and

lack of stimulation at home may result in slow development which is reversible if the parents can change their practices at an early stage. Prolonged understimulation (neglect) can cause persistent delay.

DISABILITY

Terminology

The language of disability is dynamic, depending on the perceptions of affected individuals, their representatives and society. Definitions currently used are as follows:

Impairment. Any loss or abnormality of psychological, physiological or anatomical function.

Disability. Any restriction or lack, resulting from impairment, of ability to perform an activity in the manner or within the range considered normal for a human being.

Handicap. A disadvantage for a given individual, resulting from an impairment or a disability, that limits or prevents the fulfilment of a role that is normal (depending on age, sex or cultural factors) for that individual.

According to the above definition, handicap is related to the individual's function compared with the normal population. The view of many disabled people is that the present hostile attitude must change to one of support and active help for disabled people. This anti-discrimination view was formalised in the Disability Discrimination Act (1996) which obliges all public services and premises in the UK to become fully accessible to the disabled population. The lack of understanding and tolerance of disability by a large section of the general population remains, however, the biggest obstacle to progress.

The British Association for Community Child Health (BACCH) proposed that disability be classified under 11 headings in order to clarify functional analysis of individual competencies (Box 4.2). These headings could be used for the Disability Register which is held by Social Service Departments with multi-agency co-operation under the Children Act 1989. This is part of the Register of Children in Need, which

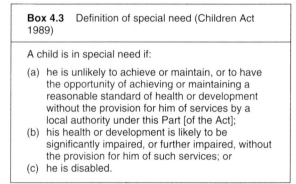

Box 4.2 The dimensions of disability (BACCH, 1994)
1. Locomotion
2. Fine motor
3. Personal care
4. Continence
5. Hearing
6. Vision
7. Communication
8. Learning
9. Behaviour and social integration
10. Physical health
11. Consciousness

Box 4.3 Definition of special need (Children Act 1989)
A child is in special need if:
(a) he is unlikely to achieve or maintain, or to have the opportunity of achieving or maintaining a reasonable standard of health or development without the provision for him of services by a local authority under this Part [of the Act];
(b) his health or development is likely to be significantly impaired, or further impaired, without the provision for him of such services; or
(c) he is disabled.

has a wider definition (Box 4.3). The Disability Register is voluntary and therefore not comprehensive; nevertheless, it is useful for local epidemiology, audit and planning of services.

The implication of the term 'children in need' is that they have a 'special need' for extra resources or facilities in order to be able to function with other, 'normal', children.

Learning disability

Some children at the lower end of the 'normal' category (IQ 71–85) have great difficulty accessing the 'normal' national curriculum and experience social problems when mixing with other children.

Moderate learning difficulties (MLD)— intelligence quotient (IQ) of 50–69

Children with moderate learning difficulties usually acquire adequate communication and basic academic skills such as reading, writing and arithmetic. They are socially competent and after leaving school can perform simple non-intellectual jobs and be generally independent.

Severe learning difficulties (SLD)—IQ less than 50

Children with severe learning difficulties often have very limited communication skills and cannot make significant academic achievements. They remain dependent on others for general care and are unlikely to perform any useful occupation.

These children are usually not able to learn in a mainstream school and are placed in a special school which is resourced to provide an appropriate learning environment. However, many local authorities now have an 'inclusion' policy and divert resources to mainstream schools that can support such children.

Statement of Special Educational Needs

The Warnock Report (1978) introduced the term 'special educational needs' (SEN) for children who require extra help in school in order to access the national curriculum. Up to 20% of children may require additional resources at some time during their school years, and 2% have needs severe enough to require statutory help under a legally binding statement.

The Education Act 1981 first proposed a system of formal multidisciplinary assessment for children suspected of having SEN. The procedure is led by the educational psychologist, and the parents can nominate other professionals involved with the child, such as a paediatrician or therapist, to supply evidence.

The local education authority (LEA) may then decide to issue a Statement of Special Educational Needs which includes:

- a detailed description of the child
- a programme for addressing his or her needs
- a list of educational and non-educational (e.g. speech therapy) resources required
- a recommended school.

The provision of educational support should specify the number of hours of support from a special needs teacher or a classroom assistant (often another parent or non-teaching member of school staff) and whether the child is supported individually or in a group. LEAs are obliged to provide the resources included in the Statement but may try to minimise the support because of limited funding. Nevertheless, they have a statutory responsibility to enable every child to access the educational system. Parents often need support to challenge the LEA if the provision does not appear to meet the needs and this is a legitimate role for a doctor and other health professionals.

Health authorities must co-operate with LEAs in assessing and providing for children with SEN. If a child is suspected of being likely to have SEN by school age, the LEA should be notified as soon as possible, and in any event by the age of 2 years. These children are usually first identified through the child health surveillance programme: the doctor or other professional should discuss the situation with the parents, inform them of any other help available (e.g. voluntary agency) and notify the LEA (usually via the educational psychologist).

Parents have considerable rights to be consulted about the statementing procedure and have to agree the final document before it can be implemented. The Education Acts of 1993 and 1996 updated the 1981 Act and introduced a system of tribunals so that parents have a formal mechanism for appealing against a statement that they feel is inappropriate or against an LEA's refusal to perform a statutory assessment of SEN. The Code of Practice (Table 4.14) introduced a series of stages for the provision of support for a child with learning difficulties.

Services for disabled children

Social Services Department (SSD)

The local authority has the primary responsibility under the Children Act 1989. It must maintain the Disability Register and ensure that co-ordinated services to support the child

Table 4.14 Stages under the Code of Practice

Stage	Trigger	Action
1	Registration of concern by teacher, parents or other professional	Class teacher collects information, identifies special educational needs, devises and implements an Individual Education Plan (IEP)
2	Stage 1 review shows that child is not improving	Special Educational Needs co-ordinator (SENCO) takes on child, reviews IEP and arranges remedial support
3	SENCO and headteacher decide that Stage 2 help is insufficient	School calls in external services—e.g. educational psychologist, specialist teacher, therapist, social worker
4	Child not responding to Stage 3 help and likely to need a Statement of Special Educational Needs	a. LEA works with school, parents and other agencies to consider need for Statement b. If necessary, conduct statutory assessment of special educational needs`

and family are available. The health authority must co-operate with the local authority SSD.

Child Development Team (CDT)

A CDT is a multidisciplinary service specifically for children. There is one in almost all areas of the UK, though the age range varies: some are responsible for pre-school children only (age 0–5 years), others cover pre-school and school age groups (age 0–19 years). In the former case, there must be a school health service capable of caring for children with special needs.

Child Development Centre (CDC). Many districts now have a CDC for multidisciplinary assessment and treatment of disabled children. This is best situated in a dedicated purpose-designed centre to offer a 'single front door' to all the appropriate professionals, which many parents find easier than having to go to different places for each consultation (Box 4.4). Ideally the CDC should have access to an assessment nursery where children can be placed for a short period (up to 8 weeks) for diagnostic observation.

Site for the CDC. The best place is probably in dedicated community premises—children and parents dislike visiting an acute hospital with its implicit aura of illness and disease. This is a major factor which significantly affects the rate of compliance with appointments and thus the effectiveness of the service. The disadvantages of a CDC not being in a hospital setting include lack of immediate access to investigation facilities, hospital records and pharmacy.

Box 4.4 Facilities in a CDC

- Medical examination rooms
- Assessment and treatment space for physiotherapy, occupational therapy (including sensory integration therapy) and speech and language therapy (sound treated room)
- Room for visual assessment (6 metre length)
- Room for hearing assessment (sound proofed)
- Administrative areas—reception, record storage, secretarial space
- Offices for professionals
- Meeting/teaching room
- Waiting area with play, changing, toilet and weighing facilities

---

The decision on the site for the CDC often depends upon whether the service is run by a community or hospital provider and what premises are available.

CDT staff. The structure varies from one team to another—a model constitution is shown in Box 4.5. It is essential to have close working relationships with representatives from the local education authority and SSD (special needs section), relevant local voluntary agencies and parents.

Assessment

Screening is a rapid procedure performed in primary care; it is designed to separate a population into two groups according to whether or not each individual is likely to have a disorder. Assessment is a secondary procedure to look at those children who have had a positive screening

---

Box 4.5 CDT staff

Core
- Developmental paediatrician
- Specialist health visitor
- Clinical psychologist
- Speech and language therapist
- Physiotherapist
- Occupational therapist
- Secretary
- Administrator

Associated
- Medical specialists:
  —neurologist
  —geneticist
  —ophthalmologist
  —audiological physician
  —child psychiatrist
  —orthopaedic surgeon
- Child psychotherapist
- Orthoptist
- Educational psychologist
- Social worker

---

result (true and false) to make a firm diagnosis. From a neurodevelopmental point of view, this often entails a detailed examination by several members of the CDT. It is therefore lengthy, expensive and stressful for the CDT and tedious and exhausting for the child (Box 4.6). Many services have developed a second tier developmental clinic or special advisory clinic (SAC) to carry out an intermediate assessment on children who need a second opinion after their primary screen but whose condition may not be severe enough to warrant immediate CDT assessment (Figure 4.2).

Medical assessment (Box 4.7)

The paediatrician is responsible for making the medical diagnosis and co-ordinating care of the whole child and family.

Family support

Keyworker

Some families have difficulty relating to a team of professionals: communication between them and the CDT can be improved by appointing one person to talk with them. This person should be

---

Box 4.6 Models of assessment procedure

Combined multidisciplinary assessment. The family is invited to the CDC for a half or whole day to be seen by a predetermined set of professionals working alone or in pairs. Each part of the assessment may last from approximately 10 minutes (e.g. orthoptist) up to 1 hour (e.g. psychologist).

Advantages
- The whole assessment is completed on a single visit to the CDC
- Inconvenience for the family is minimised
- Multidisciplinary results are immediately available and a management plan given to the family
- Multidisciplinary assessment is facilitated by observing other professionals' examination
- The 'team work' process is emphasised

Disadvantages
- The child may be anxious and exhausted by such concentrated examination
- Hence the child's performance may be compromised
- Failure to attend by a child is very expensive as the time of several professionals is wasted
- The procedure is artificial and may not represent how the child functions in a 'normal' environment

Separate assessment by each professional. Individual appointments are offered; when they have all been completed, the CDT meets to share the information and plan further management.

Advantages
- There is no time pressure to do everything on one visit to the CDC
- The child is less stressed and hence probably performs better
- Each professional can work at his/her own pace
- Assessment can be done outside the CDC, e.g. at home, nursery or school
- A failure to attend only wastes one professional's time

Disadvantages
- The whole assessment process may be prolonged and so the family has to wait for feedback
- There is less opportunity for consultation between the whole CDT
- It is a less efficient method of using a CDT and CDC

Assessment nursery
Advantages
- The child gets to know the personnel and environment and relaxes
- Several professionals can observe the child playing and interacting with other children over a longer period of time
- Observations by experienced nursery workers over several weeks can be highly valuable

Disadvantages
- May not be available
- Consistent attendance may be difficult

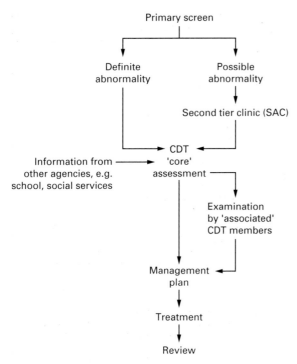

Figure 4.2   CDT assessment protocol.

well known and acceptable to the family and be their advocate in discussion with other professionals. An important role for the keyworker is to monitor the management plan and ensure that the family understands it. In some CDTs the keyworker is called the 'care manager' for the child.

Functional diagnosis

Doctors like to have clear diagnostic labels that define what is wrong in pathological terms and to understand the aetiology. Parents and children are less worried about the 'fancy' medical words but are desperately keen to know how the child's life will be affected and what the child will be able to do compared with other children. Common questions are: will children be able to walk, talk, feed, go to normal school, look after themselves as children or adults, get a job, live on their own and have children? It is often very difficult to answer these questions, especially if they relate to a distant prognosis; the most important aspect is to be open and honest and to admit ignorance when necessary.

Breaking bad news (Box 4.8)

All doctors should know how to do this by the time they qualify; however the process is often learnt only by trial and error.

Most parents go through a bereavement

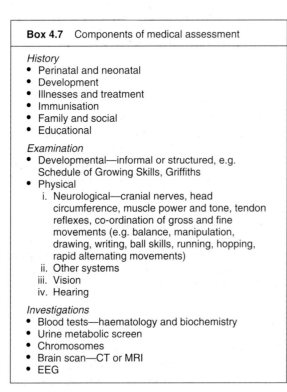

Box 4.7   Components of medical assessment

History
- Perinatal and neonatal
- Development
- Illnesses and treatment
- Immunisation
- Family and social
- Educational

Examination
- Developmental—informal or structured, e.g. Schedule of Growing Skills, Griffiths
- Physical
  i. Neurological—cranial nerves, head circumference, muscle power and tone, tendon reflexes, co-ordination of gross and fine movements (e.g. balance, manipulation, drawing, writing, ball skills, running, hopping, rapid alternating movements)
  ii. Other systems
  iii. Vision
  iv. Hearing

Investigations
- Blood tests—haematology and biochemistry
- Urine metabolic screen
- Chromosomes
- Brain scan—CT or MRI
- EEG

Box 4.8   Guidelines for breaking bad news

- Allow adequate time (at least 30 minutes)
- Eliminate interruptions (telephone, bleep, etc.)
- Do it as soon as possible
- Tell both parents together
- For a single parent suggest that another close relative or friend is present. Try to speak also to the other parent
- Use simple language
- Give full information, including doubts about diagnosis if appropriate
- Allow parents to talk
- Arrange another consultation soon after and encourage parents to prepare and write down a list of questions
- Be honest
- Offer a written report

process when they learn that their child is permanently disabled. The classic components of shock, grief, guilt and anger usually evolve and parents need to be helped through each of these stages. The time scale may last from weeks to years and more than one component often co-incides. Frequent associated emotions and reactions include rejection of the child, depression, panic, blame, seeking alternative advice, over-protection and, rarely, litigation.

The best interests of the child are paramount and the family must not be abandoned because the parents are hostile. Some parents are helped by contact with other affected families and parents' support groups. Voluntary organisations exist for most conditions and can be found through the Contact a Family (CaF) association or should be known to the local CDT health visitor or children's social worker.

Alternative therapies (Box 4.9)

Most parents wish to leave no stone unturned in their search for help for their disabled child. A vast range of techniques is available, some of which are offered by trained personnel in good faith while others are sold by charlatans. If parents ask advice about having one (or more) of these therapies they should be told that there is no scientific evidence that they help, but it is usually not appropriate for the doctor actively to discourage them. Harmful 'side-effects' include financial hardship and diversion of attention from siblings, which may be very important and should be monitored.

Child abuse

Disabled children are abused more frequently than normal children (up to 30% in some studies). They are vulnerable to abuse because:

- they have poor communication skills—they are less likely to complain or raise the alarm
- they have low self-esteem
- they are physically weak—they cannot defend themselves against attack
- they are easy to pick on—'scapegoat'

> **Box 4.9** Alternative therapies
>
> - Homoeopathy
> - Acupuncture
> - Massage
> - Cranial osteopathy
> - Aromatherapy
> - Auditory integration therapy
> - Reflexology
> - Brushing
> - Conductive education*
> - Doman–Delacato therapy (British Institute for Brain Injured Children)#
> - Hypervitamin therapy
> - Chinese/herbal medicine
> - Behavioural therapy
>
> *Conductive education was pioneered at the Peto Institute in Budapest, Hungary; some British children still go there although there are now centres in the UK. The 'conductor' spends all day with the child teaching motor skills, and some children with cerebral palsy have learnt to perform activities that they may otherwise have not.
> #The Doman–Delacato method started in Philadelphia, USA, but is now available in Somerset. It requires a team of helpers to work on the child for most of the waking hours going repeatedly through a structured programme of exercises and tasks (patterning).
> Both the above methods can produce short-term developmental progress but this is not usually maintained when the therapy stops. If conventional methods were given to a similar intensity it is likely that the results would be at least as good.

- parents have mixed emotions about them which may include rejection and anger
- they have a poor understanding of what is morally acceptable or expected
- they are more often institutionalised (abuse is more likely in these circumstances than at home).

All professionals involved in the care of disabled children must have a high level of suspicion. If any signs of abuse emerge, appropriate action should be taken without delay (see Chapter 17).

Statutory benefits

There are no benefits of childhood disability but there are a few schemes for giving moderate financial compensation to a family for the

---

Box 4.10   Disability benefits

Disability living allowance (DLA)
- Care component available from age 3 months: 3 rates—lowest (some help in day), middle (help day or night) and highest (help day and night)
- Mobility component available from age 5 years: 2 rates—lower (can walk but needs some supervision) and higher (cannot walk or needs constant help)

Invalid care allowance
- For adults caring for at least 35 hours a week for a severely disabled child in receipt of middle or highest rate of DLA
- Means tested (earnings less than £50 per week)

Orange badge scheme
- Available for a child over 2 years old in receipt of higher mobility component of DLA
- Enables car to be parked close to destination
- No time limit in official parking bays
- Up to 3 hours on single or double yellow lines (no time limit in Scotland)
- Scheme does not apply in central London

Family Fund
- Originally the Joseph Rowntree Trust
- Distributes money on behalf of Department of Health
- Families with severely disabled children can apply
- Medical support is needed
- Capital grants given according to the needs of the child
- £21.4 m allocated in 1997/98
- 95 356 families received an average sum of approximately £490
- Grants given towards holidays, beds and bedding, clothing, transport, washing machines and dryers, driving lessons, recreation and furniture. Larger grants, e.g. for home adaptations, are considered if supported by social services
- Means tested (income and capital)

General means tested benefits may apply, e.g. income support, housing benefit and council tax benefit

---

substantial expense, stress and inconvenience they suffer in looking after a disabled child (Box 4.10).

LEARNING DIFFICULTIES (LDS)

The incidence of global learning difficulties is 3–4% of the population; there are about 10 times as many cases in the moderate learning difficulties (MLD) subgroup as in the severe learning difficulties (SLD) subgroup.

Aetiology

An identifiable cause can be found in approximately 75% of severe cases but only in around 10% of the moderate group.

Chromosomal abnormalities. These account for approximately half the diagnoses in children with severe learning difficulties:

- Down's syndrome—the most common (see Chapter 7)
- fragile X syndrome
- trisomies, e.g. XXY, XYY.

Single gene defects. These are relatively rare:

- dominant, e.g. tuberous sclerosis
- recessive—metabolic disorders, e.g. neuronal, lysosomal storage diseases (Gaucher's, Batten's disease). These cause progressive development regression rather than stable developmental delay. Phenylketonuria has virtually been eliminated through the neonatal screening programme.

Intrauterine infections, e.g. rubella, CMV, toxoplasmosis.

Dysmorphic syndromes. Learning difficulties are a feature of many syndromes, e.g. Cornelia de Lange, Williams, Sotos, Prader–Willi, Beckwith–Wiedemann.

Perinatal problems (see also Chapter 3). Learning difficulties may be associated with cerebral palsy, especially the more severe types such as spastic quadriplegia. Factors include:

Intrapartum asphyxia in term infants (more than 37 weeks' gestation). The babies show severe birth asphyxia and are difficult to resuscitate. They go on to have severe hypoxic ischaemic (neonatal) encephalopathy (see p. 45); ultrasound head scan shows deep white matter damage, possibly with cyst formation.

Hypoglycaemia. The brain depends on an adequate supply of oxygen and glucose; low levels of glucose are not well tolerated especially if there is simultaneous hypoxia. If the hypoglycaemia causes clinical illness the risk of permanent brain damage is 50%; if it is asymptomatic, the risk is only 6%.

Extreme prematurity. These babies are more

likely to have predominantly motor problems. However, long-term follow-up has shown that up to 50% have subtle learning problems in school.

Developmental brain abnormalities. These are defects of structure which arise between about 6 and 20 weeks' gestation, e.g. neuronal migration defects, agenesis of the corpus callosum, hydrocephalus, microcephaly.

Acquired brain illness, e.g. meningitis, encephalitis, encephalopathy, head injury, uncontrolled epilepsy.

Investigation

It is important to find a diagnosis in order to counsel the family appropriately (including genetic advice) and give a prognosis. The yield from routine investigation of isolated learning difficulties is small, but selected tests may be justified if there are specific clues or parental anxiety is high. The following should be considered:

Chromosomes. Fragile X culture or DNA studies, especially in boys.

Brain scan. MRI gives better definition than CT (which involves irradiation), however young or restless children require a general anaesthetic as they must lie still inside the noisy, frightening machine for about 20 minutes (the time will reduce with improving technology). The yield of brain scanning is better if there are associated neurological abnormalities.

Blood biochemistry. Calcium, thyroid function, amino acids, liver function. Certain circumstances dictate other possibilities, e.g. ammonia, lead (poisoning), creatine kinase (in a young boy).

Urine biochemistry. Organic and amino acid chromatography, reducing substances.

Serology. For children less than three years old (especially under one year), antibodies against toxoplasma, rubella, CMV and herpes (TORCH screen). IgM antibody under 6 months of age is diagnostic of congenital infection. IgG without IgM indicates either passive maternal transmission (in the first year of life) or past infection at any time.

EEG. This is unlikely to help unless epilepsy or specific neurological disease is suspected.

It must be remembered that children with learning difficulties have an increased incidence of other impairments. As well as laboratory investigations, assessment should therefore include:

- full paediatric examination
- hearing test
- vision test
- occupational therapy assessment
- speech and language therapy assessment
- psychological assessment.

Microcephaly

This is usually defined as a head circumference two or more standard deviations below the mean (< 3rd centile). Some individuals may be normal but the majority have learning difficulties.

Causes

Primary (present by the seventh month of gestation):

- genetic
- developmental anomaly of the brain
- chromosomal abnormality, e.g. Down's syndrome and other trisomies
- dysmorphic syndromes (non-chromosomal), e.g. Shprintzen, Cornelia de Lange, Bloom, Dubowitz
- intrauterine infection—rubella, CMV
- intrauterine toxins, e.g. fetal alcohol syndrome, maternal irradiation and anticonvulsant therapy
- craniosynostosis—a developmental anomaly of the skull. Premature fusion of a skull suture prevents growth in that dimension and the growing brain causes excess expansion across the non-fused sutures. This results in an abnormal head shape, e.g. scaphocephaly (long and narrow), brachycephaly (short and broad), turricephaly (tall), plagiocephaly (asymmetrical). Many children with craniosynostosis do not have learning difficulties, and mild plagiocephaly is a common normal variant. Craniosynostosis may be associated with other craniofacial abnormalities, e.g. Apert and Crouzon

syndrome. Surgical treatment before the age of 6 months can give good cosmetic results.

Secondary (onset after the seventh month of gestation):

- severe maternal and infant malnutrition
- perinatal brain damage.

Clinical features

These are variable and the smallness of the head size does not correlate closely with the degree of learning difficulties. The most severe cases usually have other major neurological problems, e.g. cerebral palsy, epilepsy.

Specific learning difficulties

This is a completely different situation from global learning difficulties—the children usually have good general intelligence and can respond well to appropriate specific help. The key to correct management is accurate diagnosis, which usually requires multidisciplinary assessment.

Dyslexia (specific reading disability)

Definition. Dyslexia is usually what is meant when educationalists use the term 'specific learning difficulty'; many do not like the word 'dyslexia' because they consider it to have inappropriate negative emotional implications. In fact it simply means 'difficulty with words' and is therefore a correct diagnosis for a child who has problems with written language.

There is no simple criterion for dyslexia: a practical guide is performance in literacy skills that is at least 2 years behind chronological age. This clearly means different things at different ages—a discrepancy of 2 years in primary school is more severe than in secondary school. Another major factor is the general cognitive ability: a child who is delayed by 2 years in all learning fields does not have a specific learning difficulty, whereas one who is managing to keep up with the age group in literacy skills but has a general IQ in the superior range may well suffer from dyslexia. Unfortunately children in the latter group are often denied appropriate help by education authorities because it is argued that they do not fall into the lowest 2% of children and therefore do not need assessment for special educational needs.

Aetiology:

Neurological. It is now accepted that dyslexia has a biological basis. Structural abnormalities have been demonstrated in language and vision areas of the brain using sophisticated imaging technology.

Genetic. Studies have shown abnormal gene loci on chromosome 6 in families with dyslexia.

Auditory. Processing studies have found temporal difficulties of sound perception in dyslexic children.

Language. A high proportion of children with dyslexia have phonological difficulties on detailed language processing assessment.

Visual. Abnormalities in some children include lack of a reference eye on the Dunlop test which prevents normal lateralisation of the visual image and visual tracking difficulties which interfere with steady scanning of lines of writing.

Dyspraxia. There is an overlap between dyspraxia and dyslexia. There may be a common neurological defect of sensory processing.

Attention deficit. ADHD is another common association, possibly for similar reasons as dyspraxia because ADHD may arise from an inability to distinguish trivial from important sensory inputs and to respond appropriately (see Figure 4.5).

Epidemiology. Estimates vary but the general incidence is between 5 and 10% of school-children; in some areas up to 20% of children have literacy difficulties. There is a strong male predominance (as in all language disorders) and the family history is often positive, consistent with a dominant type of inheritance with variable penetrance.

Role of the doctor. The parents have probably already spoken to the class and head teacher at school, who may have arranged some help. Often parents find that the support available is insufficient and seek further advice from their GP. Sometimes the school and education authority refuse to recognise the problem at all, and the medical route is a last resort. Whatever the situation the doctor must respond sympathetically and assess the child.

History. Developmental, educational, social and emotional.

Examination. Neurological, including motor co-ordination and laterality, language, vision, hearing and literacy (reading and writing).

Management:

- Obtain a school report.
- Refer to the educational psychologist.
- Support the child and parents. The doctor may have to act as the child's advocate.
- Multidisciplinary assessment—speech and language therapy, psychology, occupational therapy.
- Formulate a diagnosis. It is helpful if this is contained in a written report which the parents can take to school.
- Continue to support the family if they come into conflict with the school or education authority.

Treatment:

Education. Following assessment by a dyslexia-trained special needs teacher and educational psychologist, a remedial programme should be implemented. The child will need individual teaching and additional support in the class-room, probably every day, so that he can understand and keep up with lessons. These can often only be provided through a Statement of Special Educational Needs. Dyslexic children find written examinations difficult as they can neither read the questions nor write the answers, even though their knowledge may be good. Most examination boards make concessions for dyslexia, consisting of the provision either of extra time or of someone to read the questions and/or write down the answers dictated by the child.

Technology. A computer with a good word processing package which includes a spell check program may be of great benefit.

Emotional support. Dyslexic children are at high risk of losing their self-esteem and becoming socially isolated. They need encouragement and teaching in social skills. Referral to a child and family therapy service may be necessary.

Visual therapy. Specific treatment from an orthoptist or optometrist may be helpful if reference or tracking abilities are defective. Coloured filters are sometimes offered but any benefit is probably placebo mediated.

Prognosis. Children with dyslexia have to work much harder than their peers to achieve what is often an inferior result. They frequently get left behind in class and become socially isolated. The longer the difficulties continue, the further behind they fall as school work becomes progressively demanding. This results in a high incidence of emotional disturbance as well as educational failure. Modern job prospects often depend strongly on literacy ability, and badly managed dyslexia in childhood can therefore have lifelong consequences.

MOTOR DIFFICULTIES

Cerebral palsy (CP)

Definition

Cerebral palsy is an inclusive diagnosis for a group of non-progressive motor disorders caused by brain disease.

Epidemiology

The total incidence is approximately 2 per 1000 live births. CP is much more common in premature babies—around 15–20% of survivors weighing under 1 kg and 10% of infants with birth weight between 1 and 1.5 kg. Related to gestational age, approximate risks are 12% for babies between 24 and 28 weeks and 4% from 28–30 weeks.

The overall incidence of CP in developed countries has increased in the last 20 years because of a greater number of survivors of neonatal care. The increase is mainly in the number of children with diplegia.

Classification

There are several methods of classification, going as far back as Little and Freud in the nineteenth century. The simplest is based on the neurological abnormality (Box 4.11).

> **Box 4.11**   Classification of cerebral palsy by neurological abnormality
>
> - Hemiplegia
> - Diplegia
>   —spastic
>   —ataxic
> - Quadriplegia (tetraplegia)
> - Dyskinetic (athetoid) cerebral palsy
> - Ataxic cerebral palsy
> - Mixed cerebral palsy

Aetiology

This varies according to the type of CP.

Prenatal factors:

Developmental brain abnormalities are present in approximately 10% of all CP cases, but in 50% of the quadriplegic group.

Intrauterine growth retardation (IUGR). 13% of CP cases are small for gestational age (SGA).

Gestational age. The pattern of injury resulting from a brain insult depends upon the developmental stage of the fetal brain when the insult occurred:

- Under 20 weeks' gestation: nerve cells migrate from the germinal matrix to the cortex and nuclei; disruption of this process causes dysplasia and ectopias.
- Between about 20 and 36 weeks' gestation: white matter is vulnerable to watershed ischaemic injury as well as hypoxia. The result is periventricular leukomalacia (PVL) and haemorrhagic infarction which causes cyst formation. If this process is severe and widespread, it becomes multicystic leukomalacia. Spastic diplegia most commonly arises at this gestational stage.
- Beyond 36 weeks' gestation: the grey matter of the cortex is most susceptible to ischaemic/ hypoxic injury. Watershed areas are affected, especially in the area of the middle cerebral artery. The thalamus, basal ganglia and occasionally the brainstem are also liable to damage by severe asphyxia in term infants. The characteristic clinical picture is spastic quadriplegia or dyskinetic CP.

Perinatal factors. Approximately 15% of cases of CP are due to perinatal asphyxia or trauma.

Only 2% of children born with moderate to severe birth asphyxia go on to develop CP. Some of these have predisposing prenatal brain abnormalities.

Postnatal factors account for approximately 5% of cases. The most common are infection (meningitis), trauma, drowning, suffocation and status epilepticus. The usual type is spastic quadriplegia, and there are often associated learning difficulties.

Clinical types

Hemiplegia—approximately one third of all cases of CP.

Pathology. Hemiplegia is due to prenatal causes in 75% of cases. Imaging shows infarction— usually in the distribution of the middle cerebral artery. Subcortical lesions are seen in pre-term infants following periventricular leukomalacia.

Diagnosis. Asymmetry may present early, e.g. in the Moro reflex, but is often not apparent until the age of 6 months. Fisting and a clear hand preference in the first year of life are suggestive of hemiplegia. The arm is affected more than the leg and shows a characteristic posture of abduction at the shoulder, flexion at the elbow and wrist, pronation of the forearm and extension of the fingers (Figure 4.3). The arm and leg have increased muscle tone and brisk tendon reflexes.

Prognosis. All hemiplegic children can achieve walking, although it is moderately delayed in 50%. Weakness is inevitable, and joint contractures are frequent even with adequate physiotherapy. The limbs on the affected side grow more slowly and become small compared with the normal scale. Sensory deficits, hemianopia, epilepsy and learning difficulties are frequently associated.

Spastic diplegia. This is the most common type of CP.

Pathology. Neonatal ultrasound may show intraventricular haemorrhage, ventricular dilatation and periventricular leukomalacia.

Diagnosis. The cardinal feature is weakness and spasticity in the legs which, however, may be hypotonic for the first 3 months. There is also hypertonicity of the hip adductors, which

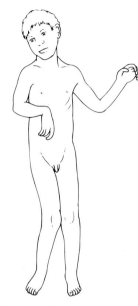

Figure 4.3 Right hemiplegia.

causes scissoring of the legs and of the hip and knee flexors. The arms are usually also moderately affected, with muscle hypertonia and brisk tendon reflexes. 70% of children with spastic diplegia have normal intelligence.

Prognosis. The vast majority will walk with a characteristic gait showing flexion at the knees, toe-walking and adducted hips. The Achilles tendons tend to become progressively shorter despite physiotherapy, ankle–foot orthoses and tendon release surgery.

Ataxic diplegia. This is often associated with hydrocephalus. Infants have marked muscle hypotonia developing into spasticity after approximately 6 months. Ataxia becomes more prominent, affecting the legs and arms, and delays sitting and walking. There are associated learning difficulties in 30–50% of cases.

Quadriplegia. This is the most severe type of CP.

Pathology. The condition is due to prenatal causes such as widespread bilateral brain lesions, e.g. neuronal migration defects, major malformations and multicystic encephalomalacia in 30% of cases. These may be seen on neonatal scanning or later MRI imaging. 20% of affected children are born small for gestational age. Quadriplegia

is due to a postnatal cause e.g. encephalitis, in 15% of cases.

Diagnosis. All four limbs are spastic, the arms more than the legs. There are abnormalities of tone, paucity of movement, abnormal primitive reflexes and fisting in the first few months of life (Figure 4.4). Feeding difficulties with tongue thrust and eventually speech difficulties are common. Disabilities such as epilepsy and learning difficulties are frequently associated.

Prognosis. The outcome in severe cases is very poor. The children invariably have severe or profound learning disability and very poor motor control and so are often totally dependent for their routine body care. Joint contractures, dislocation of the hips and kyphoscoliosis are common. Bulbar palsy causes major feeding difficulties with impairments of swallowing and gag reflex, and inhalation pneumonia is a frequent cause of death. Life expectancy in quadriplegia is significantly reduced; the most important predictive factors are lack of mobility and feeding problems.

Dyskinetic (athetoid) CP. This accounts for 10–15% of cases of CP.

Pathology. Infarction is followed by atrophy, sclerosis and calcification of the central grey matter (basal ganglia, thalamus and globus

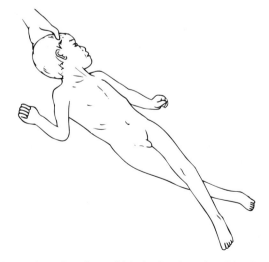

Figure 4.4 Spastic quadriplegia showing scissoring of legs and persistent asymmetrical tonic neck reflex in arms.

pallidum). Approximately two thirds of cases are due to perinatal factors including hyper-bilirubinaemia (kernicterus). Dyskinetic CP is a frequent end result of severe asphyxia in term infants, especially if it is acute and they are small for gestational age.

Diagnosis. Progress is usually normal in the first 6–9 months of life but then dystonia of the legs, trunk and mouth progressively appears. Poor truncal control delays and may prevent walking. The dystonia is exaggerated by voluntary movement which causes grimacing of the face and athetoid (writhing) and/or choreic (jerking) move-ments of the limbs. These are especially marked in hyperkinetic cases. There are invariably speech and feeding difficulties with drooling. Intelligence is usually within the normal range.

Prognosis. Life expectancy is good but quality of life is often poor as everyday tasks such as dressing, feeding and communication are very tedious and frustrating. Many children do not walk independently and the hips may become dislocated.

Ataxic CP. This accounts for approximately 10% of cases of CP.

Pathology. Dysplasia of the cerebellum is the most frequent abnormality due to prenatal factors. Asphyxial damage is rare.

Diagnosis. Many infants are very hypotonic—motor milestones are delayed. There is truncal ataxia, which interferes with sitting and standing, and ataxia of the limbs is noted on reaching out and attempting to grasp objects. Moderate learning difficulties are common.

Prognosis. Most children achieve walking though it is often delayed (up to 5 years old) and needs support with crutches.

Management

- Referral to a multidisciplinary CDT for assessment.
- Ongoing treatment, which will usually require physiotherapy, occupational therapy, speech therapy and provision of orthoses as well as medical care.
- Gait analysis in a specially equipped labora-

tory can be very helpful for initial assessment and continuing monitoring.

Physiotherapy. It is important to start therapy as soon as possible to try to pre-empt com-plications and to establish an early relationship with the child and parents (Box 4.12). There are several 'schools' of physiotherapy; the most common in the UK is the Bobath method. This is a neurodevelopmental approach which aims to promote function in the most efficient way possible for the child. There must be close co-operation between therapists and carers who are expected to continue the techniques at home and in nursery or school.

Aids and appliances. Splints, crutches, walking frames, positioning devices (e.g. wedges, boards, seats), wheelchairs, etc., are prescribed by the physiotherapist and occupational therapist. They will only be accepted by the child if they improve comfort and function. The gait laboratory can be very helpful in identifying the impairments that need correction. A skilled orthotist should also be involved at the assessment stage and not just when the appliance is made.

Orthopaedic surgery. A child with CP should be seen by an orthopaedic surgeon at an early stage. The aim of surgery is to improve function or to correct deformity. Techniques include:

Tendon lengthening. The most frequent opera-tion performed for CP is Achilles tendon length-ening for treatment of toe walking which persists despite adequate physiotherapy and splinting.

Tenotomy. This weakens muscles and is most often performed on the hip adductor muscles to try to prevent dislocation. Obturator neurectomy may also be performed at the same time.

Tendon transfer. This changes the direction of an excessive force exerted by a particular muscle.

Box 4.12 Primary aims of physiotherapy
<ul><li>Improve motor function</li><li>Prevent contractures</li><li>Minimise postural deformity due to muscle imbalance</li><li>Encourage independence</li><li>Support parents and carers</li></ul>

It is used mainly in the forearm to transfer a flexor to the dorsum of the hand to reduce the deformity and increase useful power.

Arthrodesis. An unstable or deformed joint can be permanently fixed into a functional position by fusing the bones. This can be done on the ankle joint to correct valgus or varus deformity or on the spine to treat scoliosis.

Neurosurgery. The use of the neurosurgical techniques below is controversial.

Dorsal root rhizotomy is selective division of motor spinal roots to reduce muscle spasticity. It is most effective in spastic diplegic children with normal intelligence.

Stereotactic brain surgery can be performed on basal ganglia structures to reduce severe disabling dystonic movements.

Drugs for spasticity:

Baclofen is widely used and reduces painful muscle spasms. Side-effects include sedation and weakness; these may be reduced by giving the drug intrathecally.

Diazepam can be given in small doses as it has a specific effect (GABA-agonist) as well as being a general relaxant.

Botulinum toxin can be injected into individual muscles and is effective for about 6 months.

Treatment of drooling (a common problem in spastic quadriplegia):

Oral training by a speech therapist to encourage tongue control and regular swallowing.

Anticholinergic drugs (e.g. benzhexol, scopolamine) can be tried.

Electric stimulation of swallowing reflex.

Oral surgery. This consists of moving the salivary ducts further back so that saliva tends to be swallowed rather than spilling out of the mouth.

Feeding difficulties. These can be severe in quadriplegic or dystonic CP. Several measures may help:

Speech therapy to encourage efficient chewing and swallowing.

Dietary advice. A paediatric dietician will review the nutritional intake and recommend ways to optimise it.

Physiotherapy. The danger in feeding difficulties is that food and/or liquids may be inhaled and cause pneumonia. Chest physiotherapy should be given and taught to the parents to attempt to encourage drainage from the lungs.

Nasogastric tube feeding. This is unpleasant and should only be used as a short-term measure.

Gastrostomy should be considered if prolonged oral feeding is not possible.

Other difficulties which may need active management include:

- dental care
- gastro-oesophageal reflux—especially common in children with quadriplegia. It is an important risk factor for inhalation pneumonia, even if a gastrostomy is in place. If medical treatment is not successful, oesophageal surgery (fundal plication) should be considered.
- epilepsy
- constipation.

DEVELOPMENTAL DYSPRAXIA— 'CLUMSINESS'

Clumsiness is the motor manifestation of dyspraxia—a central defect that causes impairment of organisation, sequencing and processing of information. These difficulties may affect input (receptive pathways) and/or output (executive pathways) and thus have an adverse effect on many skills such as language, motor control and perception. This combination of impairments comprises the clinical picture of developmental dyspraxia and explains its pervasive nature and the overlap with dyslexia and attention deficit disorder (ADHD), see Figure 4.5.

Clinical features

Motor milestones may be slightly delayed but are often in the normal range. However, the quality of motor control may be impaired so that, for example, feeding is messy and manipulation is poor. Children run and jump as usual but trip and fall over frequently and are often 'covered in bruises' and labelled as 'accident prone'.

School problems are common, especially if there are learning difficulties. It is quickly

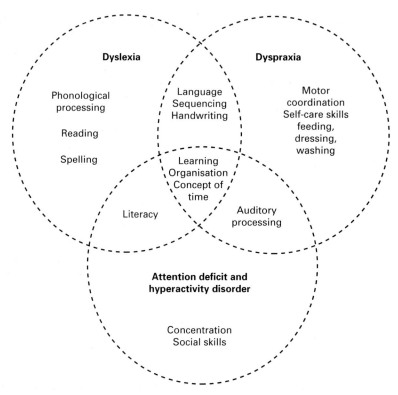

Figure 4.5 Skills adversely affected in dyslexia, dyspraxia and ADHD, showing overlaps.

apparent to other children that a clumsy child is not good at games and they are left out of team activities. Efficient undressing and dressing is impossible and PE, physical games and sports are avoided. Thus the child becomes ignored and isolated and may develop major secondary problems such as loss of self-esteem and social withdrawal.

Unfortunately such children often also have difficulties with pastimes such as painting, modelling, playing musical instruments, reading and writing, and they end up preferring to spend their time listening to music or watching television. Many can use a computer competently and find it an enjoyable and useful occupation if they can be directed to educational programs and not just games.

The sense of time is often distorted: clumsy children usually find it difficult to tell the time from a clock face, judge the passage of time, or anticipate. Teasing and bullying are common and must be managed quickly and firmly by teachers and parents.

Associated factors

• Gender. Males outnumber females in a ratio of approximately 3:1 (similar to language difficulties).

• Social class. Dyspraxia is diagnosed more commonly in upper than lower socio-economic groups but this probably reflects a greater awareness by parents.

• The term 'minimal brain dysfunction' (MBD) is no longer used, but there is an increased incidence of perinatal difficulty without brain damage severe enough to cause major motor or cognitive sequelae.

• Left-handedness is more common. A child who is left-handed, left-footed and left-eyed, reflecting a dominant right hemisphere, is no more likely to be disabled than a right-handed child. Crossed laterality or a tendency to ambidexterity, however, may be associated with a lack of efficient cerebral organisation. Alternatively the child may have been developing a naturally dominant left hemisphere but suffered a brain insult which affected the left more than the right hemisphere; the more efficient right hemisphere would then take over some functions from the left hemisphere in order to optimise central processing and control. This is the basis of brain plasticity which works better the earlier it happens in relation to brain development; however the brain circuitry is less efficient than normal following this process because of the resulting 'faulty wiring'.

Management

Assessment

Medical. History and neurological examination, paying special attention to motor co-ordination and control. Visual function should also be checked.

Occupational therapy. This is the key discipline involved with clumsy children. Occupational therapists (OTs) are expert at assessing motor co-ordination, visuo-motor skills, perceptual integration and routine self-care functions (activities for daily living—ADL). There are several test methods available to them which give structured information and standardised results, e.g. the movement ABC, the Beery test of visual–motor integration and the Bruininks–Oseretsky test of motor proficiency.

Investigation

It is rare for neurological investigations to yield useful results in the absence of other clinical abnormalities. However, the technology for functional brain imaging is still improving and in the future MRI, PET or other types of brain scanning may be helpful.

Treatment

Occupational therapy. Following assessment, the OT will design an individual programme of therapy for the child, to be carried out collaboratively with parents and teachers. Ideally the OT will continue to see the child regularly until function is satisfactory. Unfortunately, however, in practice there is a shortage of suitably trained paediatric OTs and children are usually seen less often or for intermittent intensive courses.

Sensori-integration therapy. This technique is used by OTs and involves subjecting the child to multiple sensory inputs in a structured way so that the child learns how to process and integrate the information and respond appropriately. A specially equipped gymnasium is required so that the child can do different manoeuvres in varying positions including suspension.

Recreational activities which require motor co-ordination should be encouraged. Examples are martial arts (for boys) and ballet dancing (for girls) but any activity that needs good co-ordination, e.g. painting, model making, cycling, swimming or ball games, will help.

Emotional development. The child should be reassured that there is no medical disease and that he or she will improve. If there are problems in peer relationships these should be addressed at school. Severe emotional problems may necessitate referral to a child and family therapy service.

COMMUNICATION DIFFICULTIES

Language is a system of communication by symbols. Animals have simple signalling systems for communicating basic needs and emotions such as hunger, danger, pleasure and anger. However, high level language which allows communication of complex thoughts from one individual to another is unique to humans. It has evolved over millennia and is the main reason for human dominance on earth.

Epidemiology

Speech and language abnormalities are the most common impairments found on child health surveillance. Approximately 1% of children have a severe language delay or disorder and a further 3% have moderately severe difficulties. At school entry age around 7% of children have a language difficulty severe enough to interfere with education.

Factors

- Gender—about twice as many males as females.
- Social class—more common in lower socio-economic groups.
- Ethnicity—more common in children whose first language is not English.

Classification

Language is a very complex function and there is no simple system for classifying abnormalities. A linguistic and a medical model are described below.

Linguistic model

First level. Receptive (comprehension), or expressive.

Second level:

Semantic difficulties. Poor concepts of words and meaning of language. Example: limited comprehension of vocabulary and word finding difficulty.

Syntactical difficulties. Lack of understanding of the rules of language. Poor use of grammar in speech and misinterpretation of receptive language. Example: Subjective/objective nouns or passive/active verbs are confused.

Phonological difficulties. Impairment of the ability to distinguish between similar sounds (phonemes). Example: inability to generate rhymes or to distinguish between words like 'mat' and 'cat' or 'ship' and 'sheep'.

Pragmatic difficulties. Pragmatics is a central

Box 4.13 Components of pragmatics
• Grammar • Syntax • Phonology • Semantics • Lexicon • Morphology

process and embraces all linguistic (including non-verbal) functions (Box 4.13). Impairment interferes with the social use of language. Communicative intent is impaired both expressively and receptively and therefore the basic concept of using language for communication is compromised.

Example: 'cocktail party syndrome'—words are used and speech may be fluent but there is little communicative content.

The difficulties listed above often co-exist; for example autistic children usually have a semantic–pragmatic language disorder. A language problem should be analysed according to the grid in Figure 4.6. This usually requires referral to a paediatric speech and language therapist (SLT).

Speech difficulties:

Phonological disorder.

Impairment of phonetic articulation due to structural abnormalities or oro-motor dyspraxia (incoordination of motor control of the muscles of speech). Poor articulation interferes with intelligibility and can lead to major social and emotional problems for affected children. Language is often normal.

Medical model

Language difficulties can also be classified on

	Semantics	Syntax	Phonology
Expression			
Comprehension			
Pragmatics			

Figure 4.6 Analysis of language difficulty.

medical lines according to the cause of the prob-lem (this system is, however, less satisfactory from a functional and management point of view):

- anatomical defects of the speech apparatus, e.g. cleft palate, malocclusion, vocal cord abnormality (dysphonia)
- central neurological pathology affecting muscle control for speech production, e.g. cerebral palsy, sequelae of head injury, stroke (dysarthria)
- developmental neurological control dysfunction, e.g. oro-motor dyspraxia
- peripheral neurological abnormality, e.g. vocal cord paralysis, bulbar palsy
- deafness
- learning difficulties
- emotional disorders, e.g. elective mutism, persistent stammer
- understimulation
- ideopathic—specific language impairment.

It is important to distinguish between a language delay, in which the pattern of language develop-ment is normal but is behind the expected level for chronological age, and language disorder, in which the language pattern is one which would not occur in normal children. The prognosis for the former condition is much better than for the latter, even without intervention, although it is likely that catch-up will be speedier with the help of speech and language therapy. The ceiling of performance for language delayed children is determined by their cognitive ability.

Specific language impairment (SLI)

This term is used for children whose language disorder has no known underlying cause or asso-ciation. It may affect any or all of the linguistic components previously described. The prognosis for severe cases is poor, particularly for literacy skills; hence the overall educational, social and emotional outlook for these children is limited. Early structured help with regular speech and language therapy is essential. Consideration must be given to placement in a language unit and alternative technologies for communication, e.g. sign language, computer systems.

An important cause of specific language im-pairment may be an auditory processing defect which compromises the function of the decoding device in the language centre (Figure 4.7). How-ever, expressive language is mainly affected in some SLI children and the encoding device may be similarly defective.

Clinical features

Children suspected to have SLI must be assessed by an experienced paediatric SLT in order to identify the pattern of difficulties requiring help.

Verbal dyspraxia. Speech is dysfluent, very difficult and requires great effort. Words tend to be short, distorted and incomplete, and are usually unintelligible to strangers and sometimes familiars. Not surprisingly, the child becomes extremely frustrated and may stop trying to talk and develop severe social and behavioural problems. The condition is often associated with oro-motor dyspraxia which affects other oral

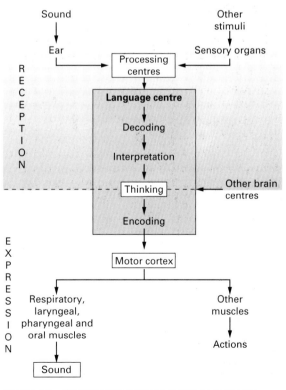

Figure 4.7 Central and peripheral language pathways.

functions; there is a history of feeding difficulties as a baby and dislike of chewing in later childhood. Intensive speech therapy is required.

Lexical-syntactic deficit—severe word-finding difficulties. The word is stored in the memory bank (lexicon) but cannot be retrieved in the instant it is required. It causes erratic speech with long pauses, fillers ('er'/'em' etc.) and circumlocutions.

Semantic-pragmatic deficit—difficulty in using language for social intercourse. The vocabulary may be large and such children may be 'chatterboxes'. Their sentences are often grammatically correct but the words may be wrong and the content irrelevant. Social skills are often poor and there is difficulty in appropriate turn-taking in conversation. These children may fall into the autistic spectrum.

Phonological-syntactic deficit—sentences are grammatically incorrect with words missed out or wrongly formed. The sounds of the words are distorted and mixed up producing spoonerisms and malapropisms. Comprehension may be affected as well as expression. There is usually a long history of slow speech development which may not have been taken seriously at first.

Phonological programming deficit—speech is fairly fluent but words are mispronounced and so intelligibility is poor. Consonants are usually affected more than vowel sounds, particularly at the end of words. The prognosis is good, especially with the help of speech therapy.

These subtypes of language difficulty are common in minor forms in the general adult population.

Stammer (stutter/dysfluency)

This causes erratic delivery of speech with blockages, prolongations and repetitions of sounds. Approximately 4% of children stammer between the ages of 2 and 4 years but in about 1% the stammer persists. These children should be referred to a SLT; treatment is speech therapy combined with a behavioural programme which may involve the whole family as frequently there are complex emotional factors which need to be addressed.

Non-oral communication systems

Children who had good cognitive capacity but were unable to talk used to be regarded as mentally retarded, however the use of sign language has gradually evolved to give them the ability to express themselves. Now there are several sophisticated language systems that do not require speech and these are supplemented by a growing number of increasingly accessible and useful computerised communication aids.

The Department of Health sponsors several Communication Aid Centres across the UK and there are others attached to special schools or research units. Children can usually be referred to an appropriate centre for assessment via a Child Development Team or speech and language therapy department.

Communication technologies

Bliss symbols. These consist of simple diagrammatic pictures which are usually mounted on a board to which the child points. This system is mainly used for children with cerebral palsy and learning difficulties. Pointing can be performed by many means including digits, head mounted pointer, eye pointing, etc. Most children now are better helped by a more sophisticated device but Bliss boards remain an easily used, cheap communication aid.

Makaton. Signs are based on gestural body language and are easy to learn. They are very suitable for young children and those with learning difficulties. They are mostly hand positions and convey approximately 350 functions, objects and ideas.

Paget–Gorman. This is a word based signing system and includes grammar to enable more complex communication. The signs require good hand control so Paget–Gorman presents problems for children with motor difficulties.

British Sign Language (BSL). This is mainly used by deaf people but can improve communication in a child with good comprehension, cognitive abilities, and expressive language and dexterity but unintelligible speech.

Computerised communication aids. At present a variety of systems exist in which words or other communication symbols are presented on a screen. These can be selected by many methods, e.g. keyboard, joysticks, pressure pads for head or other body parts, eye movement. They can then be put into text on screen, typed or processed into sound via a speech synthesiser.

Information technology to enhance communication is steadily gaining in its accessibility and efficiency. Computers are becoming faster and are able to process more information input. They can therefore take limited clues and make decisions about interpretation after 'getting to know' the operator. Speech synthesisers and recognition systems are also becoming more 'intelligent' and may eventually allow language disabled people to participate in conversation. Computers in general are also getting smaller (the largest component is the display unit, which may be dispensable for this purpose); in the foreseeable future, it is possible that a complete computerised communication system could be mobile enough for a child to carry it around. In this way, the handicap of biological communication difficulties may be greatly reduced.

FURTHER READING

Bellman M, Lingam S, Aukett A 1996 The Schedule of Growing Skills II. NFER-Nelson, Windsor
British Association for Community Child Health 1994 Disability in childhood: Towards nationally useful definitions. Royal College of Paediatrics and Child Health, London
Illingworth R S 1987 The development of the infant and young child, 9th edn. Churchill Livingstone, Edinburgh

USEFUL ADDRESS

Contact a Family (CaF), 170 Tottenham Court Road, London W1P 0HA. Tel. 0207 383 3555 – publishes the CaF directory of specific conditions and rare syndromes in children with their family support networks (4th edn, 1997).

Internet addresses

Development
http://www.luhs.org/health/topics/chil/index.htm

Cerebral palsy
http://www.scope.org.uk

5

Cardiovascular and respiratory disorders

Michael Bamford

CARDIOVASCULAR SYSTEM

Heart disease in childhood presents as an unusual problem in primary care and is suitably managed in conjunction with a local paediatrician. It will often require referral to a tertiary centre, however the emphasis should be on minimising disruption to the child's life, and shared care clinics offer a suitable setting for the majority of reviews and non-invasive treatment where possible. Developments in imaging, interventional cardiological techniques, paediatric anaesthesia, surgical techniques and supportive care have greatly improved the outlook in children's heart disease in the last 20 years, and the need for hospitalisation has been much reduced.

DEVELOPMENT OF THE HEART

The major structure of the heart is formed by the end of the sixth week of gestation. A number of fetal problems and maternal medical conditions or drugs can interfere with development of its normal anatomy and function.

Fetal abnormalities

Major chromosomal disorders—particularly Down's syndrome, trisomy 13 and 18 and Turner's syndrome—are associated with characteristic cardiac abnormalities. The trisomic syndromes may be picked up by maternal triple screening,

Table 5.1   Chromosomal abnormalities associated with heart disease

Abnormality	Associated heart problem
Trisomy 21 (Down's syndrome)	Aortic stenosis (AS), atrial septal defect (ASD), atrioventricular septal defect (A/VSD)
Trisomy 18 (Edwards' syndrome)	Ventricular septal defect (VSD), patent ductus arteriosus (PDA), pulmonary stenosis (PS)
Trisomy 13 (Patau's syndrome)	VSD, PDA, dextrocardia
XO (Turner's syndrome)	Coarctation, AS, ASD

or by screening with ultrasound, where typical associations such as the atrioventricular septal defect in Down's syndrome may prompt diagnostic ultrasound scanning and amniocentesis. Despite these screening tests, children with Down's syndrome may be born unexpectedly with heart disease.

A number of infant malformation syndromes are typically associated with heart disease (Table 5.1).

Heart disease should be considered in any child born with a congenital abnormality as there are a large number of rarer associations between congenital abnormality syndromes and heart disease (Table 5.2). In all cases the heart should be examined, and, if doubts remain, echocardiography performed. Some of these syndromes are known to be associated with specific chromosomal microdeletions (e.g. Williams' syndrome—chromosome 7, Di George syndrome—chromosome 22) and can be diagnosed with techniques such as fluorescent in-situ hybridisation (FISH) cytogenetic tests.

Maternal factors

Many maternal conditions are associated with

> **Box 5.1**   Maternal causes of congenital heart disease
>
> - Diabetes (especially if poorly controlled)
> - SLE—complete heart block
> - Autosomal dominants—Marfan's syndrome, Noonan's syndrome, HOCM, prolonged Q-T (Romano–Ward) syndrome
> - Infections—rubella, CMV, herpes
> - Drugs—anticonvulsants, amphetamines, warfarin

an increased risk of cardiac malformation in the fetus; Box 5.1 lists some of the more common.

FETAL CIRCULATION AND NEONATAL CHANGES

Dramatic changes in the infant circulation occur at birth, with the removal of the placental circulation immediately on clamping of the umbilical cord. The systemic arterial pressure rises and pulmonary resistance falls with a consequent increase in pulmonary blood flow. The rise in blood oxygen tension causes relaxation of the pulmonary arteries. The ductus arteriosus and the foramen ovale close functionally in the first 24 hours of life in term infants; obliteration of the ductus subsequently takes place over 2 months.

Table 5.2   Syndromes associated with heart disease

Syndrome	Associated heart problem
Williams' syndrome	Supravalvar AS
Di George syndrome	Hypoplastic aortic arch
Noonan's syndrome	Pulmonary valve dysplasia
Marfan's syndrome	Aortic and mitral valve regurgitation
VACTERL association (Vertebral defects, Anal atresia, Congenital heart disease, Tracheo-oesophageal fistula, Renal dysplasia, Limb defects)	VSD most common

These events may be disturbed by perinatal hypoxia, acidosis or premature birth, septicaemia (particularly with group B streptococcus) or anatomical underdevelopment of the lungs, as in diaphragmatic hernia, hypoplastic lungs in prolonged amniotic fluid leak, or other thoracic dystrophic conditions.

Persistent fetal circulation

Persistent raised pulmonary vascular resistance results in cyanosis and may mimic cyanotic cardiac malformation. Investigation of the heart reveals normal anatomy with raised pulmonary artery pressures. Management is by treatment of the cause, correction of acidosis and appropriate ventilatory support. In severe cases newer treatments such as ventilation with additional nitric oxide, or extracorporeal membrane oxygenation (ECMO) may improve survival.

In premature infants the ductus arteriosus may remain patent and complicate medical progress. Pharmacological closure with indomethacin is commonly effective, particularly if given early. Occasionally surgical closure is required.

EXAMINATION OF THE CARDIOVASCULAR SYSTEM

Infant

The heart should be examined as part of the general examination of the newborn. This is best achieved with the infant relaxed (e.g. after a feed). The breathing and colour should be noted with the child undressed in a warm environment; auscultation with a warm paediatric stethoscope should be an early part of the examination before the child has been distressed by any other procedure. In particular, once breathing is established, cyanosis should be recognised, if present. Circumoral cyanosis after feeds is a common harmless finding, otherwise any suggestion of central cyanosis should be investigated. Murmurs heard in the first day should be reviewed after 4–6 days if the child appears otherwise well, and again at around 6 weeks unless the child develops symptoms (particularly breathlessness or poor feeding). The presence of femoral pulses should be confirmed by gentle palpation at the mid-inguinal point with the forefinger, with the infant's hips partly abducted. The timing should be compared with the radial pulse. Any delay of the impulse or difficulty in feeling the pulses should be investigated by measuring the blood pressure in arms and legs. A gradient of more than 20 mmHg is suggestive of coarctation. The heart should be reviewed by full examination at 4–6 weeks as many shunt-dependent murmurs may not be obvious in the first few days of life. In later childhood opportunities should be taken to examine the cardiovascular system as they present. The blood pressure should be measured as part of this process.

Older children

Formal examination of the cardiovascular system should involve *inspection* of the child's colour and the shape of the chest, noting any prominence of the precordium or surgical scars. Anaemia, if present, may be associated with flow murmurs. The fingers should be examined for clubbing (Figure 5.1) or splinter haemorrhages. Tachypnoea in the absence of respiratory problems may suggest cardiac failure, as may the scrawny appearance of a child that is failing to thrive.

Palpation should begin with the pulses, noting the timing and quality of the pulses at the wrist and at a major artery, preferably at the groin. If there is a suspicion of a bounding pulse, the

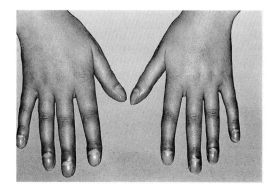

Figure 5.1 Finger clubbing.

strength of the impulse at the dorsalis pedis may confirm this. The rate and rhythm should be measured. Any irregularity of the rate should be timed in respect of the breathing pattern. Sinus arrhythmia, with an acceleration of the pulse as the child breathes in, and a corresponding deceleration with breathing out, is a common and often misinterpreted finding. The quality of the cardiac impulse at the sternal edge should be felt with the flat of the hand, and the location of the apical impulse confirmed with the finger tips. Cardiac thrills should be felt for at the precordium and at the sternal notch. Auscultation should usually be with the bell of the stethoscope, and the principal areas of the precordium—the sternal edge, the apex, the aortic and pulmonary areas—examined. The sites of extra-cardiac murmurs—the lung fields, the back, and the neck—should also be examined with the child lying and sitting or standing. The normal heart sounds should be recognised, particularly the splitting of the second sound in the pulmonary area and its physiological variation. Any murmurs should be timed in the cardiac cycle and the intensity (on a scale of 1–6, see Box 5.2) and quality noted. Finally the abdomen should be palpated for hepatic and/or splenic enlargement.

BENIGN MURMURS

Cardiac murmurs are commonly heard in early childhood, particularly in early newborn examination, at the time of a febrile illness or in the course of a routine examination, as in a pre-school examination. If a murmur is discovered, attention should be focused on a full cardio-vascular examination including the colour of the child, peripheral pulses, liver size and breathing rate. The *timing, character, intensity, site of maximum intensity, radiation of audibility, and any associated thrill* should be noted, together with the character of the heart sounds, particularly the second sound or the presence of an ejection click. The benign heart murmurs are typically characterised by the 10 Ss—see Box 5.3.

If the murmur seems benign the child should be re-examined at a later date. An intermittent murmur is almost certainly benign. Referral for specialist opinion may be required if there is doubt or excessive parental anxiety. A confident clinical diagnosis of a benign murmur will very rarely overlook a significant abnormality. The benign murmur which causes most uncertainty is the systolic murmur in the aortic area, giving rise to concern about the possibility of mild aortic stenosis or a bicuspid aortic valve.

Investigation with chest X-ray and ECG rarely adds much to the certainty of the diagnosis, but may be reassuring. An echocardiogram performed by an experienced paediatric examiner is usually conclusive.

If a benign murmur is diagnosed the parents should be given strong reassurance that the child's heart is normal and that the finding is harmless and should not be re-investigated. Persistent re-examination and speculation carries a real risk of exacerbating and perpetuating parental anxiety, resulting in inappropriate handling of the child.

Box 5.2 Murmur intensity

1. Just audible in ideal conditions
2. Readily audible to most examiners
3. Loud murmur, widely transmitted, without a palpable thrill
4. Loud murmur, widely transmitted, with an associated thrill
5. Murmur heard with the stethoscope only partly applied to the chest, and with a thrill
6. Very loud murmur heard with the stethoscope off the chest

Box 5.3 10 'S' characteristics of benign murmurs of childhood

1. *S*oft (grade 2/6 at most)
2. *S*hort (mid systolic, ejection murmurs)
3. *S*ystolic
4. *S*mall in area (confined to one location)
5. Heard at the *S*ternal edge, though other typical sites are the pulmonary or aortic area
6. The *S*econd sound should be normal in intensity, with normal variation with breathing
7. *S*itting/lying postural variation may be noted
8. *S*tops with the child performing a Valsalva manoeuvre, or taking a deep breath and holding it
9. The child should have no cardiac *S*ymptoms of breathlessness, cardiac pain or syncope
10. No additional abnormal *S*igns should be noted

METHODS OF INVESTIGATION

Chest X-ray

This gives information on cardiac size and configuration, and may also give information on the perfusion of the lungs in the presence of left–right or right–left shunts. Problems of interpretation may arise when, as is often the case, the timing of the films in respect of a young child's breathing is inappropriate. Care should also be taken in interpreting the upper mediastinal shadow of the thymus which is commonly evident in the first year of life (Figure 5.2).

Electrocardiograph

The paediatric ECG differs from the adult pattern, reflecting the more or less equal sizes of the ventricles at birth and gradually evolving with a shift of the QRS axis to the normal adult values in the teens.

Echocardiography

In experienced hands the echocardiograph gives valuable information on the structure and function of the heart (Figure 5.3). In conjunction with Doppler studies it allows diagnosis and first line evaluation of many childhood cardiac disorders, and is a useful tool in the follow-up of their

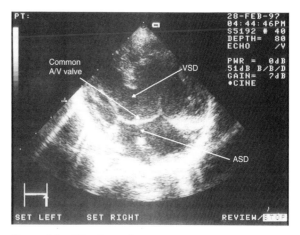

Figure 5.3 2D echocardiogram—apical view. Atrioventricular septal defect in an infant with Down's syndrome.

evolution. It is a relatively non-invasive investigation but may be difficult in lively or uncooperative children. If it is deemed essential that it be undertaken in these circumstances, it may be necessary to sedate the child to allow an adequate assessment.

Magnetic resonance imaging (MRI)

MRI and data from radionuclide scanning may contribute to the evaluation of defects.

Cardiac catheterisation

This gives direct and accurate structural and haemodynamic information, and allows non-surgical intervention in a wide variety of conditions (Box 5.4). In childhood it is normally carried out under general anaesthetic, with an attendant small risk.

ARRHYTHMIA

Perinatal arrhythmia

Arrhythmia may be identified on a cardiotocograph (CTG) and interpreted as fetal distress.

Tachyarrhythmias (normally supraventricular) usually exceed 200 bpm. If noted, they require evaluation of the fetus with ultrasound exami-

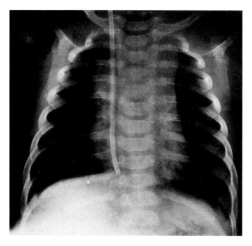

Figure 5.2 Chest X-ray showing enlarged mediastinum due to normal thymus.

Box 5.4 Current transcatheter interventional techniques

- *Rashkind septostomy* of the atrial septum is still used to increase systemic oxygenation, usually as a temporising measure in transposition of the great arteries (TGA)
- *Balloon dilatation.* Commonly used in pulmonary stenosis, selected patients with aortic stenosis and discrete coarctation
- *Shunt occlusion.* A variety of devices are available including umbrella and coil devices for occlusion of a patent ductus arteriosus, and increasingly devices for the occlusion of ASDs and VSDs are becoming regularly used
- *Stents* may be inserted to maintain dilatation achieved by balloon in a narrowed vessel
- *Radiofrequency ablation* of abnormal conducting tissue may be used in persistent arrhythmias

nation for cardiac anatomical abnormality and signs of heart failure (fetal hydrops). Persistent tachycardia for more than a few days may result in fetal heart failure and severely threaten the infant's survival. In a very pre-term infant, treatment of the mother with digoxin may cause reversion of the arrhythmia. Nearer term, elective delivery may be considered, followed by medical treatment and subsequent prevention with digoxin for the first year of life. After this age digoxin may be withdrawn, and most tachyarrhythmias do not recur.

Bradycardias have a poor prognosis if associated with structural anomalies. Otherwise, complete heart block may be a marker of maternal lupus (SLE). In such children the bradycardia is usually remarkably well tolerated—the child can be delivered normally and subsequently does not require pacemaker insertion.

Paroxysmal tachycardia

This may present at any age with either recurrent symptoms of identifiable palpitations, or episodes of pallor or lethargy in a young child. Parents may observe a rapid heart beat, or persistent tachycardia may cause heart failure, with tachypnoea, lethargy, pallor and hepatomegaly. In such circumstances the diagnosis should be considered if the pulse rate by auscultation is in excess of 200 bpm (typically, faster than can be comfortably counted). This is a medical emergency requiring immediate referral for treatment.

A small proportion of children presenting with tachycardias have structural cardiac anomalies. The majority have normal gross anatomy, but aberrant conduction. Evaluation of the resting ECG shows Wolff–Parkinson–White (WPW) syndrome in 10–20% of cases with short P-R interval and delta wave (slurred upstroke of the R wave) in some leads (Figure 5.4). Otherwise a short P-R interval may be an isolated finding. A 24-hour tape may reveal the tachyarrhythmia or, if the episodes are infrequent, the family may be loaned an event recorder device to record the child's heart rhythm during the suspect episodes. The large majority of tachycardias are *supraventricular* in origin (SVT), and show narrow complex QRS complexes during the episode. Such events are not life threatening in the short term, and the treatment can be considered according to the severity of the symptoms of the arrhythmia, the duration of the episode, the precipitating causes, and the frequency of the events. A prolonged SVT may be treated by *vagal stimulation* with carotid sinus massage or initiation of the diving reflex by the application of an ice pack to

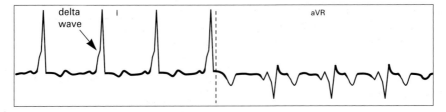

Figure 5.4 Wolff–Parkinson–White syndrome. ECG lead 1 and AVR showing short P-R interval and delta wave.

the bridge of the nose (with ECG monitoring). Inpatient treatment includes intravenous *adenosine* in incremental doses, *digoxin* and *DC cardioversion*.

Recurrent tachycardia

If only mildly inconvenienced by the episodes, the child may be left untreated. Self-induced physiological manoeuvres such as breath holding or swallowing ice cream may allow the child to control the episode. Digoxin remains an option, particularly in the first year of life; after this time it may be withdrawn without recurrence of episodes. Children older than 5 years at presentation are unlikely to lose the tendency for further episodes; if treatment is elected, beta blocking agents (propranolol, atenolol or sotalol) are the usual first choice. Severe or refractory arrhythmias may be treated by surgical or transcatheter ablation of aberrant conducting pathways.

Ventricular tachycardias (VT)

Rarer than SVT, these are usually associated with structural abnormalities, particularly right ventricular dysplasia or Romano–Ward syndrome (long Q-T syndrome). The ECG during the arrhythmia shows broad complexes, and the pulse rate may be high (> 300 bpm) and rapidly lead to cardiogenic shock. If the diagnosis is certain, emergency treatment should be DC cardioversion (0.5–2 J/kg) or lignocaine infusion. A trial of adenosine may be offered if SVT with aberrant conduction is suspected. Recurrent VT may be prevented by beta blockade or amiodarone. Radiofrequency ablation of abnormal foci may be effective.

Isolated ectopic beats

These are common but may cause concern. Children and their families should be strongly reassured that no intervention or precaution is necessary.

Bradycardia and heart block

Congenital complete heart block may be well tolerated and need no treatment. Acquired heart block may be symptomatic with blackouts and a risk of asystole.

Syncope may be vagally triggered, as in reflex anoxic seizures (see Chapter 9), or associated with situations causing hypotension, such as prolonged standing in a warm environment or getting out of bed rapidly, particularly in adolescence. An accurate history will usually clarify the nature of the event. Unexplained syncope should be investigated with ECG. Findings may include abnormal P-R intervals, or sinus arrest, or complete heart block. Myocardial disease should be suspected; complete heart block may be a sequel to cardiac surgery. Recurrent symptomatic bradycardias may be treated by pacemaker implantation.

CONGENITAL HEART DISEASE

Incidence

This remains approximately 8 per 1000 live births (Table 5.3), although some of the more serious conditions may now be detected prenatally and termination offered after counselling.

Severe cyanotic heart disease

This should be picked up in early infancy and requires urgent evaluation and treatment. Early medical care may involve maintaining the patency of the ductus arteriosus by prostaglandin infusion pending definitive treatment.

Lesions causing early severe cyanosis

Transposition (TGA) is now commonly treated by an anatomical correction after initial investi-

Table 5.3 Common conditions presenting in early childhood

Ventricular septal defect	28%
Patent ductus arteriosus	12%
Atrial septal defect	10%
Coarctation	9%
Transposition of the great arteries (TGA)	8%
Fallot's tetralogy	7%
Pulmonary stenosis	6%
Aortic stenosis	4%
Others	16%

gation and stabilisation, commonly with a temporising balloon septostomy (Rashkind procedure). In this the distal great arteries are switched, together with the coronary arteries. Older children may have been treated by procedures which divert blood in the atria to the appropriate ventricles (Senning or Mustard repairs). These procedures continue to use the morphological right ventricle to sustain the systemic circulation, with an attendant risk of long-term problems, particularly arrhythmias.

Tricuspid or pulmonary atresia may be treated by palliative surgery to divert blood to the lungs (e.g. Blalock–Taussig shunt) pending longer-term palliation. The Fontan operation, whereby the right atrium or the vena cava is directly anastomosed to the pulmonary arteries, may be used. Depending on the size of the pulmonary arteries and the right ventricle, complete repair of pulmonary atresia may be possible. Less severe cyanotic disease usually results from defects causing common mixing of oxygenated and deoxygenated blood within or outside the heart. These children may not be recognised early and may present with failure to thrive and poor feeding. Clubbing of the fingers is a late clinical feature of cyanotic heart disease.

Fallot's tetralogy. This is the most common cyanotic condition. Here the cyanosis is progressive, with worsening infundibular pulmonary stenosis associated with a VSD. The other components of the tetralogy are right ventricular hypertrophy and aortic override of the VSD. The child may also show spells of worsening cyanosis and pallor from infundibular spasm. There is an obvious loud systolic murmur over the pulmonary area radiating to the lung fields and a prominent right ventricular impulse. Investigation by ECG, chest X-ray and echocardiography should confirm the diagnosis. Frequent spells may require treatment by beta blockade, pending complete surgical correction. Following surgery it is usual for there to be a residual systolic and early diastolic murmur, due to pulmonary outflow turbulence and regurgitation.

Other cardiac problems which may be associated with moderate cyanosis include *total anomalous pulmonary venous drainage, persistent truncus arteriosus, double outlet right ventricle,* and *Ebstein's anomaly.* A useful measure of the severity of continuing cyanosis is haemoglobin estimation as continued arterial desaturation causes a progressive rise in red cell production and a raised packed cell volume.

Pulmonary hypertension. Cyanosis is also a late feature of pulmonary hypertension and occurs as a consequence of longstanding high pulmonary blood flow, e.g. in an uncorrected large VSD or A/V septal defect in Down's syndrome. This situation is called *Eisenmenger's syndrome* and at this stage the lesion is inoperable and progressive. Complications of long-term cyanotic heart disease include intravascular thrombosis due to polycythaemia, and cerebral abscess.

Acyanotic heart disease

Ventricular septal defect

This is the most common congenital heart problem, its presentation and prognosis depending on the size and haemodynamic effect of the lesion. The large majority tend to get smaller or close with time.

Clinical features. The presentation may be delayed until after the first few days of life, when the fall in pulmonary vascular resistance allows an increasing flow from left to right across the defect. The usual presentation is with a cardiac murmur, typically harsh, pansystolic and loudest at the left sternal edge. A thrill may be palpable and an early diastolic flow murmur may be heard in VSDs with a large left to right flow. If the defect is in the muscular part of the septum the systolic murmur may be short and stop before the second sound. A delayed and loud second sound may indicate developing pulmonary hypertension. Patients with small lesions typically have normal chest X-ray and ECG findings.

Lesions with a large left to right shunt may present with the onset of cardiac failure in the first weeks of life. Symptoms include breathlessness, poor feeding, restlessness and excessive sweating (the *sweaty, surly* and *scrawny* infant). A key feature in the history is the duration of feeds—the baby will pause frequently and typically take over 30 minutes to feed.

Examination will show a tachycardia with a hyperdynamic precordium and an enlarged liver.

Investigation. Chest X-ray shows an enlarged heart with plethoric lung fields, and ECG may show left ventricular or biventricular hypertrophy. Echocardiography with Doppler studies is helpful in determining the size, position and the blood flow across the defect. Smaller lesions with high pressure gradients between the ventricles show a high velocity flow (a restrictive defect). A large left to right shunt results in a rise in right ventricular pressures and low Doppler flow velocity.

Management. Small restrictive defects without symptoms can safely be followed up intermittently, with optimism that they may close. The child should be encouraged to lead an unrestricted life. Children presenting with heart failure may be treated medically, with diuretics and with captopril. Calorie intake may be increased with feed supplements. If there is any clinical or echocardiographic concern in respect of the development of pulmonary hypertension, investigation by cardiac catheter is indicated. Surgical closure is reserved for children developing pulmonary hypertension, or for children with heart failure refractory to medical treatment. Complete closure may not be achieved, particularly with multiple lesions, and a residual murmur is common. Recently, catheter implantable devices have been developed for the closure of some defects, and their use may become more widespread.

Patent ductus arteriosus

The ductus arteriosus normally closes as a response to physiological changes in the first 24 hours of life. In the pre-term or ill neonate this closure may be delayed and may complicate management. Indomethacin may close the duct but occasionally urgent surgical closure may be required. In a proportion of otherwise normal infants the duct may not close spontaneously.

Clinical features. A persistent patent ductus commonly presents with a murmur. Before the fall of pulmonary arterial pressure this may be a systolic ejection murmur, but as the pressure drops the classic systolic and diastolic machinery murmur may be heard in the pulmonary area. Peripheral pulses are prominent. Occasionally a large duct may present with heart failure.

Investigation. On chest X-ray the heart may be enlarged with plethoric lung fields, and the ECG may show left or biventricular hypertrophy. An echocardiogram is used to confirm the presence of the duct, and Doppler studies will show the flow and pressure gradient between the aorta and pulmonary arteries. In the small infant treatment is usually conservative, with medical treatment of heart failure if required, unless there is evidence of pulmonary hypertension. Catheter closure with coil or umbrella devices may be undertaken in a child of over 10 kg. Surgical closure is an option if closure is urgently required at any stage.

Atrial septal defect

Clinical features:

Ostium secundum defect is the most common. It is usually asymptomatic, presenting with a systolic ejection murmur in the pulmonary area. A key finding is wide fixed splitting of the second sound.

Chest X-ray may show cardiomegaly and increased pulmonary blood flow. ECG shows right bundle branch block pattern, and right axis deviation and mild right ventricular hypertrophy may be present. Echocardiography confirms the diagnosis; radionuclide studies may be used to quantify the flow across the lesion and confirm the need for closure. This is usually undertaken electively in childhood because of the long-term prospect of arrhythmias in adult life. It is normally performed at around 4 years of age, before entry to school. Catheter introduced clam-shell devices are becoming more widely used as an alternative to surgical closure, which remains a low risk option.

Ostium primum defects may be part of a complete atrioventricular defect or an isolated finding. They are a typical finding in Down's syndrome. The lesion may involve the mitral valve and thus may be associated with mitral incompetence. The clinical findings are as in secundum defects, but the ECG shows a superior QRS axis (predominantly positive voltages in AVR) with right bundle branch block. First degree AV block may be present. Echocardiography and Doppler studies confirm the diagnosis. The prognosis is for progression to pulmonary hypertension, and surgical correction is indicated in the second year of life or earlier if there are severe symptoms. Surgery may be complicated by complete heart block.

Complete atrioventricular septal defect is a problem typically associated with Down's syndrome. The lesion involves contiguous atrial and ventricular septal defects and is commonly associated with atrioventricular valve abnormalities with mitral regurgitation. This results in a large obligatory left to right shunt and inexorable progression to pulmonary hypertension. Presentation is with a pansystolic murmur heard in the first week of life, or with symptoms and signs of heart failure. The X-ray findings are of cardiomegaly with increased pulmonary blood flow. ECG findings are as in ostium primum ASD. Echocardiography confirms the defect. Surgical correction is required, and may be complicated by complete heart block.

Obstructive lesions

Coarctation

This occurs more frequently in males than females and is commonly found in Turner's syndrome. There are two main modes of presentation:

1. In the newborn, critical coarctation is commonly associated with other defects, either VSD or hypoplastic left heart. The onset of heart failure with tachypnoea, tachycardia, pallor and hepatomegaly is found, associated with reduced or absent femoral pulses. There may be a systolic murmur in the precordium, together with a gallop rhythm, and a murmur audible in the back. Blood pressure recorded in the legs is reduced by more than 20 mmHg compared with the arms. Chest X-ray shows cardiomegaly and pulmonary oedema. ECG shows right ven-

tricular hypertrophy and, in the presence of hypoplastic left heart, reduced left ventricular voltages in the lateral chest leads. The diagnosis may be confirmed by Doppler echocardiogram. Treatment is urgent, with diuretics, correction of metabolic acidosis, and maintenance of the patency of the ductus arteriosus by prostaglandin infusion. Urgent surgical treatment is indicated where possible. Follow-up is required to monitor for re-coarctation and residual hypertension.

2. Asymptomatic coarctation may be picked up incidentally with reduced femoral pulses at routine examination, with hypertension or with a murmur. This may be a systolic murmur at the apex and aortic area from the bicuspid aortic valve, which is a frequent concomitant abnormality, and a systolic murmur audible over the central back. Blood pressure recorded in the arms and legs shows a reduction in the legs. Chest X-ray in the older child may show rib notching from dilatation of the intercostal arteries, dilatation of the descending aorta, or may be normal. ECG may show left ventricular hypertrophy in the presence of hypertension. Doppler examination shows accelerated flow in the descending aorta. MRI scan may be used to confirm the anatomy of the lesion. Balloon dilatation of a discrete coarctation may be successful, but surgical treatment is usually indicated. Hypertension may persist postoperatively and require treatment, and re-coarctation may occur.

Pulmonary stenosis

Severe pulmonary stenosis may present with cyanosis in the newborn period, otherwise presentation is usually with a murmur. This is an ejection systolic murmur, heard over the pulmonary area and radiating into the lung fields. If the stenosis is at the valve, an ejection click may be heard. Chest X-ray may be normal or show a post-stenotic dilatation of the pulmonary arteries. In severe stenosis the heart may be large with reduced pulmonary vascularity. Doppler echocardiography shows a gradient which may be infundibular, valvar, post-valvar or peripheral. Mild stenosis may be monitored and remain unchanged or regress. Progressive or severe stenosis may require treatment, usually with balloon dilatation in the first instance. Occasionally surgical treatment by valvotomy or valve replacement may be required.

Aortic stenosis

Severe stenosis may present with heart failure in the first weeks of life, as in coarctation. Otherwise the child is usually asymptomatic and presents with a murmur. This is an ejection systolic murmur heard at the cardiac apex and the aortic area, radiating into the neck; it may be associated with a precordial, suprasternal or carotid thrill. If the stenosis is valvar, there may be an ejection click. Chest X-ray is usually normal; the ECG may be normal or show left ventricular hypertrophy (Figure 5.5). Doppler echocardiography confirms a gradient which may be at subvalvar,

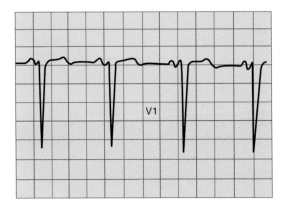

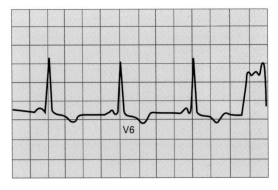

Figure 5.5 ECG showing left ventricular hypertrophy due to aortic stenosis.

valvar, or (particularly in Williams' syndrome) supravalvar levels. Aortic stenosis, if severe, may lead to symptoms of syncope, chest pain and sudden death on exertion. If severe stenosis is suspected, cardiac catheterisation is usually required to confirm the gradient, and surgical valvotomy or valve replacement may be required. Balloon dilatation is less often successful than in pulmonary stenosis.

Bicuspid aortic valve

This is a frequent anatomic variation of the valve with an incidence of up to 2% of the population. It may be associated with coarctation. It presents with a systolic ejection murmur at the apex and in the aortic area. There may be an ejection click. In the child there are no symptoms and investigation is normal apart from confirmation of the anatomy and possibly mild stenosis on echocardiography. In adult years the valve may calcify and become stenotic. Antibiotic subacute bacterial endocarditis prophylaxis is indicated (see below).

Hypoplastic left heart syndrome

This presents in the newborn period with heart failure, or may be detected antenatally. The left ventricle is underdeveloped in association with other defects and cannot sustain the systemic circulation. The condition was formerly universally fatal, but heroic surgical approaches may now be offered (Norwalk operation or heart transplant) after discussion with parents.

Antibiotic prophylaxis against subacute bacterial endocarditis

Children with a structural abnormality of the heart run a continuing but very small risk of bacterial endocarditis (see below). Organisms which commonly cause this are commensal in the mouth (*Streptococcus viridans*) and the risk is increased when a bacteraemia is produced by oral or dental surgery. Other procedures with a significant risk are adenoidectomy and tonsillectomy, genito-urinary surgery or instrumentation, and gastrointestinal surgery. Such procedures should be covered by prophylactic administration of antibiotics (Figure 5.6).

Children with simple secundum ASD, spontaneously closed VSD or closed PDA do not require antibiotic prophylaxis.

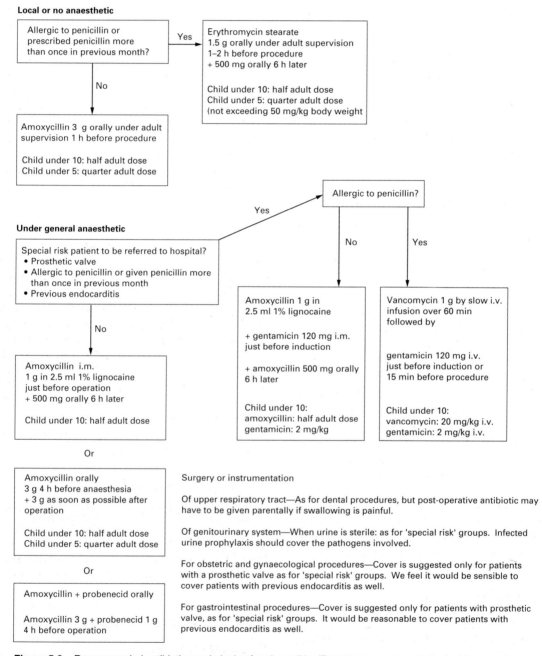

Figure 5.6 Recommended antibiotic prophylaxis of endocarditis. (Based on recommendations of the Endocarditis Working Party, BSAC, Lancet 1990: 335; 88–89, with permission.)

Congenital heart disease and exercise

Children with heart problems should usually be allowed to exercise without external restraint; no harm will accrue, and children will be aware of their physiological limitations. Parents and carers should be encouraged to allow them to exercise to the limits of their capability. The exceptions to this rule are children with severe aortic stenosis, who should be discouraged from competitive or isometric exercise, and children with hypertrophic obstructive cardiomyopathy. Occasionally children with exercise induced arrhythmias may need restraint if the arrhythmias are not pharmacologically controlled.

Other anxieties and heart disease

The suggestion of heart problems in a child is a potent cause of anxiety for parents.

Possible symptoms

Fatigue is rarely a symptom in heart disease, and more commonly is associated with infections or is emotionally determined.

Chest pain should be evaluated but commonly arises from the chest wall, as in pleurodynia, or from the oesophagus. Cardiac pain is unlikely, except in severe aortic or pulmonary stenosis.

Peripheral cyanosis is a common symptom in childhood relating to environmental temperature and occasionally neglect (acrocyanosis). In the absence of central cyanosis, it is not likely to indicate a cardiac abnormality.

Isolated palpitations caused by ectopic beats are almost universal, and may be increased by anxiety or caffeine. Both child and parents should be strongly reassured as to their normality.

CARDIOMYOPATHY

Disease of the heart muscle is a result of a large number of inherited or acquired conditions. There are three main anatomical consequences of such disease, with differing presentations.

Dilated cardiomyopathy

This may result from viral myocarditis, auto-immune disease or anthracycline chemotherapy, or it may be a consequence of persistent tachy-arrhythmias. A proportion of cases are familial, but a specific cause is often not found. Children present with cardiac failure, failure to thrive, pallor, breathlessness and hepatomegaly. There is tachycardia with a thready pulse and quiet heart sounds and a gallop rhythm. Treatment is with diuretics, digoxin and ACE inhibitors such as captopril, under close supervision. The prognosis is poor in up to 50% of patients, and inexorable deterioration may result in death, or possibly heart transplantation. Approximately half of the survivors will recover completely, the remainder requiring continued medical support.

Hypertrophic cardiomyopathy

This may be a transient finding in infants of diabetic mothers, or may present with a family history of premature sudden death. There may be a history of exertional syncope or chest pain, or a systolic ejection murmur as a result of left ventricular outflow tract obstruction. Clinical findings include a jerky pulse and additional third and fourth heart sounds. Treatment is with beta blockers or long-term amiodarone. Surgery may be required. There is a risk of sudden premature death, particularly in those children with early presentation or exertional syncope. Up to 6% of sufferers die each year in childhood and severe exertion is contraindicated.

Restrictive cardiomyopathy

In this rare cardiomyopathy the ventricle fills poorly because of stiff ventricular walls but retains normal contractility. It results in congestive heart failure. Patients may benefit from treatment with diuretics and may require anticoagulants to prevent thrombosis.

INFECTIVE HEART DISEASE
Rheumatic fever

This condition declined in incidence after the

Box 5.5 Modified Jones criteria

Major criteria
- Carditis
- Polyarthritis
- Erythema marginatum
- Subcutaneous nodules
- Chorea

Minor criteria
- Fever
- Arthralgia
- Previous rheumatic fever
- Neutrophilia, raised CRP or ESR
- Prolonged P-R interval (1st degree heart block)

Second World War but may now be increasing. It follows a group A streptococcal throat infection, typically in the 5–15-year age group, and most commonly presents with painful migratory arthritis affecting large joints. The modified Jones diagnostic criteria (Box 5.5) remain the guide for diagnosis: the presence of two major criteria, or one major and two minor criteria, with supporting evidence of a preceding streptococcal infection, strongly supports the diagnosis. Evidence of infection may be obtained from a positive throat swab culture or a high or rising antibody titre (anti-DNAase B titre or ASOT).

Clinical features

Rheumatic carditis occurs in about 50% of children with rheumatic fever. It presents with an inappropriate tachycardia and a murmur, usually the pansystolic apical murmur of mitral incompetence or an aortic regurgitant diastolic murmur at the left sternal edge. It may progress to congestive cardiac failure or pericarditis, with chest pain and a pericardial rub.

Investigations

Chest X-ray may reveal cardiomegaly, and ECG may show a prolonged P-R interval. Echocardiography may demonstrate cardiomegaly and impaired ventricular function in severe carditis; Doppler studies show mitral incompetence and possibly aortic regurgitation. Carditis may last up to 6 months and carries the attendant risk of permanent valve damage.

Management

Rest is advised in patients with carditis; aspirin in anti-inflammatory doses (100 mg/kg/day) is specific treatment. The dose should be monitored by serum levels. In severe carditis, steroids (prednisolone 2 mg/kg/day) are indicated in the first instance. Heart failure should be treated with diuretics and complete bed rest. Aspirin is continued until there is evidence of resolution of acute inflammation, and then tapered. Penicillin is given in the first instance to clear any residual streptococcal infection, and then continued twice daily indefinitely in the presence of confirmed carditis to prevent further attacks. Children allergic to penicillin should have alternative prophylaxis (e.g. sulphadiazine). Affected children should remain under cardiological review and be advised about the need for prophylaxis against subacute bacterial endocarditis.

Treatment is similar in children without carditis, with penicillin and high dose aspirin until inflammation resolves. Penicillin prophylaxis may be discontinued after 5 years, as the risk of recurrence with carditis is much reduced.

Chorea may be treated with chlorpromazine, haloperidol or valproate. The signs may be subtle but can result in significant school difficulties and may be misinterpreted as a behavioural problem. Schools should be counselled appropriately.

Kawasaki's disease

Since its description and endemic occurrence in Japan, Kawasaki's disease has been recognised sporadically in all countries. It is postulated that it occurs as a consequence of immune mechanisms following an infection. It usually affects children in the first 4 years of life, but occasionally occurs in older children.

Clinical features (Box 5.6)

The acute phase may be complicated by sterile meningitis, arthritis or mononeuropathy. There may be gastrointestinal symptoms: diarrhoea, vomiting and hydrops of the gallbladder. The

---

Box 5.6 Clinical features of Kawasaki's disease

- Persistent high *fever* lasting more than 5 days
- *Sterile conjunctivitis*
- Generalised *macular rash*
- *Hands and feet* may be *swollen and red*
- *Reddening of the mouth and tongue* may be evident with *strawberry tongue*
- *Cervical lymph node enlargement* is typical
- The condition gradually resolves with *characteristic peeling of the skin of fingers and toes*

A combination of four of these symptoms is considered to be diagnostic.

---

cardiac complications include coronary artery aneurysms which may thrombose and cause sudden cardiac arrest. There may also be evidence of myocarditis during the acute phase of the disease.

Investigations

Features supporting the diagnosis include anaemia, a marked neutrophilia, raised acute phase reactants and a significant thrombocytosis. The liver function may be disturbed and triglyceride levels may be elevated. The ECG may show a prolonged P-R interval, reduced QRS complexes and S-T changes. An echocardiogram is mandatory and may show proximal coronary artery aneurysms.

Management

Treatment with intravenous high dose pooled gamma globulin in the early stages of the disease is thought to reduce the likelihood of cardiac complications. Otherwise anti-inflammatory doses of aspirin are used until the acute phase of the illness is over. If there is evidence of coronary aneurysm, low dose aspirin is used to prevent thrombosis and continued while evidence persists. Follow-up echocardiograms are undertaken to document the progress of the cardiac lesions; a significant proportion resolve in the year or two following the acute illness. Persistent evidence of coronary artery disease may require coronary angiography and exercise ECG testing.

Myocarditis

This may present following a recognised viral infection or may appear without evident prior illness. Usually the myocardial damage is immune mediated. A wide variety of precipitating viruses have been implicated, although enteroviruses (Coxsackie and echoviruses) are most common. Presentation is typically with lethargy and breathlessness. Clinical findings include tachycardia, gallop rhythm, tachypnoea and hepatomegaly, and arrhythmia may be present. The chest X-ray reveals cardiomegaly, and ECG may show low voltage complexes, S-T segment changes and ectopic beats. Echocardiography demonstrates ventricular dilatation and reduced function. Further investigations include viral culture and antibody studies, and may involve radionuclide studies and myocardial biopsy. Treatment consists of appropriate anti cardiac failure drugs, including diuretics, and captopril. Immune suppression with azathioprine and steroids has been tried, without clear benefit. The majority of mildly affected children make a complete recovery, although those who are more severely affected may continue to have impaired myocardial function and arrhythmias.

Pericarditis

This may be caused by direct bacterial infection (e.g. *Staph. aureus*, *Haemophilus influenzae* or *Streptococcus pneumoniae*) or be a long-term consequence of tuberculous infection (restrictive endocarditis). Viral causes are similar to those of myocarditis. Pericarditis may be part of a multisystem disease such as juvenile rheumatoid arthritis or rheumatic fever.

Clinical features

Presentation is with chest pain that is central and may be worsened by movement and eased by sitting forward. There may be fever, breathlessness and lethargy in acute infection, or a history of a related infection or other systemic symptoms. Signs include raised jugular venous pressure and hepatomegaly, tachycardia and a friction rub audible in the precordium. Heart sounds may be muffled, and in acute effusion there may be pulsus paradoxus (pulse volume that lessens with inspiration).

Investigations

The chest X-ray shows cardiomegaly, and ECG may show low voltages and S-T segment changes. Echocardiography delineates the size and location of the effusion.

Management

Needle or surgical aspiration of the effusion is performed as a diagnostic measure and to drain the fluid to prevent tamponade. Treatment is then directed towards the primary disease. Restrictive pericarditis may require formal surgical pericardectomy.

Endocarditis

This usually occurs as a rare complication of structural heart disease, but may occur in a structurally normal heart in intravenous drug abusers or in the presence of indwelling intravenous long lines used for medical treatment, as in malignant disease, cystic fibrosis or thalassaemia major. Infection settles at the site of intracardiac turbulence and more usually at the site of a high pressure gradient as in VSD, PDA or AS. Children with indwelling foreign material in the heart, such as prosthetic valves or pacemakers, are also at risk. The infective organisms are usually streptococci such as *Strep. viridans* or *Strep. faecalis*. Other faecal organisms may be involved. *Staphylococcus aureus* may cause a particularly aggressive acute bacterial endocarditis. Organisms may enter the circulation at the time of surgery or instrumentation, particularly oral surgery that causes gingival trauma, or gut or genito-urinary surgery. In children with known heart abnormalities, prophylaxis at the time of such surgery is recommended (Figure 5.6). Frequently, however, there may be no history of such an event.

Clinical features

The presentation is usually with gradual onset of lethargy, weight loss, recurrent fevers, rigors and anorexia. Children with cyanotic heart disease or aortic valve disease may present with peripheral embolic abscesses, particularly cerebral abscesses. Examination shows fever, pallor and splenomegaly. Petechial haemorrhages may be evident anywhere on the skin or in the fundi. Subungual splinter haemorrhages may be seen, as may clubbing of the fingernails. Cardiac findings include a tachycardia and a changing heart murmur.

Investigations

Investigations should include multiple blood cultures before treatment. Urinalysis may show haematuria. A blood count shows normochromic anaemia, and neutrophil and acute phase reactants will be raised. Echocardiography may confirm the presence of vegetations at the site of the infection.

Management

Confirmation of the infection by positive blood culture will reveal the sensitivity pattern of the organism and guide antibiotic treatment. Usually this will be with penicillin and flucloxacillin together with an aminoglycoside (e.g. gentamicin) in the first instance, in high doses intravenously until the organism is known, and then continued for 4–6 weeks, usually with two agents, guided by the clinical progress of the patient and the return of the haematological findings to normal. It may be necessary to remove long lines, and surgical replacement of affected heart valves may be required. The echocardiogram appearance of vegetations may persist after treatment. The child should be monitored closely on stopping antibiotics for signs of a recurrence.

Endocarditis may cause further damage to the original heart lesion and a change in management may be required.

THE MANAGEMENT OF HEART FAILURE

It is useful to consider three categories of presentation:

- *high output failure*, as in children with a large left to right shunt, e.g. with a VSD
- *low output failure* (pump failure, e.g. in dilated cardiomyopathy)
- *right ventricular failure* (congestive cardiac failure, e.g. in severe pulmonary stenosis).

Management of acute heart failure

In acute heart failure from any cause, treatment measures include sitting the patient upright and administering oxygen; a short acting diuretic may be given. Distress may be reduced by giving morphine sulphate (0.01 mg/kg, i.m. or s.c.). The child should be admitted to hospital.

High output failure. Symptoms of high output failure include tachypnoea, dyspnoea, poor feeding and poor weight gain. Treatment is with diuretics. In refractory failure, an angiotensin converting enzyme (ACE) inhibitor such as captopril may be added. This is usually undertaken in hospital. If such treatment is unsuccessful, surgery to correct or palliate the defect may be indicated.

In **low output failure** the heart may be supported by intravenous inotropic agents or with digoxin. Diuretics should be used with caution.

In **right heart failure** diuretics are used and captopril may be added.

HYPERTENSION

Recording of blood pressure should be part of the pre-school medical examination, where these are performed, or if the child presents with significant systemic illness, and particularly in the event of suspected kidney disease or urinary infection. Blood pressure rises with age; in childhood it is most closely related to height (Fig. 5.7). Readings should be taken with the child as relaxed as possible. If the manual method is used a direct reading mercury sphygmomanometer is desirable; aneroid devices may be inaccurate.

Otherwise an oscillometric device (Dinamap) is helpful, particularly in smaller children. The cuff used should be the largest that fits comfortably round the upper arm. Diastolic readings should be taken at the point of muffling and of disappearance of the Korotkoff sound; if these are close together the point of disappearance should be used. Occasionally the sounds do not disappear completely, and the point of muffling is then taken. If hypertension is suspected on an initial reading it is advisable to take several readings, discard the highest and lowest, and average the remaining figures. Blood pressure tends to follow the same centile with age, and is influenced by family history and obesity. Hypertension (blood pressure exceeding the 95th centile for height) should be investigated. Coarctation and renal disease are the most common causes of secondary hypertension. Occasionally other conditions such as neuroblastoma, neurofibromatosis or hyperaldosteronism may present with raised blood pressure.

Minimum investigation should include the examination of femoral pulses and leg blood pressure to exclude coarctation, and urinalysis, urine culture, blood electrolytes and creatinine, renal ultrasound and some other renal imaging such as DMSA scanning for renal scarring.

Treatment

Suspected hypertension should be monitored prospectively. Advice on weight control and exercise may be helpful. In acute hypertensive emergencies infused labetalol is the drug of choice, although diazoxide, hydralazine or sublingual nifedipine may be used. In longer term control, beta blockers (propranolol or atenolol) may be used as first line treatment, although with caution in asthmatic patients. ACE inhibitors such as captopril may be added, with particular caution in renal impairment. Creatinine levels should be monitored. Further drugs occasionally used in refractory hypertension include thiazide diuretics, methyldopa and nifedipine. The hypertensive child should be monitored through puberty and into adult life and particularly advised about the additional risk of other

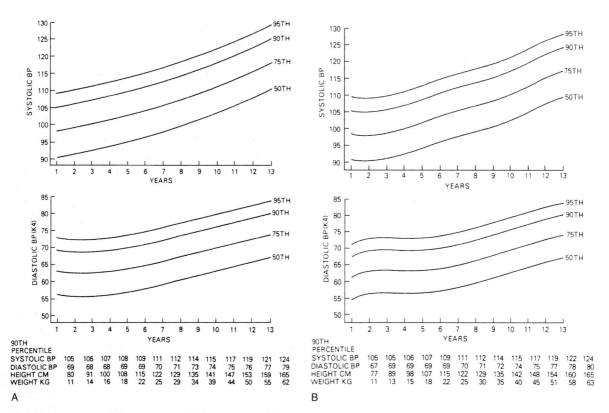

Figure 5.7 Age specific percentiles of BP measurements. A. in boys aged 1–13 years. B. in girls aged 1–13 years. Reproduced with permission from the American Academy of Pediatrics.

lifestyle factors such as smoking, obesity and excessive alcohol intake.

CARDIAC ARREST

Unexpected cardiac arrest occurring outside hospital in childhood is rare. Extreme trauma, smoke inhalation and drowning are the most usual causes in older children. Infants with apparent cot death are another important group. At the scene a rapid evaluation of any compounding problem such as neck injury, electrical contact, foreign body in the airway or evidence of medical problems (e.g. Medicalert bracelet) should be undertaken and acted upon if appropriate. Without advanced equipment, resuscitation with attention to the airway, artificial ventilation by mouth to mouth ventilation, and external cardiac massage may be initiated whilst help is summoned (Airway, Breathing and Circulation). A

wide awareness of resuscitation techniques in parents should be encouraged and has been advocated as part of school and antenatal education. Immediate resuscitation upon confirmation of cardiorespiratory arrest offers the best chance of a successful outcome. Paramedically trained emergency aid may be summoned, or the child transported urgently to hospital while resuscitative efforts continue, unless the child is clearly unresuscitatable.

Advanced resuscitation may be started after evaluation of the pulse and breathing effort. Once the airway is secured in the first instance, bag and mask ventilation may be offered in the short term, but endotracheal intubation should be undertaken as soon as is practicable. A breathing rate of 40–60 breaths per minute should be sustained. Cardiac rhythm should be evaluated by ECG monitor. In the event of asystole, adrenaline should be given by intracardiac injection

(0.1 ml/kg 1:10 000 solution) or via the endotracheal tube (0.1 ml/kg 1:1000 solution). Ventricular fibrillation should be treated by DC shock (2–4 Joules per kg). Atrioventricular dissociation should be treated with adrenaline or atropine. Cardiac output should be monitored by palpation of a large artery—the carotid or femoral. Vascular access through a large vein or with intraosseous needle should be established as rapidly as possible to allow infusion of sodium bicarbonate (1 ml/kg 8.4% solution) if the child is not responding rapidly, followed by colloid or crystalloid infusion to sustain the circulation once it has been established. If resuscitation is successful, the child should be transferred to an intensive care area for further support and evaluation.

Resuscitation should be terminated when the outcome is clearly hopeless—no effective circulation established within 25 minutes, and fixed dilated pupils. Agreement should be sought from all attendants that resuscitation should be withdrawn. Accurate records of circumstances, observations and procedures should be made.

Advanced life support training should be part of medical postgraduate training for all doctors in clinical practice.

SUDDEN INFANT DEATH SYNDROME (SIDS, COT DEATH)

The cardinal findings are that a previously apparently well child, usually between 4 weeks and a year of age, often with a preceding history of a mild viral illness, has been put down to sleep and found dead without warning. Post mortem examination reveals no abnormal findings other than perhaps a few pericardial and thymic petechiae. Epidemiological predisposing factors include social disadvantage, a family with a large number of young children, low birth weight, infant of a multiple birth, male sex, young maternal age and parental smoking (both during pregnancy and afterwards). More recently, sleeping position and overheating of the infant have been emphasised as factors; the campaign to advise a supine lying position and to avoid overwrapping

the infant appears to have had a real and lasting effect on the incidence of cot death in the United Kingdom, with a drop from 2 per 1000 live births in the 1980s to around 0.6 per 1000 in the mid 1990s. A wide variety of causal mechanisms have been suggested, with disease processes and environmental agents being blamed. It is likely that the syndrome is an endpoint of a number of coincident factors. A few rare diseases have been identified that may contribute: cardiac arrhythmia due to the prolonged Q-T syndrome (which may be associated with a history of sudden death in other members of the family), and the congenital metabolic defect LCAD (long chain acyl-CoA dehydrogenase) deficiency.

Management of a cot death

An infant found dead in the home or the community may be declared dead at the scene. If there were no preceding evident causes, a presumption of cot death may be made and discussed with the parents. However a coroner's inquest (in England, or investigation by the procurator fiscal in Scotland) is always held. These officials should be informed at the earliest opportunity and the parents warned that there will need to be an enquiry by the police into the circumstances, that this is routine, and that no blame attaches to them in this process. The body may be released to a mortuary, but a post mortem examination will be required. The registration of the death will follow the decision of the coroner as to the cause of death. Following this the funeral of the child may proceed.

In some cases the child may not be observably dead in the initial circumstances, and resuscitation may be attempted. The child will be transferred urgently to hospital where the emergency paediatric team should be alerted of the impending arrival. Paediatric departments and accident and emergency departments should have protocols for the management of this situation, with appropriate support and advice to parents.

The loss of a child through cot death causes immense distress to families, and entails prolonged, profound problems of adjustment. Support may be offered to the family by keeping in touch with them on a regular basis. In the first instance a discussion of cot death and its implications and of the post mortem report should be offered. This may be undertaken by a paediatrician or GP. Contact with the local parents' group of the Foundation for the Study of Infant Death should be made. This organisation offers lay support from other parents who have suffered the same loss (often the most valuable direct support available) and provides literature and a continued outlet for their grief. Professional support should be offered on a continuing basis, and it is to be expected that the bereavement will result in continued questioning and the accompanying reactions of anger and longer term depression. Other bereavement support agencies may be able to offer help.

Subsequent infants in the family will be the subject of intense anxiety. Counselling should be offered again on the risk of recurrence and the management and supervision of the newborn infant. A widely used protocol—the CONI programme (care of the next infant)—is a useful model in which a package of support to the parents is agreed antenatally. This consists of close monitoring of the child's symptoms through a parent held symptom diary, together with regular visits from a health professional, usually a health visitor. Easy access to medical advice should be encouraged through the primary care team and paediatrician. The family may be offered scales to weigh the baby frequently and/or an apnoea monitor in the home (with warning about their attendant technical limitations). Resuscitation advice is also offered. Support should continue through the age of the preceding child's death and until anxieties have abated. Families vary considerably in their need for support and reassurance, which may appear irrationally profound on occasion.

APPARENT LIFE THREATENING EVENT (ALTE)

In these episodes a child, usually an infant, may appear to the carer to have had a sudden change in breathing which may be associated with a change of colour or state of consciousness and which causes the carer to experience significant concern for the life of the child. The initial response to such events should be immediate, both in regard to attention to the child's welfare and to the anxieties of the carer. Often the child will be admitted to hospital through involvement of the emergency services. If the well-being of the child is secured the evaluation of the episode will depend heavily on the *history* of the event and will be coloured by the circumstances and the experience of the observer. Particular attention should be paid to the timing of the event, the position and posture of the infant, the pattern of attempted breathing (if any), the relationship to a feed, the presence of vomit or mucus in the airway, the tone and colour of the infant, and the intervention needed before the child resumed normal breathing. If the doctor is involved in the resuscitation of the infant, some of these details may be apparent at the time.

The child should usually be admitted to hospital for observation of any further events, to reduce the family's inevitable anxiety and to allow appropriate monitoring and investigation. Common causes are listed in Box 5.7.

Once admitted to hospital, the child should be examined for evidence of intercurrent illness and for underlying abnormality. It is usual to undertake cardiorespiratory monitoring for 24–48 hours; if the reason for the episode is not evident, a number of baseline investigations should be undertaken, including chest X-ray, ECG (and possibly a 24-hour ECG tape), urine

---

Box 5.7 Causes of apparent life threatening events

- Observation of a normal sleep variation (e.g. a pause in REM sleep)
- Gastro-oesophageal reflux
- Choking episode with mucus or feed
- Breath-holding attack
- Convulsion (febrile or otherwise)
- Cardiac arrhythmia
- 'Near miss' cot death
- Apnoea as part of a respiratory illness (e.g. bronchiolitis)
- (Occasional) imposed airway obstruction— suffocation

culture, blood count, electrolytes and blood glucose. If a convulsion is considered possible, an EEG may be requested together with oeso-phageal pH monitoring if reflux is likely. Apart from treating any evident cause (e.g. reflux with feed thickeners), there remains the need to advise and reassure the parents—by explanation, by offering to teach cardiopulmonary resuscitation techniques and, in some cases, the offer of a home breathing monitor, although this latter is usually of no benefit other than as an adjunct to reassurance, and may cause more anxiety than it allays, through false alarms and technical problems. Once it is established that the child is stable, it is possible to return to the home environment. It is likely however that there will be a need for an increased level of support for a time, and hospital follow-up. The role of the health visitor in these circumstances is particularly valuable.

RESPIRATORY DISEASE

RESPIRATORY INFECTION

Bronchiolitis

In 80% of children with clinical bronchiolitis there is evidence of infection with the respiratory syncytial virus (RSV), an RNA virus. It typically occurs in winter epidemics and usually occurs in the first year of life. Up to 2% of affected infants require hospitalisation. It presents with a history of 2–3 days of coryza and mild fever, often in a household where older members of the family have symptoms of a cold.

Clinical features

The child develops a cough and rapidly progressive breathlessness and feeding difficulty. Severely affected children may become cyanosed and occasionally present with apnoea. They may also have diarrhoea. Clinically, the child has a mild fever, tachypnoea and a congested cough. The chest is hyperexpanded and there may be subcostal recession and nasal flaring. Coarse crackles and a wheeze may be heard on auscultation, and the liver edge may be prominent because of the descent of the liver with the diaphragm. Mildly affected infants may be nursed at home but hospital admission should be considered if the child is feeding poorly, cyanosed or apparently exhausted.

Investigation

Confirmation of the presence of RSV may not be required, particularly in an epidemic. Immunofluorescent techniques are available which give a rapid result on nasopharyngeal secretions. Other investigations include a chest X-ray, which may show increased expansion of the lung fields, with a flattened diaphragm and sometimes segmental lung collapse. Blood electrolytes should be checked as there is a risk of hyponatraemia due to water overload and inappropriate antidiuretic hormone (ADH) secretion. Oxygen saturation should be monitored by pulse oximetry,

where available. Blood gases are checked when there is concern that the child is developing respiratory failure.

Management

In most children management is supportive, pending the resolution of the illness after 4–5 days. Sitting the child up may lessen the work of breathing. Oxygen should be given if the child is measurably desaturated or cyanosed. Feeding should be via nasogastric tube or with intravenous fluids when the child is struggling with feeds. Fluids are moderately restricted (80–100 ml/kg/day) to avoid the risk of water overload. There is no good evidence that steam tents, physiotherapy, bronchodilators or antibiotics have any effect on the course of the disease. Antibiotics may be given if there is evidence of secondary bacterial infection. Mechanical ventilation may be required in the child with respiratory failure; it is difficult because of the hyperinflated lungs—a result of air trapping.

Ribavarin, an antiviral agent, has a virostatic effect on RSV. There is evidence that it shortens the course of the disease in severely affected infants. It is administered by an aerosol generator into a head box or ventilator circuit over extended periods. The drug is expensive and is commonly reserved for the most ill children or those with pre-existing cardiorespiratory conditions which may additionally compromise the child, such as severe congenital heart disease or bronchopulmonary dysplasia.

As the child recovers, oxygen dependency lessens and feeding improves. Hospital discharge is possible when the parents are confident that the child is coping with feeds, however they should be warned that the child will continue to cough for many days after the acute illness. The infection causes prolonged airway lability, and the child may wheeze and cough with succeeding upper respiratory infections for many months.

Croup

Croup is a result of a viral laryngotracheobronchitis. It occurs in children largely under

GP Overview 5.1 Cough

ACUTE
Common causes
Upper respiratory tract
- Coryza
- Pharyngitis/tonsillitis
- Sinusitis/laryngitis/otitis media
- Measles/pertussis
- Foreign body

Lower respiratory tract
- Tracheobronchitis
- Bronchiolitis
- Asthma
- Pneumonia
- Foreign body

CHRONIC
Respiratory
- Post-nasal drip, with or without adenoidal hypertrophy—common
- Allergy, asthma, bronchitis—common
- Cystic fibrosis
- Bronchiectasis
- TB, HIV, CMV
- Foreign body

Cardiac
- Heart disease
- Heart failure

Gastrointestinal
- Hiatus hernia
- Achalasia

Congenital anomalies
- Laryngeal stenosis, cysts
- Sequestrated lobe
- Bronchogenic cyst
- Tracheo-oesophageal fistula
- Vascular ring

Features in history
- Is the cough dry or productive?
- Is the sputum mucoid, purulent or blood stained?
- Character of cough
- Possible triggers, e.g. exercise, cold, emotion or allergy, ?nocturnal
- Consider smoking
- Consider psychological state
- Any associated symptoms, e.g. failure to thrive, diarrhoea

Investigations
- FBC/immunoglobulins/possibly allergy testing
- Sputum culture mc+s (consider TB cultures)
- Chest X-ray
- Lung function tests
- Consider bronchoscopy, laryngoscopy and upper GI endoscopy

the age of two years and is epidemic in winter. The most common agent is parainfluenza virus.

Clinical features

The affected child develops symptoms of a cold with a slight fever, then a cough which rapidly becomes harsh and barking. The voice becomes hoarse. The child develops an inspiratory stridor and may become distressed and dyspnoeic, with rapid breathing, a tracheal tug and subcostal recession. A severely affected child prefers to sit up, leaning forward, and may become cyanosed. Otherwise the child appears well, with good peripheral perfusion and an appropriate tachycardia. Throat inspection is not advised. A mildly affected child may be nursed at home, with instruction to the parents to contact the doctor if the child becomes more distressed. Humidification of the environment with steam is commonly recommended. There is no evidence that this is beneficial, except as a placebo.

Management

If there is evidence that the child is very distressed or tired, or if there is a suggestion of cyanosis, the child should be referred for hospital observation and treatment. The treatment of choice for the moderately severely affected child is nebulised budesonide or oral dexamethasone. These drugs have been shown to accelerate recovery, which normally takes less than 24 hours. Treatment may be given in an accident and emergency department, provided there are facilities to monitor the child thereafter. During admission the child should be closely monitored and adequate fluid intake ensured. In a severely ill child, nebulised adrenaline may give short-term benefit but a cyanosed child with croup should be considered for endotracheal intubation in order to protect the airway. Administration of oxygen may mask worsening respiratory failure. Intubation should be undertaken by an experienced anaesthetist in controlled conditions in an operating theatre. There is little place for tracheotomy except in extreme circumstances. The intubated child should be nursed in an intensive care area, by staff experienced in the care of the paediatric airway. The child may be managed sedated, with appropriate analgesia, or may require short-term ventilation. Steroids (dexamethasone) are usually given to accelerate recovery. It is usually possible to extubate the child in 24–48 hours. The child may go home when there are no longer signs of respiratory distress, as the stridor resolves. Parents should be warned of a possible worsening of symptoms, and readmission offered. A small proportion of children, usually those who are atopic, have a tendency to recurrent croup.

Occasionally croup arises with acute laryngeal oedema caused by trauma to the vocal cords, prolonged overuse of the voice, or chemical or smoke inhalation.

Epiglottitis

Epiglottitis results from an acute infection of the epiglottis and surrounding tissues with *Haemophilus influenzae* type B. It usually affects children up to five years of age, but may affect any age. It occurs sporadically with no seasonal pattern. It was a relatively rare condition and, since the adoption of Hib immunisation, has become extremely rare, occurring only in the non-immunised or the exceptional immunisation failure (e.g. the immune compromised child).

Clinical features

Epiglottitis may arise without pre-existing symptoms, though it is commonly associated with a viral illness. The child develops a high fever and an intensely sore throat, and may have difficulty swallowing. A low pitched gurgling stridor develops. The child may be inhibited from coughing by pain, may prefer to sit up, leaning forward, and may become lethargic and drowsy. Examination reveals an ill, toxic child with a high fever, stridor and a tachycardia. Peripheral perfusion may be poor, and the child is cyanosed and drooling saliva because of swallowing difficulties.

Management

If suspected, the condition should be treated as a medical emergency. Throat inspection is abso-

lutely contraindicated until the child is in a controlled environment in hospital, because of the risk of acute airway obstruction and cardiac arrest. Receiving hospitals should have a protocol whereby a senior paediatrician, an experienced anaesthetist and an ENT surgeon are called to receive the child on admission. If the diagnosis is still suspected, the child is taken to an operating theatre and the airway is examined under anaesthetic. The cardinal finding is an intensely inflamed, oedematous epiglottis (the cherry-red epiglottis) with a narrowed airway. If the diagnosis is confirmed, endotracheal intubation is undertaken, bacteriological cultures taken and an antibiotic to which *Haemophilus* is sensitive (e.g. cefotaxime) given intravenously. The child is nursed in an intensive care area and is usually extubated after 48 hours when the clinical condition has improved and the temperature settled. Extubation should only be undertaken in controlled circumstances that will allow reintubation if required.

Rarely, acute infective stridor may be caused by staphylococcal tracheitis, which may mimic epiglottitis.

Pertussis

Whooping cough (pertussis) is a highly infectious illness usually caused by *Bordetella pertussis*, a Gram-negative rod bacterium. Immunity is not transmitted from the mother to the newborn infant, and therefore very young infants are vulnerable. It has an incubation period of 6–20 days (mean 7).

Clinical features

Pertussis presents with symptoms of coryza, slight fever and a trivial cough for up to two weeks. Coughing spells develop and become forceful and paroxysmal. Typical coughing spasms consist of a prolonged volley of coughs, without intake of breath. The child becomes red, then blue, finally drawing breath with a gasp through a narrowed glottis, causing a crowing whoop. The whoop may not be evident in infants under 8 months of age. Coughing spasms frequently cause vomiting and may result in syncope. They can be triggered by mild stimuli such as exertion, cold air or drinking. If suspected, the diagnosis may be confirmed by the isolation of the organism, from a pernasal swab, or getting the child to cough onto a plated out Petri dish with specific (Bordet–Gengou) medium. The peripheral blood count may show an absolute lymphocytosis ($> 12 \times 10^9$/l).

In infants the coughing spasms and vomiting result in failure to thrive. The spasms are exhausting at any age, continuing through the night and waking the child and family. They may continue for up to four months, justifying the Chinese description 'One hundred days cough', and may recur with further colds. Apart from nutritional problems and the family disruption caused by the illness, complications include secondary pneumonia, otitis media, and rarely cerebral haemorrhage, convulsions and hernias. There is a significant mortality rate, particularly in infants.

Management

Once the disease is established there is no specific effective treatment. Antibiotics (macrolides) hasten the clearance of the organism from the respiratory tract, thus reducing the infectious period which otherwise lasts up to a month. Erythromycin in the prodromal phase may limit the duration of the illness and may be used in unimmunised contacts of an index case, particularly young infants, if they develop symptoms. Young children need hospitalisation when exhausted or failing to thrive. Treatment consists of nutritional support, with intravenous fluids, minimal disturbance, antibiotics for secondary infections and, occasionally, mechanical ventilation.

The illness may occur in apparently fully immunised children as a result of immunisation failure, or from infection with *Bordetella parapertussis* which may cause a very similar illness.

Pneumonia

Infection of the lung parenchyma can be caused by a large number of agents in childhood: bacterial, atypical bacterial, mycobacterial, viral and fungal. This section deals with those most commonly encountered.

Bacterial pneumonia

Lobar pneumonia, caused by the Gram-positive *Streptococcus pneumoniae*, is a relatively common illness that usually follows a viral upper respiratory tract infection.

Clinical features. After a mild prodromal illness, the child develops a high ($> 39°C$) swinging fever and, typically, rigors. Delirium is common. Older children may complain of chest pain and breathing is rapid and shallow. There may be an expiratory grunt and at the start of the illness there may a slight dry cough only, which becomes more obvious later. Basal pneumonia may present with abdominal pain, mimicking an acute abdominal problem. Upper lobe pneumonia may cause meningism, and mimic meningitis. In the infant presentation may be as a non-specific high fever with anorexia and diarrhoea, mimicking dysentery.

On examination the child is feverish and toxic with tachycardia, tachypnoea and sometimes cyanosis and drowsiness. Examination may reveal asymmetric chest wall movement, deviated trachea, localised dullness due to consolidated lung or an associated effusion and reduced air entry with bronchial breathing. Signs may be hard to elicit, however, and a chest X-ray should be part of the infection screen in any young child with an unexplained high fever. This usually shows a segment or lobe of lung which is consolidated (Figure 5.8). Blood investigations show a neutrophil leukocytosis and raised acute phase reactants (e.g. ESR, CRP, plasma viscosity). Blood culture should be performed if the diagnosis is suspected, and may grow *Strep. pneumoniae*.

Management. Treatment, in the uncomplicated case with typical findings, is with intravenous benzyl penicillin. In young infants, or where the diagnosis is uncertain, broad spectrum antibiotics are appropriate. Otherwise the child should be supported with intravenous fluids, oxygen and fever control. The fever usually resolves rapidly

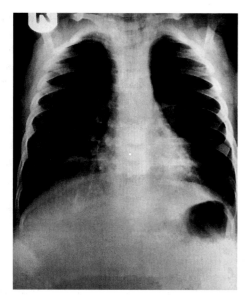

Figure 5.8 Chest X-ray showing right middle lobe pneumonia.

and the child may be treated with oral antibiotics after 48 hours, allowing discharge from hospital. Physiotherapy may help to clear the lungs in the recovery phase. Late diagnosis may result in an empyema. This may respond to prolonged antibiotic treatment, however a persistent empyema may require aspiration or formal surgical drainage. Follow-up with a repeat X-ray at 4–6 weeks to confirm complete clearing of the changes is usual, but not mandatory.

Other bacterial causes of pneumonia in childhood include *Haemophilus influenzae*, Klebsiella and group A streptococci, which tend to cause bronchopneumonia rather than lobar changes and should be treated with appropriate antibiotics. *Staphylococcus aureus* causes a particularly aggressive infection with severe systemic symptoms, lung abscess formation and empyemas, and has a high mortality. Prolonged treatment is required, and the infection causes long-term lung damage with pneumatoceles and bronchiectasis. It is a particular complication of cystic fibrosis.

Atypical pneumonia

Infection with *Mycoplasma pneumoniae* is a common cause of pneumonia in children of school age. The organism is a free living organism without a cell wall. The disease affects all ages and presents insidiously with a progressive cough and dyspnoea, following a prodromal illness of fever, headache and sore throat. The child is usually not toxic, but has widespread crepitations audible in the lung fields.

An X-ray reveals widespread patches of pulmonary infiltration and consolidation, and may show hilar lymphadenopathy. Blood investigations show a neutrophil leukocytosis and moderately raised acute phase reactants. Cold haemagglutinins occur in about 60% of patients. Serological confirmation may be obtained with IgM antibodies in the acute illness, or retrospectively with rising titres of specific IgG. Treatment with erythromycin or other macrolide antibiotic is usually offered, although proof of benefit is not certain. Complications include post infectious arthritis, haemolytic anaemia, erythema multiforme and meningoencephalitis.

Viral pneumonia

This may complicate many viral infections, including adenovirus, influenza virus, varicella and measles. Typically a child with a prodromal upper respiratory tract infection (URTI) will develop a progressive cough and breathlessness. Symptoms vary in severity, there may be audible crepitations and wheeze evident in the lung fields. X-ray may show patchy infiltrates or diffuse fine increased markings. Treatment is supportive with oxygen and nasogastric or intravenous fluids as required. Recovery is usual but is occasionally complicated by prolonged wheeze.

Chlamydial pneumonia

This is a cause of persistent cough and respiratory distress in newborn and pre-term infants. It is acquired from the maternal genital tract. Treatment with macrolide antibiotics is recommended.

Pneumonia in the immune compromised child

These infections are increasingly prevalent with the advent of HIV infection and treatment of malignant and other diseases with immune sup-pressant drugs. The causative organisms tend to be opportunistic agents with otherwise low pathogenicity. *Pneumocystis carinii* is a protozoal organism which causes a progressive tachypnoea and cough, superseded by cyanosis. Systemic symptoms are mild. Fine crepitations may be audible over the lung fields and X-ray shows diffuse generalised infiltration of the lung fields. In a child with known immune problems it may be suspected and treated prospectively with cotrimoxazole, but if firm diagnosis is required the organism must be recovered by broncho-scopic alveolar lavage, open lung biopsy or needle biopsy. It is usual to treat children on prolonged immunosuppressive therapy for leukaemia with prophylactic cotrimoxazole.

Cytomegalovirus may be congenitally acquired or arise in the immunodeficient or immuno-suppressed. Other organisms which may cause pneumonia include Pseudomonas, Aspergillus, and candida. Giant cell pneumonia is particularly associated with the measles virus.

Tuberculosis (TB)

TB is an uncommon illness in the developed world because of widespread BCG inoculation and improvement in living standards, but it remains endemic in developing countries. With the increase in travel and the spread of HIV infection it has increased again everywhere. The organism, *Mycobacterium tuberculosis*, is spread by droplet infection. In the previously non-immune child it causes an initial focal infection in the peripheral lung with a local hilar lymphadeno-pathy (the primary complex).

Clinical features

Systemic symptoms may be minimal; in the fit child the lesion may heal, leaving calcified scarring that may be evident on a chest X-ray as the Ghon focus. Sensitisation to protein in the bacterial cell wall occurs and forms the basis for the tuberculin test. At the time of sensitisation, other symptoms such as erythema nodosum or phlyctenular conjunctivitis may occur.

Dissemination of the disease is in part related to host factors such as nutritional state and social environment as well as immune status. Media-stinal lymph node enlargement may compress the bronchi causing distal lung collapse, particu-larly of the middle lobe. The initial infection may spill into the lungs, causing a tubercular bronchopneumonia, or spread haematogenously, causing miliary TB, meningitis or other distal infections of the kidneys or bones, particularly the spine, with vertebral collapse causing an acute angular kyphosis (Pott's spine).

The classic illness of late adolescence or young adulthood results from reactivation of the initial focus, with progressive lung destruction and systemic symptoms, productive cough and haematemesis.

Symptoms in young children with progressive disease consist of malaise, intermittent fever, weight loss, and possibly symptoms of cough and haematemesis. TB should be suspected parti-cularly when there is a history of family contact or travel to an area or community where the disease is endemic.

Diagnosis

The diagnosis may be suspected from typical X-ray findings. Blood investigations may show a normochromic anaemia and raised acute phase reactants. Indirect investigation by tuberculin test can support the diagnosis. In the Mantoux test, 0.1 ml of 1:1000 solution is injected intra-dermally in the forearm. If the disease is strongly suspected, 1:10 000 solution may be used initially to avoid an extremely florid response. The test is read at 48–72 hours: induration with erythema greater than 10 mm in diameter is diagnostic of present or previous infection; 5–10 mm reactions are equivocal, and further diagnostic tests should be sought; less than 5 mm reactions are non-specific. False negative tests may arise in immune suppression or in miliary TB.

A specific diagnosis is confirmed by the finding of acid fast bacilli, obtained in young children by gastric lavage, usually on three successive days. In older children, the bacilli may be found in sputum which may be obtained by bronchial lavage with saline. Culture of the organism is slow, requiring a specific medium (Lowenstein–Jensen), and may take up to 6 weeks. The organism may be sought by local aspiration in extrapulmonary disease, e.g. in spinal fluid, splenic puncture, or in the urine.

Management

Treatment is usually with a combination of agents over an extended period—a minimum of 6 months. The choice is governed by the sensitivity of the organism and the potential or actual side-effects of the drugs. Normally treatment is with isoniazid, rifampicin and pyrazinamide for two months, followed by four months of rifampicin and isoniazid. Resistant organisms may require longer treatment with different agents, e.g. ethambutol or streptomycin. All these agents have significant side-effects (e.g. hepatotoxicity in isoniazid and rifampicin, and ototoxicity with streptomycin) and the child should be closely monitored.

Prevention

Inoculation with BCG (Bacille Calmette–Guérin), an attenuated strain of *M. bovis*, is a long established means of immunisation against TB. It is given as a subcutaneous injection. Studies have shown that it confers a varying degree of protection. Its use varies with the epidemiological setting. In endemic communities, immunisation at birth has been shown to be beneficial. Infants in families where contact with active TB is likely should also be offered immunisation except when there is a risk of HIV positivity. When prophylactic treatment with isoniazid is contemplated, isoniazid resistant strains of BCG are available. Currently, in the UK, children aged 13 years are given a tuberculin test by the Heaf method and offered BCG if they are not immune. Where cases of TB are identified, close contacts should also be offered immunisation. Complications of inoculation include BCG abscess and extensive local reactions if an already sensitised individual is inoculated.

Atypical tubercular disease

Infections with atypical strains of mycobacteria may occur. They most typically present with an indolent cervical lymphadenitis, eventually resulting in abscess formation. The usual organisms include *M. kansasii* and *M. avium–intracellulare*. These may be resistant to commonly used antitubercular drugs. The infection commonly regresses, and after drainage of a cervical abscess the infection may need no further treatment.

Antitubercular treatment should be offered only with progressive disease, according to the sensitivity of the organism, if identified.

Bronchiectasis

Bronchiectasis is a condition of chronic infective disease of part or parts of the lungs, with dilatation of the bronchi and persistent cough and production of purulent sputum. It may have no identifiable underlying cause, or be the result of a number of pathological processes including cystic fibrosis, immotile cilia syndrome, immune deficiency, bronchial obstruction due to foreign body or bronchial stenosis, or following pneumonia, particularly staphylococcal pneumonia.

It usually presents with a chronic cough, with associated symptoms depending on the etiology and severity of the condition. Clinical signs include finger clubbing and localised areas of fixed rales audible in the lung fields, often at the lung bases. The diagnosis may be suggested by plain X-ray, but is confirmed by bronchogram or high resolution CT scan. Treatment is by physiotherapy with postural drainage, and appropriate antibiotics for exacerbations. If the disease is localised, segmental or lobar surgical resection of the lung may be appropriate.

RESPIRATORY FUNCTION TESTING

The testing of lung function in the child who is unable to co-operate needs a specialised laboratory. Once a child can co-operate, useful information may be gained from peak flow rate determination and spirometry.

Peak flow rate (PFR)

This may be measured with a Wright meter that may be used in the surgery or at home, and is available on prescription in the UK. It requires a maximal effort in blowing out and is usually measured as the best of three attempts, after teaching the child the use of the meter. Reliable measurements are usually possible after the age of 5 years. Its major use lies in the detection of airway obstruction. Normal values are related most directly to height in childhood, and centile charts are available. In diagnosis PFR may be particularly useful if asthma is suspected or where dyspnoea is a symptom. In conjunction with exercise, either informal or on a treadmill, it may demonstrate exercise induced asthma. A fall of 20% or more during or following exercise is significant. In diagnosed asthma the PFR may be documented on a regular basis in a patient diary in order to assess symptom severity or treatment benefit. Care is needed in interpreting these diaries, as compliance may be questionable and they are open to manipulation.

In spirometry the child breathes out with maximum effort into a spirometer. Flow and expired volume is measured throughout the expiratory effort. A number of measurements may be made.

Vital capacity (VC)

This is the volume of lung available to the largest possible voluntary breath. It is reduced in mechanical restriction of the lung, neuromuscular disease, and in air trapping.

Forced expiratory volume in one second (FEV₁)

This can be related to the vital capacity, and as a ratio gives a measure of airways obstruction. Normally it exceeds 70% of the VC. It may be used in the ill child, after provocation with exercise or inhaled allergens, or before and after treatment with beta agonists, to demonstrate reversible airway obstruction.

The maximum expiratory flow volume curve (MEFV) records the flow rate at all points of the expiratory effort and, if flow is recorded at

---

GP Overview 5.2 Wheezing

Common causes
- Wheezing with viral infection
- Asthma
- Bronchiolitis
- Cystic fibrosis

Rarer causes
- Lobar emphysema
- Foreign body
- Vascular ring
- Reflux
- α₁-antitrypsin deficiency
- Tracheal/mediastinal tumours/cysts
- Tracheomalacia

Features in history
- Age at onset
- Possible triggers, e.g. emotion, exercise, infection
- Duration
- Family history (?atopic background)
- History of gastro-oesophageal reflux
- Failure to thrive
- History of choking ?foreign body
- Passive smoking history

Examination
- Chest wall deformity, Harrison sulcus
- Peak flow pre/post bronchodilation
- Peak flow pre/post exercise
- Growth measurements (height/weight)
- Skin ?signs of eczema
- Check for nasal polyps, rectal prolapse, cardiac murmurs

Investigations
- FBC + eosinophil count
- Sputum culture
- CXR
- Consider allergy tests (RAST), sweat test (CF)
- Consider bronchoscopy, upper GI endoscopy and pH monitoring

---

a fixed proportion of the VC, gives a sensitive method of detecting airways resistance.

ASTHMA

Asthma may be defined as a disorder characterised by varying reversible obstruction to air flow in the lung, and is most typically recognised by clinical evidence of episodic wheezing, coughing and hyperinflation of the lungs. The pathological process involves narrowing of the airways by inflammatory response, excessive mucus production and variable constriction of the airway through bronchoconstriction. It presents in a variety of clinical settings.

Asthma appears to be increasing in prevalence in the developed world. This is possibly because of increased recognition and partly because of other factors such as environmental pollution and changing early feeding practices. Up to 20% of children are known to wheeze at some time during their childhood; 7–10% have recurrent wheeze and therefore fulfil the diagnostic criteria for asthma. It is the most common cause of health related school absence, and the most common medical reason for hospital admission in childhood. Sudden death rates from asthma have remained unchanged despite advances in treatment; these deaths largely occur in adolescents and young adults, possibly related to problems of compliance with treatment. The debate about whether wheezing with viral illness in young children represents asthma is irrelevant—the treatment principles are similar, and other diagnostic terms may be misleading and distract from appropriate treatment.

Clinical features

The symptoms of asthma vary with the age of the child. In taking a history, details of the duration of symptoms and their variability are important in view of the episodic nature of asthma; precipitating situations such as viral infections, seasonality (in respect of airborne allergens) and exertion or emotional stress should be sought. The child with constant symptoms is less likely to be suffering from asthma. The cardinal symptoms are recurrent cough and breathlessness (or fast breathing). A family history of asthma or other atopic symptoms (hay fever, eczema) may be an important pointer to the probability of atopy in the child.

In the younger child, cough is usually the dominant symptom, commonly following a viral illness. In early episodes it is often assumed to be due to secondary infections and is treated with antibiotics. Thus the child may present with the parental complaint that the child is 'always on antibiotics, and that they are not doing him any good'. The cough is frequently more evident at night and may be associated with vomiting of mucus. The parents may not be aware of wheeze, but may describe noisy breathing from upper airway catarrh. Diagnosis may be delayed until an episode of wheezing becomes severe enough for the child to be admitted to hospital. The differential diagnosis includes chronic cough due to recurrent aspiration, inhaled foreign body, or abnormal lung immune defences.

Older children more typically present with cough on exertion, or breathlessness and wheeze with a variety of precipitating circumstances. The differential diagnosis includes hyperventilation, panic attacks, and aspiration, together with rarer lung diseases and very occasionally cardiac problems such as paroxysmal tachycardia. In any history of recurrent symptoms suggestive of asthma, a history of the social, emotional and educational effect of the symptoms is most important, including missed schooling, the ability of a child to take part in sports and social activities and the parental response to the illness, in allowing the child access to normal childhood activities and diet.

Examination

Examination starts with the height and weight centiles. Severe chronic asthma and its treatment, particularly with steroids, can interfere with growth and delay puberty. The fingers should be examined for clubbing in case the asthma is complicating another condition such as cystic fibrosis. The chest shape should be examined for symmetry, hyperexpansion, and the presence of a Harrison's sulcus. The tracheal position is noted and, in the acute episode, cyanosis, respiratory rate, use of accessory muscles and costal and suprasternal recession. The pulse should be felt in the ill child, and pulsus paradoxus (a decrease in pulse volume with inspiratory effort) noted. Percussion of the chest will usually show a hyper-resonant chest and the area of liver dullness pushed down. Listening to the chest may reveal a generalised expiratory wheeze, with a prolonged expiratory phase, although in the severely ill child this may not be evident (the silent chest). In the young infant the wheeze may be obscured by transmitted rattles from the upper airway. In a child old enough to co-operate, an attempt at peak flow rate measurement will show a reduction on the centiles or compared to a previous known best effort.

None of these clinical markers may be evident in the currently well child, and the doctor must rely on the history to suggest the diagnosis. In an older child an exercise test, with the child performing peak flows during and after significant exertion, may be helpful in confirming asthma. The response to beta agonists (such as salbutamol, and terbutaline) may give useful supporting information, particularly in the older child, where demonstrable benefit supports the diagnosis.

Investigation

In the initial assessment of a child presenting with probable asthma, a chest X-ray is usual in order to exclude other major pathology. In the acute episode it may show hyperinflation. This may be difficult to assess in younger children. Segmental collapse/consolidation may be present due to mucous plugging of the bronchi. A blood count may show eosinophilia. It is helpful to ask for a symptom diary, together with a peak flow diary to document changes over an extended period; this is useful as a reference point to evaluate treatments. When treatment with inhalers is contemplated, or is already established, an evaluation of technique and tuition in the use of different devices, either by the doctor, respiratory nurse or physiotherapist, is essential.

Treatment

Following the initial evaluation, environmental or lifestyle changes should be considered, e.g. avoidance of provoking factors such as pets, house dust mite and cigarette smoke. House dust mite allergy is very frequent in atopic children in the developed world, and asthmatic symptoms have been shown to be reduced by avoidance techniques. These include covering mattresses and pillows in plastic, frequent vacuuming with a filtering dust collection system, hot washing of bedding, and removal of carpets and other dust retaining furnishings from the bedroom. Acaricides are of no proven benefit. Cat dander is another important provoking factor, and families should be advised accordingly.

Drug treatment is tailored to minimise disruption to the child's life and potential side-effects, whilst aiming at an unrestricted lifestyle. It should be accompanied by education of the child and the family in the use of medications, and the child should be followed up to monitor the effects of the condition and to optimise treatment. Treatment is offered with a hierarchy of drugs and methods of administration according to the chronicity and severity of the symptoms. There are a number of classes of drug.

Beta 2 agonists. These stimulate the receptors in the smooth muscle of the bronchi and relax the bronchial walls. Short acting stimulants such as salbutamol and terbutaline are used in the short-term control of symptoms. Longer acting beta stimulants such as salmeterol may be useful in maintenance preventative treatment. Side-effects include tachycardia, tremor and hyperactivity. Tolerance may occur if these drugs are used very regularly.

Anticholinergic drugs such as ipratropium bromide block cholinergically mediated bronchoconstriction and may be used as an adjunct to beta agonists in the management of the acute episode. In some younger infants the response may be better than to beta agonists. Paradoxical bronchoconstriction may occur.

Theophyllines have a central stimulant effect on breathing. Aminophylline may be used intravenously in the acute attack. Slow release preparations may be given orally in control of chronic symptoms, and should be monitored with serum levels. Side-effects include gastric irritation, tachycardia, and arrhythmia, particularly in acute administration, which should be monitored by ECG.

Sodium cromoglycate is an inhaled preparation that stabilises mast cells. Used regularly it reduces attack frequency and severity. There are no known side-effects.

Steroid drugs. These have an anti-inflammatory action and potentiate the action of beta agonists. In the acute attack, intravenous hydrocortisone may be used, or oral prednisolone in short courses, e.g. 4–5 days (1–2 mg/kg/day). In severe chronic asthma, unresponsive to other therapies, longer term oral treatment may be necessary. Dosage at all times should be minimised to reduce the side-effects of growth restriction, Cushingoid appearance, immune depression, osteopenia, hyperphagia, behavioural problems, adrenal suppression, and glucose intolerance. Alternate day therapy may minimise these effects.

Inhaled steroid preparations, e.g. beclomethasone, budesonide and fluticasone, act as local anti-inflammatory agents in the respiratory tract. They are used in prevention of chronic symptoms by regular inhalation. Usually they are not absorbed in sufficient quantities to cause steroid side-effects, although beclomethasone in high dose has been implicated in growth restriction and adrenal suppression in some children. They may promote oro-pharyngeal thrush, and lowering of the timbre of the voice.

Leukotriene receptor antagonists. These recently introduced oral preparations may improve symptoms and reduce steroid dosage in persistent asthma.

Methods of administration should be tailored to the ability of the child and family to use the preparation effectively. Inappropriate expectation by the clinician or poor tuition of the family and child are common reasons for treatment failure.

Oral preparations of beta agonists may be the only medication tolerated by some younger children and may be appropriate in children with occasional mild symptoms. Disadvantages include large dose and therefore potential for side-effects, slow onset of action, and short shelf life. Tablet slow release formulations, e.g. theophylline drugs, may be difficult to take. Spansule preparations of slow release theophylline can either be swallowed whole by older children or separated and the contents given as granules on food to the younger child.

Inhaled methods include metered dose aerosols which require co-ordination of breathing effort and timing of delivery and are rarely suitable under the age of 7 years. Breath actuated aerosols are simpler and acceptable to some younger children. Aerosols may be delivered through spacer systems which contain the aerosol pending inhalation; in infants these may be used in conjunction with a round, soft face mask. These have the disadvantage of being cumbersome and wasteful, and the delivered dosage is unpredictable. Dry powder inhalers require little inspiratory effort and are convenient and portable, but some children tolerate them poorly. Nebulisers deliver a suspension of active agent in liquid, usually saline solution, and require no effort on the part of the patient. They are particularly useful in the acute attack and in the infant requiring regular treatment. They are not yet prescribable in the UK. The equipment is often obtained on loan from a practitioner or hospital. Steroids, aminophylline and beta agonists are used in intravenous form in the acute attack.

Management

Protocols for the management of acute attacks and recurrent asthma have been agreed by the International Paediatric Asthma Consensus Group, published in 1988 and revised in 1992, giving guidelines for the primary and hospital care of children with asthma. Additional similar guidelines for recognition and management in asthma have been formulated by the British Thoracic Society (Thorax 1997).

Acute attack. In the previously untreated mild attack management may be started with beta agonists such as terbutaline or salbutamol, given preferably by inhalation 4-hourly, either with a standard device or a nebuliser. Treatment started at home should be accompanied by instruction to the parents regarding the potential danger signals of severe asthma, such as cyanosis or breathlessness too severe to allow the child to talk. If the episode persists the child may be started on a short course of oral prednisolone. In severe asthma requiring hospital admission, beta agonists are usually started by nebuliser, driven by oxygen and monitored by peak flow measurement and pulse oximetry. In this setting they may be given at an increased frequency, continuously in severe cases. Oral prednisolone or intravenous hydrocortisone should also be started in these circumstances, and intravenous aminophylline may be used as an adjunct with cardiac monitoring. If the asthma is worsening despite these measures, intravenous beta agonists may be given, blood gases should be monitored, and attention paid to adequate hydration. In respiratory failure, mechanical ventilation should be considered. The majority of acute attacks respond to beta agonists and steroids, which should be continued for 4–5 days. With recovery, the longer term management of the child's condition should be reviewed, with attention to regular therapy and mode of delivery of treatment.

Continuing asthma:

Intermittent mild symptoms: inhaled intermittent beta agonists.

Occasional severe symptoms: additional provision of oral prednisolone at home, to be started after discussion with the primary care doctor. Such treatment should not be given more than 2–3 times in a year.

Frequent beta agonist use (more than 3 times per week): prophylaxis should be started. Sodium cromoglycate given 4 times per day is traditional and safe but has the disadvantage of compliance problems because of the need for frequent administration. It is administered by dry powder device, spacer or nebuliser.

Cromoglycate not effective after 6 weeks (or increasingly as an initial move): prophylaxis with low dose inhaled steroids. These should be given regularly, with careful instruction to the child and family regarding the need for their continuation. A symptom diary and peak flow recordings may be used to monitor the benefit of treatment.

Adequate control is not established: additional therapy with slow release theophylline monitored with plasma levels, long acting beta agonists or ipratropium should be tried sequentially, or occasionally in combination.

Severe, disabling asthma: high dose inhaled steroids, e.g. becloforte or alternate day oral steroids. Leukotriene receptor antagonists may be tried.

Children with asthma should be monitored prospectively with regard to asthma control,

physical growth (particularly those children on oral or high dose inhaled steroids), exercise capability, school attendance, and social and emotional adjustment. The treatment should be reassessed periodically and adjusted up or down the therapeutic ladder depending on the degree of control. Treatment should be kept as simple and as straightforward as is possible, in keeping with the objective of keeping the child's life as normal as possible. The education of the child and family about the condition and its treatment should be continued, with the aim of giving the child autonomy and appropriate responsibility for his or her own management as social independence is achieved. This may be helped by involvement of support groups and specialised supervised holidays, particularly for the severe asthmatic. Appropriate exercise should be encouraged with the expectation that a child should be able to enjoy most sporting activity, with the possible exception of long distance running. Schools and other carers should also be involved in understanding the child's condition and in the appropriate use of and access to medication, e.g. before sporting activity. School medical officers may liaise with teachers to increase confidence and awareness and to establish appropriate school protocols.

It is to be expected that adolescents will go through periods of denial of their illness and of poor compliance. With continued good humour and engagement by the doctor such periods can usually be overcome, but more formal counselling or residential supervision may occasionally be required.

Of children presenting with asthma in the first 3 years of life, 40% lose their symptoms, 34% improve to the point of requiring occasional treatment only, 25% persist with symptoms through adolescence into adult life and approximately 0.5% die. A proportion of those losing their symptoms in childhood regain symptoms in later life.

The infant with wheeze

A recurrent wheeze with succeeding viral infections is common following bronchiolitis. The response of young infants to bronchodilator drugs may be poor. Ipratropium may be more effective in this group than beta agonists. Oral steroids may be effective in the short term; regular nebulised budesonide is effective if symptoms are causing serious interference with day to day health.

The 'happy wheezer'. A group of infants, typically thriving babies, persist with noisy wheezing breathing, more or less continuously. This frequently causes the parents significant concern but, if the child is feeding well and conspicuously thriving, no treatment other than reassurance may be required. The description of such babies as happy wheezers is apt, and may be helpful to parents.

UPPER AIRWAY OBSTRUCTION

In the infant, compromise of the airway is more critical than in the larger child, because of the small diameter of the airway and the necessity of co-ordinating breathing and sucking as the principal means of feeding. The very young infant is an obligatory nose breather and the airway is particularly threatened by slight nasal blockage, as in colds. If feeding difficulties arise, it may be necessary to clear the nose mechanically, with saline nose drops or with gentle suction.

Chronic airway obstruction presents with inspiratory stridor which may be associated with signs of increased inspiratory effort, with tachypnoea and subcostal recession. In extreme circumstances it may be a cause of poor feeding, failure to thrive and respiratory failure.

Causes

Infancy

Laryngomalacia is the most common cause. It is a congenital anatomical abnormality with increased laxity of the epiglottis and arytenoids, which tend to collapse during inspiration. It presents with persistent stridor from birth which varies with the state of the child and may be quieter in sleep or when the child is crying. Feeding is rarely compromised. It is usual to confirm the diagnosis by laryngoscopy and to

exclude other more progressive problems. The natural history is for improvement with age; the problem is rarely evident after a year. Occasionally surgery may be required in severe cases.

Vascular ring around the trachea. This may be identified by the compression of the oesophagus evident on barium swallow; it requires surgical treatment.

Laryngeal papillomas may be acquired at birth and cause progressive narrowing of the airway. They can be identified at laryngoscopy and treated by surgical removal or laser therapy, but usually require a tracheostomy initially to protect the airway.

Laryngeal haemangiomas similarly cause progressive stridor and symptoms, and may require laser treatment after protective tracheostomy.

Subglottic stenosis secondary to prolonged endotracheal intubation in the pre-term infant requiring prolonged ventilatory support is an increasing cause of persistent obstruction. This may require treatment with tracheoplasty, but management may be very difficult and require prolonged endotracheal intubation and tracheostomy.

Muscular weakness from neuromuscular disease or cerebral palsy may also cause airway obstruction which may be compounded by swallowing difficulty due to bulbar palsy and require tracheostomy.

The older child

Obstruction may be caused by adenoidal and tonsillar hypertrophy. This problem commonly starts in the second year of life. The child develops a tendency to mouth breathe, and to snore at night. Typical adenoidal facies develop and the child may have difficulty in swallowing lumpy food. If the obstruction is severe and persistent the child may fail to thrive and show sleep apnoea, with recurrent waking at night, struggling to breathe. This may cause sleepiness in the day, headaches and poor concentration. The diagnosis may be confirmed with sleep studies, during which oximetry, breathing effort, snoring, body movements, nasal airflow, and

ECG trace are monitored. If the diagnosis is confirmed, adenotonsillectomy is indicated.

FOREIGN BODY ASPIRATION

Small objects such as peanuts and plastic toys may be inhaled, particularly by children under two years of age. The child should be protected from such environmental hazards where possible.

Larger objects may cause acute upper airway obstruction with the rapid onset of choking, respiratory distress and cyanosis. See Box 5.8 for first aid.

Smaller objects may be inhaled into the small airways and commonly lodge in the right main or lower lobe bronchus. Inhalation may be marked by the acute onset of choking, coughing or a fixed stridor, but may go unnoticed at the time. When a choking episode is noted, immediate assessment may show differential chest wall movement, with the object being responsible for a ball-valve effect. Auscultation may reveal a fixed rhonchus. The object may be radio-opaque and revealed directly on X-ray or inferred from the associated finding of an overinflated area of lung. An expiratory film should be requested to reveal this. Treatment should be by bronchoscopic removal of the object; this may be difficult— peanuts are particularly likely to fragment. Occasionally thoracotomy may be required.

If the inhalation is overlooked, subsequent lobar or segmental lung collapse and recurrent infection ensues. The child may present with recurrent coughs and examination may show persistent localised chest signs. The X-ray may reveal recurrent or persistent local collapse and consolidation. Ultimately bronchiectasis may develop. Diagnosis is aided by high resolution CT scanning and bronchoscopy, at which time the removal of any persistent foreign body may be attempted. Lobectomy may be required if irreversible damage has occurred.

Recurrent aspiration

Aspiration of swallowed food or regurgitated stomach contents may occur recurrently if there are disorders of swallowing mechanisms, oesophageal motility problems and strictures, or gastro-oesophageal reflux. Very occasionally there may be an abnormal connection between the oesophagus and the trachea, as in the H-type gastro-oesophageal fistula or congenital laryngeal cleft. Recurrent aspiration is most frequently observed in children with cerebral palsy and other neuromuscular problems, or after oesophageal surgery. Inhalation causes infective and chemical pneumonitis, and the child presents with recurrent pneumonia, recurrent cough, or wheezing which is unresponsive to asthma treatments and possibly resulting in failure to thrive. The history may give recognisable clues such as habitual vomiting in infancy or with postural changes. The child may have feeding difficulties, particularly with liquids, and may be observed to have choking episodes and a postural related cough. The chest X-ray may show persistent or varying patchy collapse/consolidation. Further investigation is by oesophageal pH monitoring to detect frequent reflux, barium swallow to detect overspill, fistulae or oesophageal strictures, or videofluoroscopy to visualise swallowing co-ordination.

Recurrent overspill due to inco-ordination may require nasogastric tube feeding or gastrostomy. Reflux may require symptomatic treatment with feed thickening, propping the head of the cot or bed, or prokinetic medication (cisapride). In refractory reflux, surgical treatment by Nissen fundoplication may be needed. Oesophageal strictures may require endoscopic dilatation.

Box 5.8   First aid for foreign body aspiration

- Lift the child's chin and inspect the airway
- Remove any visible or removable obstruction
- If the obstruction cannot be removed, place the child head down in the prone position and give 5 hard blows to the back
- If the airway does not clear, place the child supine and administer 5 thrusts to the chest with the hand to the sternum
- If breathing is not re-established, mouth to mouth ventilation should be offered, and the cycle repeated if necessary
- In a child over one year of age, the Heimlich manoeuvre may be attempted, with the patient sitting or standing

IMMOTILE CILIA SYNDROME

Impaired ciliary function results in poor muco-ciliary clearance and in chronic lung infection, sinusitis and ultimately bronchiectasis. This condition may occur in association with situs inversus (Kartagener's syndrome) inherited by autosomal recessive transmission (Fig. 5.9). Diagnosis is confirmed by electron microscopy of ciliary structure obtained by nasal or tracheal biopsy. Males are infertile.

CYSTIC FIBROSIS (CF)

Genetics – see page 161.

In CF the transport of chloride (Cl⁻) ions and secondarily of sodium (Na⁺) ions through the epithelial cells lining sweat glands, airways, intestines and pancreas, is decreased. This results in a high level of chloride and sodium in the sweat, and causes thickened mucous secretions in lung and pancreas which are responsible for most of the pathological features of the disease.

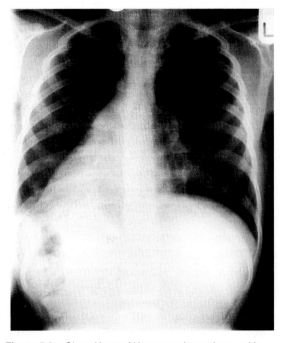

Figure 5.9   Chest X-ray of Kartagener's syndrome with situs inversus.

Diagnosis and clinical features

The diagnosis of CF is usually based on clinical criteria and the analysis of sweat chloride (> 60 mEq/l). In 10–20% of cases CF is diagnosed shortly after birth because meconium ileus leads to intestinal obstruction (abdominal distension and vomiting of bile). In the remainder the diagnosis is suggested by a history of gradually worsening cough associated with recurrent respiratory infections (especially with staphylococci and Pseudomonas) and failure to thrive. Neonatal diagnosis is possible as plasma trypsin is raised in neonatal CF, and Guthrie filter-paper blood spots are increasingly being used for the assay of immunoreactive trypsin. It is still uncertain whether diagnosis in the newborn leads to a better long-term prognosis, however it does mean that parents become aware of the genetic risk before their next pregnancy, so that they then have the option of early prenatal diagnosis. Published data indicate that most couples who have had one affected child request prenatal diagnosis and terminate an affected pregnancy.

Persistent respiratory infections are the main feature of CF. Later on chronic rhinitis and nasal polyps can occur. Pancreatic insufficiency occurs early, leading to malabsorption and causing bulky, greasy, offensive stools and failure to thrive in spite of an excessive appetite (Figure 5.10). This may result in depletion of vitamins A, D, E and K. Other complications include rectal prolapse in infancy and small bowel obstruction. Diabetes, gallstones and cirrhosis of the liver may also develop. Delay in the onset of puberty is likely in both sexes. All but a few percent of males with CF are infertile due to disturbed embryonic development of the vas deferens, epididymis and seminal vesicles. Females are more likely to be able to have children.

Many babies have frequent chest infections, but CF is rare. It is difficult for parents to accept that, in the absence of a positive family history, it is almost inevitable that diagnosis will be delayed in a rare disease that presents with common symptoms. Their anger will be more marked if they had sensed that there could be a serious problem for some months but had been repeatedly reassured by the doctor or health visitor.

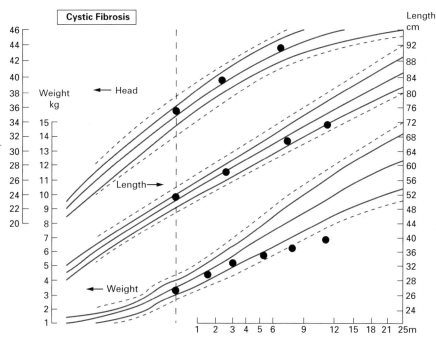

Figure 5.10 Growth chart of a child with cystic fibrosis.

Treatment and prognosis

As with all uncommon chronic childhood diseases, the family doctor may have to decide whether to refer the child to the local hospital or to a specialist unit, which may be some distance away from the family's home. The latter is preferable, though a combination of basic care provided locally and regular assessments at the specialist centre may be a reasonable compromise. Management includes an open and positive approach to the disease by health professionals, and encouragement of older children to take increasing responsibility for their own health, in order to enhance their self-confidence.

Management

Pulmonary care is centred on regular physiotherapy to assist lung drainage, and the use of antibiotics. Prophylaxis with regular flucloxacillin in early childhood is used to prevent staphylococcal infection. The bacteriological flora of the lungs is monitored and specific infections treated. Superinfection with Pseudomonas is common; it causes further damage and requires aggressive treatment. Nebulised antibiotics may be indicated; treatment with intravenous antibiotics administered via an indwelling intravenous catheter (Portacath) may also be required. Increasingly this is being organised in the home. Asthma is a common complicating problem and requires treatment. Recent advances in treatment include the use of inhaled DNAase and the possibility of inhaled gene replacement therapy. Ultimately lung or heart–lung transplant may be required. The prognosis is improving and the current median survival is around 30 years.

Nutritional support is provided with pancreatic enzyme supplementation at each meal. Calorie supplements may be required; if weight gain is unsatisfactory despite these measures, supplemental feeding by overnight nasogastric tube feeding or gastrostomy feeding may be offered. Regular supplementation with fat soluble vitamins is given.

Psychosocial support for the child and family requires a team approach. Genetic counselling of families should be offered, and antenatal screening in further pregnancies may provide the possibility of termination of affected fetuses, if desired.

Complications

Complications include the onset of diabetes mellitus in late childhood, cirrhosis, and male infertility. Poor growth and delayed puberty are common and may be treated by administration of testosterone or oestrogen if appropriate.

An increasing number of patients with cystic fibrosis are surviving into young adult life, and the handover of care to physicians dealing with adults requires careful management. Joint clinics for the review of adolescent patients are encouraged.

FURTHER READING

British Thoracic Society 1997 British guidelines on asthma management. Thorax 52: Suppl I
Dillon M J 1984 Modern management of hypertension. In: Meadow R (ed) Recent Advances in Paediatrics 7, pp 35–55
Dinwiddie R 1997 Diagnosis and management of paediatric respiratory disease, 2nd edn. Churchill Livingstone, Edinburgh
Park M K 1996 Paediatric cardiology for practitioners, 3rd edn. Mosby, London

Internet addresses

Paediatric cardiology
http://www.tc.umn.edu/nlhome/m475/bjarn001/stuff/abstract.html

Respiratory disease
http://hebw.uwcm.ac.uk/respdis/index.html

SIDS
http://dspace.dial.pipex.com/fsid/

6

Gastroenterology and nutrition

Jeffrey Bissenden

VOMITING

Acute vomiting

If a previously well child has an attack of acute vomiting, it is a worrying symptom in the absence of an obvious cause (Box 6.1). Any infection can cause vomiting, particularly in the younger child. In the presence of fever, serious infections need to be excluded.

Gastroenteritis

Globally, bacterial dysentery is a major health threat. Organisms such as cholera, salmonella and shigella cause not only profound diarrhoea and vomiting, but the children are toxic. In Europe, such illnesses are seen only in children returning from Asia or Africa. Occasionally, infection with Campylobacter or pathogenic *E. coli* presents as abdominal pain and bloody diarrhoea in children who have not been abroad. More commonly, gastroenteritis is linked with the enteroviruses such as rotavirus, echo and adenovirus. Viral gastroenteritis is a milder condition; the amount of sodium lost in the stool is much

---

Box 6.1   Causes of acute vomiting

- Gastritis/gastroenteritis
- Other infection, e.g. otitis media, urinary tract infection (UTI), meningitis
- Acute abdomen, e.g. appendicitis, strangulated hernia
- Alcohol or drug ingestion, deliberate or accidental

---

less. Whatever the infectious agent, the principle of treatment is the same—to prevent dehydration with appropriate fluid replacement. Hospital admission is warranted on medical grounds only if a child is dehydrated and vomiting, but many admissions take place for social reasons. The skill of the clinician is to assess the degree, if any, of dehydration (Table 6.1).

It is of great benefit that the modern generation of parents is taught to carry child health records. In the first year the weight is frequently recorded so, if there is a recent weight in the child health record, the percentage of dehydration can be calculated from the weight of the child in the surgery or in the casualty department (Table 6.2 and Box 6.2).

Rehydration. The oral route is preferable; for 24 hours the formula fed infant is given an oral rehydration formula. The commercial formulas (Dioralyte, Rehidrat) are mixtures of sodium, potassium and approximately 5% dextrose in a buffered solution. Wherever possible breast feeding should continue, perhaps with top-ups

Table 6.1 Degrees of dehydration

Degree of dehydration	Clinical features
< 5%	Undetectable
5–10%	Tongue dry, eyes sunken, loss of skin turgor
> 10%	Peripheral perfusion poor, consciousness impaired

Table 6.2 Fluid requirements of children at different ages

Age of child	Needs
Newborn	150 ml/kg
6-month infant	120 ml/kg
12-month infant	100 ml/kg

Box 6.2 Example of dehydrated infant

If an infant weighing 7 kg is estimated to be 7% dry, in the next 24 hours he requires:
7 × 120 = 840 ml
plus 7% of 7 kg = 490 ml
total fluid required for replacement = 1330 ml

---

of rehydration fluid given by spoon. The skill of rehydration is seen in tropical countries; there the infants are fed slowly, often by spoon—if one 5 ml spoonful is given every minute it equates to 300 ml in one hour. The mistake in the UK is to feed large volumes in a short period of time. The thirsty baby takes the whole feed and promptly vomits. If the baby is 10% or more dehydrated, intravenous fluids are safer. If there is imminent circulatory failure, intravenous colloid or saline should be given in a volume of 20 ml/kg over one hour. When an infant has been vomiting for days, ketosis causes nausea and intravenous fluids are necessary to break the cycle.

In the UK, the rehydration fluid contains approximately 30 mmol of sodium per litre. In the tropics, where sodium loss is more severe, the WHO recommends that the sodium content should be 90 mmol/l.

After initial rehydration, it is unnecessary to reintroduce full strength feeds slowly. A small minority of infants will relapse because of temporary cow's milk or lactose intolerance and they may take longer to return to normal feeds. There is no place for anti-emetics or bowel sedatives in the acute situation, and they may be positively harmful in young children. Similarly, antibiotics have little role. The only exception is when the pathogen is known and the infant is systemically unwell, e.g. Campylobacter enteritis may be treated with erythromycin. If the infant has severe dysentery with blood in the stool, the antibiotic ciprofloxacin is excellent. In practice, all the possible bacterial pathogens would be covered by this antibiotic.

Persistent vomiting

This is a problem of babies and toddlers and is unusual in the older child (Box 6.3).

Possetting (oesophageal reflux)

The mechanism of possetting or oesophageal reflux is the same. The difference is merely one of degree. Practically all babies posset a little.

Reflux is the most common cause of significant persistent vomiting in the first 6 months. The

---

Box 6.3 Common causes of persistent vomiting

- Possetting
- Oesophageal reflux
- Pyloric stenosis
- Chronic occult infection such as a urinary tract infection
- Intermittent intestinal obstruction, e.g. from malrotation or volvulus
- Raised intracranial pressure
- Migraine
- Peptic ulcer

GP Overview 6.1 Diarrhoea and vomiting

Causes
Gastrointestinal
1. Feeding problems
2. Gastroenteritis
   - Viral—rotavirus 60%
   - Bacterial—shigella/salmonella/campylobacter
   - Protozoal—amoebiasis (rare)
   - Parasitic—hookworm (rare)
3. Pyloric stenosis—less common (2–6 weeks of age)
4. Lactose intolerance
5. Cow's milk protein intolerance
6. Coeliac disease

Non-gastrointestinal
Otitis media/respiratory infections
Urinary tract infection/uraemia
Hepatitis A
Meningitis/septicaemia

Surgical causes
Appendicitis
Intussusception

Metabolic causes
Diabetic ketoacidosis
Hypercalcaemia
Galactosaemia

Others
Raised intracranial pressure
Adrenal insufficiency

History
Duration of vomiting and/or diarrhoea
Character of vomit ?blood ?altered food ?bile

Examination
Check for dehydration
Check pulse rate, temperature, respiratory rate
Examine abdomen, scrotum and other systems

Investigations
Dipstick urine for sugar/protein/blood
FBC
Urea, electrolytes, serum creatinine
Sugar
LFTs (liver function tests)
MSU for M, C + S
Stool for M, C + S ova, cysts, parasites
Surgical opinion if indicated

---

cause is incompetence of the sphincter at the gastro-oesophageal junction. It is made worse by the fact that babies spend much of the day horizontal and the main oral intake is milk. The vomiting is effortless. It may begin at birth or after a few weeks. The mild form, regarded as posseting, is a cosmetic problem. The baby thrives and the only anxiety is the state of the parents' clothes. With significant reflux, the weight may be compromised and the vomiting is severe. When the history is typical, therapy can commence without investigations. The purpose of investigation is not to prove that the child is vomiting but:

1. to exclude a hiatus hernia
2. to quantify the reflux and detect silent episodes of reflux
3. to detect reflux oesophagitis.

Hence, a barium meal will rule out a hiatus hernia as well as showing reflux. 24-hour oesophageal pH monitoring demonstrates the number of refluxing episodes. Oesophagoscopy will detect reflux oesophagitis.

If therapy is necessary, the following measures are helpful:

1. early introduction of solids, certainly by 4 months
2. agents such as Gaviscon which coat the stomach
3. milk thickeners such as Carobel or Nestargel
4. gut motility and gastric emptying drugs such as cisapride (0.1 mg/kg) given 3 times per day (also increase lower oesophageal sphincter pressure) (contraindicated in premature infants under 3 months of age)

5. sensible measures such as winding and sitting supported after a feed.

If the condition is severe and there is demonstrable oesophagitis, ranitidine should be given to lower the gastric pH. Failed medical management will lead to surgery to the oesophageal sphincter.

Pyloric stenosis

Pyloric stenosis is not difficult to diagnose in the classical form. If a 6-week-old male infant whose father had pyloric stenosis as an infant presents with relentless projectile vomiting which is not bile stained, it is 99% certain that this child has pyloric stenosis (M:F ratio 4:1). In practice, the condition takes a while to develop and become obvious. This is particularly true in premature babies. If a test feed is negative but the history is highly suggestive, an abdominal ultrasound will identify the tumour in the hands of an experienced paediatric radiologist. A barium meal would also confirm the diagnosis. It is unusual to require radiological assistance in making the diagnosis. The biochemistry may be disturbed with a hypokalaemic alkalosis. This requires correction before anaesthesia can be safely undertaken. The definitive operation of pyloromyotomy (Ramstedt operation) is very successful and the babies are returned home in days.

Vomiting in the older child

This is unusual; the cause may be one of a range of unconnected pathologies.

1. *Brain tumour.* It is every clinician's nightmare to miss or to be late in diagnosing a brain tumour. Unfortunately, brain tumours are not uncommon in children. If the history is one of vomiting in the morning or if there is a hint of neurological symptoms such as ataxia, it is very important to institute some form of cranial imaging. Magnetic resonance imaging (MRI) is replacing CT scanning.

2. *Chronic infection* such as giardiasis can cause vomiting. This should be considered in malnourished children returning from abroad.

3. *Malrotation of the gut* can occur at any age. This may be considered in the situation of subacute intestinal obstruction. An abdominal X-ray would suggest the diagnosis and a barium follow-through will confirm it.

4. *Peptic ulcer.* Occasionally a child in the early teens presents with a peptic ulcer. Helicobacter gastritis is well recognised in this age group and eradication treatment is the same as for adults.

Endoscopy may require anaesthesia but it is a better investigation than barium studies.

5. *Cyclical vomiting* or *periodic syndrome* is a condition that is not fully understood; the terms are applied to children who vomit profoundly, becoming ketotic. They settle on intravenous fluids. It is a diagnosis of exclusion and is impossible to make on the first occasion. Metabolic diseases are suspected but never proven.

6. *Migraine* is a very real problem in children. In order to make the diagnosis, recurrent vomiting would have to be accompanied by other factors such as headache, visual symptoms or a strong family history.

CHRONIC DIARRHOEA IN INFANTS

History (Box 6.4)

The two key questions about an infant with chronic diarrhoea are:

- 'What is the description of the diarrhoea?'
- 'Is the infant gaining weight despite the diarrhoea?'.

The purpose of these questions is to differentiate the four main causes of chronic diarrhoea:

1. toddler diarrhoea
2. secondary cow's milk/lactose intolerance
3. coeliac disease
4. cystic fibrosis.

In Europe, chronic infection is an unlikely cause though children returning from abroad

---

Box 6.4 Essential questions to ask at initial consultation

1. Is the diarrhoea from birth?
2. Did the onset coincide with a change of milk, e.g. breast to bottle?
3. Did the onset coincide with beginning solid feeds?
4. Do these solid feeds contain wheat?
5. Is the stool particularly greasy and smelly (mothers nearly always say 'yes')?
6. Is the baby particularly chesty?
7. Does the stool contain blood?
8. Does the stool contain undigested food particles?
9. Is there perianal excoriation?
10. Does the baby taste salty when kissed?

may still carry a bacterial bowel pathogen or organism such as Giardia. Inflammatory bowel disease can present early in life but presents as rectal bleeding.

Examination

It cannot be emphasised too strongly that paediatrics is a measuring speciality. Height and weight are the most important physical signs. The presence or absence of anaemia and clubbing is an important feature.

1. Children with toddler diarrhoea look remarkably well, considering the impressive description of the diarrhoea by the parents.
2. Infants with lactose intolerance/cow's milk intolerance may have sore bottoms with a bad napkin dermatitis.
3. In classic coeliac disease the infant has a distended abdomen and is anaemic. There is wasting around the upper thighs and buttocks.
4. Children with cystic fibrosis look hungry and wasted and have a pasty complexion, though they are not anaemic. Abdominal distension is not so pronounced but the wasting described in coeliac disease is also present.

Investigations for 'failure to thrive' are shown in GP Overview 6.2.

Toddler diarrhoea

The term 'toddler diarrhoea' is used of infants or young children who have diarrhoea containing undigested food particles, e.g. peas, carrots. The parents give an impressive account of a vast number of nappies being used every day but despite this the child thrives. There is no diagnostic test. The diagnosis lies in the history and the negative clinical findings. A gastro-colic reflex is a common feature in the older child. The growth chart must show adequate weight gain before confirming the diagnosis. The explanation is one of overactive bowels and rapid gastro-intestinal transit times. Treatment is rarely indicated but often the diagnosis coincides with potty training. If the stools are too loose and too frequent, it is reasonable to prescribe loperamide

to counter bowel peristalsis. The children often come from families with irritable bowel syndrome so there is some empathy from the parents. Most cases have resolved by the age of 5 years.

Lactose/cow's milk intolerance

Any cause of undigested sugar reaching the large bowel will lead to an osmotic diarrhoea. The congenital sugar intolerances are rare and are classified as monosaccharide (glucose, galactose) or disaccharide (lactose) intolerance. Lactose intolerance may be a primary disease but is usually secondary to a severe bout of gastroenteritis. It may be necessary to rest the bowel by using a lactose-free milk for weeks or even months. Cow's milk intolerance is associated with a patchy enteropathy. It is neither practical nor sensible to separate lactose from cow's milk intolerance. The treatment is discussed under Food intolerance (see p. 150).

Coeliac disease

Coeliac disease is common in Ireland but is less common in the UK since gluten has been excluded from the commercially available early weaning foods. The gliadin component of wheat causes a severe enteropathy in the duodenum and jejunum, with flattened villi and consequent malabsorption. The history may be classical, with the onset of offensive diarrhoea soon after the introduction of gluten, but often anaemia and poor growth are the predominant features; the bowels may be only slightly loose in the older child. Growth measurements show failure to thrive on the centile chart, weight rather than height being affected (Figure 6.1). There may be muscle wasting and loss of fat in the area of the buttocks and inner thighs. The abdomen is distended with gas. The distension is in the upper abdomen, in contrast to the apparent lower abdominal distension seen in the normal toddler with a prominent lordosis. The differential diagnosis is cystic fibrosis or lactose intolerance. Investigations will show an iron deficiency anaemia. The most helpful investigation in recent times has been the ability to measure anti-gliadin

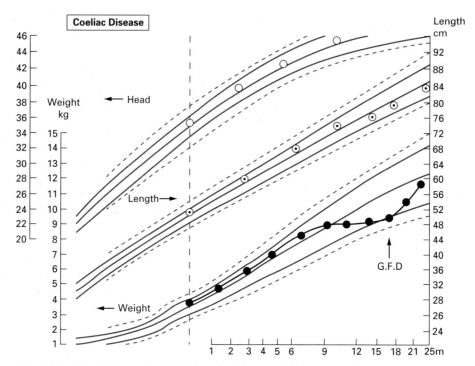

Figure 6.1 Growth chart of a child with coeliac disease. G.F.D = gluten-free diet.

antibodies. Prior to this, absorption tests such as the measurement of blood xylose one hour after a xylose load were used but there were too many false negatives for this to be reliable. In contrast, the measurement of anti-gliadin IgA and anti-endomysial cell antibodies (also IgA) is very specific and sensitive. If both of these antibodies are negative, it is extremely unlikely that the infant has coeliac disease. It is customary to measure anti-gliadin IgG antibodies at the same time; if these are positive, it is important to know that the infant is not IgA deficient. Hence it is sensible to request IgG, IgA and IgM antibodies when screening. A positive anti-gliadin IgG level alone has no significance, being found in the normal population and in other bowel insults.

If the clinical picture and the anti-gliadin antibody levels are suggestive of coeliac disease, then a jejunal biopsy is mandatory to confirm the diagnosis. This can be done with a Crosby capsule and X-ray screening or by endoscopy and direct biopsy. If the latter is feasible, it is more reliable than blind biopsy with all the practical

difficulties associated with the Crosby capsule. It is very important that the biopsy is handled correctly in the pathology department, and it is best viewed under the dissecting microscope by the pathologist and the clinician; that way, the orientation of the specimen is satisfactory.

As soon as the diagnosis is confirmed, the dietician becomes involved and the parents learn about a gluten-free diet. The Coeliac Society issues an annual booklet to its members listing all foods and whether or not they contain gluten. It is therefore important that the parents join the Society. The response to a gluten-free diet is dramatic. If the diagnosis is correct and the child is over the age of 2, the condition should be regarded as lifelong. The increased incidence of small bowel lymphoma is reduced to normal if a gluten-free diet is maintained. If the diagnosis was made when the child was under the age of 2, or if there was any doubt and the response to gluten withdrawal was unimpressive, a challenge should be made. The gluten challenge has been the subject of debate but, essentially, gluten is introduced into the diet under controlled circumstances at around the age of four years. The original protocols suggested that, before the reintroduction of gluten, a normal biopsy should be obtained, and a repeat biopsy performed after 6 weeks on gluten. The measurement of gliadin antibodies can now eliminate the need for the repeat biopsies. If the antibodies become negative on a gluten-free diet and then reappear when challenged, accompanied by clinical deterioration, there is no need to do any further biopsies. If the challenge is negative and the child continues to thrive and does not develop antibodies, then that child had a temporary gluten intolerance which has now resolved.

Cystic fibrosis (see Chapter 5, p. 134)

Other causes of chronic diarrhoea (infective)

Chronic infection with gut pathogens is unlikely, though protracted diarrhoea occurs with organisms such as Cryptosporidium. One important pathogen which causes traveller's diarrhoea in adults and malabsorption in children is *Giardia lamblia*. Giardiasis presents as chronic diarrhoea, abdominal pain and failure to thrive. The diagnosis may be made by microscopy of a fresh stool, looking for ova. Whenever a jejunal biopsy is performed for coeliac disease, it is good practice to send jejunal juice for Giardia isolation. Giardiasis can be acquired in the UK but it is more common after a visit abroad. The treatment is a 3-day course of oral metronidazole.

RECURRENT ABDOMINAL PAIN

The further away the pain is from the umbilicus, the more likely it is to be organic. Practically every child with recurrent abdominal pain who attends outpatients when asked 'where does it hurt?', points to the umbilicus. It does of course hurt; children do feel pain. The most important message to the child and parents is that you believe that there is pain, that it is not serious and that an explanation will be offered.

A detailed history, including social changes,

GP Overview 6.2   Failure to thrive

This means failure to gain weight consistently as plotted on a centile chart.
A fall across centile lines needs an explanation.

Causes
- Inadequate food intake
- Feeding problems/family deprivation
- Learning disability
- Emotional deprivation
- Chronic illness:
  —renal: urinary tract infection, chronic renal failure
  —cardiac: congenital heart disease
  —respiratory: cystic fibrosis
  —gastrointestinal: malabsorption, reflux, hiatus hernia, coeliac disease, lactose intolerance
  —malignancy

History
- Full history of pregnancy, birth and neonatal period
- When did the problem start?
- Feeding history
- Assessment of parenting skills and social history
- Consider UTIs/respiratory infection/diarrhoea and vomiting/chronic illness

Examination
- Child's demeanour
- Growth measurements (height, weight, head circumference) present and past recordings plotted on centile chart
- Check for wasting, muscle loss (e.g. buttocks in coeliac disease)
- Check CVS, RS and abdominal examination

Initial investigations (may include)
- FBC, ESR, Hb electrophoresis
- Urea electrolytes, creatinine, sugar
- LFTs (liver function tests)
- Serum Ca^{++}, PO_4^{--}
- Thyroid function
- Anti-gliadin and anti-endomysial cell antibodies
- Immunoglobulin levels incl. IGA
- Faecal chymotrypsin levels
- Sweat test
- Stools for microscopy, culture, sensitivity and ova, cysts and parasites
- Stools for reducing substances
- Stools for sugar chromatography
- Urine for microscopy, culture and sensitivity
- Urine for amino acid screen
- X-rays—CXR and bone age
- Developmental assessment
- Social/family report

---

schooling and family illnesses, is vital for accurate clinical assessment. Examination should focus on well-being and growth. Abused children can certainly have abdominal pain. Abdominal palpation may suggest constipation but a rectal examination is not routinely justified. No investigations should be done once a clinical diagnosis of non-organic disease has been made. X-rays and blood tests merely perpetuate the fear that there may be something wrong. The true explanation is that either these children have an increased autonomic nerve supply so that increased peristalsis can be perceived, or they genuinely have anxiety causing the pain. If no specific anxiety can be identified during the consultation, the child must be told that he is merely feeling the workings of his intestines. This is normal and he must not be anxious.

Organic causes

Investigations are indicated if:

- the pain is in the epigastric or loin area
- there is associated failure to thrive
- there is diarrhoea, with or without blood.

Upper abdominal pain (Box 6.5)

Peptic ulcer and Helicobacter gastritis are uncommon but not unknown in children. It is justifiable to perform an endoscopy if the child is over the age of 10 and there is pain and tenderness in the epigastrium. A general anaesthetic may be necessary. The treatment of children with gastric pathology is similar to that of adults.

Acute and chronic pancreatitis are uncommon but may occur in childhood. A form of familial pancreatitis may present as recurrent severe abdominal pain, and this may be associated with neutropenia.

Renal causes are suggested by loin pain. Routine urine tests, blood electrolytes and creatinine, a plain X-ray of the abdomen for stones and an ultrasound of the kidneys as a non-invasive screen are the initial investigations. Measurement of blood pressure should be routine.

Constipation as a cause of abdominal pain

There is no doubt that constipation can cause abdominal pain and that effective treatment can take away the pain. That having been said, constipation is one of the most overdiagnosed conditions, particularly if that diagnosis is made on the basis of a plain X-ray of the abdomen. Many children have masses of faeces demonstrated on abdominal X-ray but do not complain of pain.

Inflammatory bowel disease should be considered when generalised abdominal pain is associated with bloody diarrhoea and ill health.

Abdominal migraine

If there is a strong family history of migraine and if there are symptoms such as headache, there is a possibility that migraine is the cause. It is a very difficult diagnosis to make but if the pain is frequent and the child is over the age of 8, a trial of food exclusion or pizotifen 500–1000 µg at night is recommended.

Causes of chronic/recurrent abdominal pain outside the abdomen (Box. 6.6)

There are theoretically a huge number of causes of abdominal pain. The art of the consultation is the taking of a careful history and sympathetic reassurance to the child and family. It is important to the family that the doctor believes (or is seen to believe) that the child genuinely feels the pain. Diagrams of the gastrointestinal tract help

---

Box 6.5   Possible causes of upper abdominal pain
<ul><li>Peptic ulcer or Helicobacter gastritis</li><li>Pancreatitis—acute, chronic or familial (rare)</li><li>Renal causes such as urinary tract infection, stones or obstruction</li><li>Constipation</li><li>Inflammatory bowel disease (ulcerative colitis or Crohn's disease)</li></ul>

Box 6.6   Causes of chronic/recurrent abdominal pain outside the abdomen
<ul><li>Chronic chest disease such as asthma (pneumonia is a well established cause of acute abdominal pain)</li><li>Sickle cell disease</li><li>Porphyria</li><li>Diabetes</li><li>Lead poisoning</li><li>Psychosomatic</li></ul>

GP Overview 6.3 Abdominal pain

Common symptom, often difficult to diagnose.
Remember, the cause is often outside the abdomen.

- Acute—often periumbilical with vomiting, fever, anorexia and malaise
- Chronic—affects 10% children, but < 10% of these have organic cause

Common causes

Acute

GASTROINTESTINAL
- Gastroenteritis
- Constipation
- Mesenteric adenitis
- Appendicitis
- Irritable bowel syndrome
- Intussusception
- Volvulus
- Malrotation
- Henoch–Schönlein purpura

RENAL
- Renal tract infection
- Renal calculi

ABDOMINAL
- Trauma
- Pancreatitis
- Hepatitis
- Testicular torsion

OTHERS
- Chest infection
- Diabetes mellitus (ketoacidosis)

Chronic (N.B. 95% *not* gastrointestinal)
- Common (inorganic)
  - recurrent abdominal pain
  - constipation
- Rarer (organic)
  - peptic ulcer
  - diabetes mellitus
  - lead poisoning
  - inflammatory bowel disease
  - coeliac disease

- porphyria
- food allergy
- child abuse
- neoplasms
- sickle cell disease
- pain referred from spine, testes, pelvis

History

Pain: site, length of history, aggravating/relieving factors, presence/absence of vomiting, diarrhoea, blood in stool, rash.

- Further from umbilicus, the more likely organic cause

Examples:
- Related to meals—peptic ulcer disease, gallbladder disease/stones, pancreatitis
- Related to milk ingestion—lactose intolerance
- Nocturnal pain—peptic ulcer
- With diarrhoea—inflammatory bowel disease, giardiasis, irritable bowel syndrome

Examination

General appearance:
- ? anaemic
- ? level of hydration
- ? jaundiced
- Evidence of weight loss
- Check ear, nose, throat/respiratory system
- Check for abdominal tenderness, guarding, masses or organomegaly
- Always examine the scrotum.

Investigations include:
- FBC, ESR
- Urea/electrolytes/serum creatinine
- Blood sugar
- LFTs (liver function tests)
- Amylase
- MSU (mid stream urine for MC + S)
- Stool for MC + S
- Plain abdominal X-ray
- Chest X-ray
- Abdominal ultrasound
- Surgical opinion

---

in the explanation to the family of how a variety of factors, organic or otherwise, can affect the autonomic nervous system supplying the small intestine. The late John Apley, who devoted much time and research to this topic, unfortunately came to the conclusion that little bellyachers become big bellyachers.

CONSTIPATION

Constipation is defined as pain, difficulty or delay in defecation. The constipated child presents a difficult but important challenge to the paediatrician. Constipation is not a glamorous subject. The children are not easy to love, the families exhibit strained relationships, and unfortunately few health professionals have the time or inclination to intervene before the situation becomes critical. It is vital to nip constipation in the bud, otherwise the rectum will become dilated and atonic. The treatment depends on the cause and the cause can be found by taking a good history. The following questions are mandatory at the consultation:

- Did the problem begin at birth and, if not, when did it start?
- What exactly does the mother mean by constipation?
- Does the infant/child pass large rocks of stool resulting in rectal bleeding?
- What does the child eat?
- Is the child thriving?

The examination should concentrate on recording growth on the centile charts, looking for signs of anaemia, palpation of the abdomen and a gentle but careful rectal examination.

The definition of constipation is far from rigid but, clearly, babies who strain, go red in the face and then pass a normal stool are not constipated, despite the insistence of their mothers. At the other extreme, some children hardly pass any stool apart from a few pellets and they may have stool palpable up to the level of the umbilicus; they are indeed constipated.

It should be clear from the history and examination what causes need to be considered. Hirschsprung's disease usually presents in the neonatal period, but a short aganglionic segment may cause chronic problems later. Recurrent abdominal distension with infrequent passage of stool in the first months of life demands investigation. Rectal biopsy in experienced hands is an outpatient procedure and a better screening test for Hirschsprung's disease than a barium enema. A more common problem is simple anal stenosis, which can only be diagnosed by rectal examination. This condition responds to anal dilatation.

Constipated children may present with diarrhoea which in reality is gross constipation with overflow. These children are so obstructed that only liquid stool can slip round the impacted faeces; this is termed 'spurious diarrhoea'.

Treatment

Having excluded the above treatable causes, it is extremely important to counsel the mother, and the child if old enough. The first step to be taken is to establish a quality diet. It helps to explain that constipation is unknown in, say, African countries but that constipation is extremely common on the milk and low fibre diets favoured by European toddlers. Appropriate cereals, fruit and vegetables and pasta are acceptable foods to most children and lead to a 'good quality' stool. Many constipated children strain ineffectively, pushing hard with levator muscles but not relaxing the lower sphincter. This failure to relax may be a primary phenomenon but may also arise from fear of pain due to stretching of the anus with hard stools. This is where explanation of the role of stool softeners is needed. Each child is an individual as regards the dose but conservative use of laxatives is a cause of failure. Lactulose is the most popular stool softener, the dose ranging from 5 ml at night to 20 ml twice daily. If the stool is soft but the bowel not contractile, senna or another bowel stimulant would be appropriate. From this point onwards, if the child is impacted with faeces, a day case admission may be expedient. There are protocols for dealing with situations which have not responded to lactulose and senna. Sodium picosulphate (Picolax), which is a sachet of powder dissolved in water, is quite powerful and is used as a bowel preparation before surgery or radiology. Finally, polyethylene glycol (Klean-Prep or Go-litely) is the last resort for the oral route. The volume necessary is so great that it has to be administered by nasogastric tube. It is unlikely that further measures would be required, but enemas and manual evacuation under anaesthetic could be used in gross faecal impaction. When the dilated bowel has been emptied, lactulose and senna are restarted in good doses. The child should be seen weekly and parents must be taught to adjust the dose of laxatives to ensure the passage of a softish stool at least every other day.

It is always preferable to use the oral route to treat constipation. Children do not like the suppositories which may be appropriate for babies. They certainly do not appreciate enemas, which are an unpleasant experience for all concerned.

Constipation in the pre-school child is associated with fear by the child and stress by the parents. Overflow incontinence secondary to constipation in the school age child is socially disastrous. This is an important topic and one which the medical profession must get right.

RECTAL BLEEDING

The three most important factors which determine the significance of rectal bleeding are:

1. the age of the child
2. the period of the bleeding
3. whether the bleeding is associated with diarrhoea or constipation.

For instance, necrotising enterocolitis occurs only in the newborn, and inflammatory bowel disease principally in the older child. From a diagnostic point of view, the classification is simplified by the length of the symptoms, so the causes are divided into acute or chronic.

Acute rectal bleeding

In the newborn (GP Overview 6.5)

Swallowed maternal blood should in theory present as melaena but it is surprisingly red and dramatic. It causes temporary anxiety but the diagnosis is not difficult. There is usually a history of maternal antepartum or significant intrapartum haemorrhage. As maternal and fetal haemoglobin are chemically distinguishable, the type of blood can be distinguished in the biochemistry laboratory (Apt's test).

Necrotising enterocolitis is a condition which to all intent and purposes is restricted to the premature baby. It presents as abdominal distension with the passing of mucus and blood. The most vulnerable babies are those who are recovering from a period of intensive care and in whom oral nutrition is being established. The diagnosis is made radiologically by the finding of intramural gas in the small or large bowel. The condition may be mild and restricted to a small segment of bowel, in which case conservative management with intravenous fluids and broad spectrum antibiotic cover is sufficient. At the other extreme, the whole of the gut can be affected in which case there is no hope of recovery. At surgery, bubbles of gas may be visible to the naked eye. Death occurs from perforation and septic shock. Many cases fall between the two ends of the spectrum and present a challenge to the neonatologist and the paediatric surgeon. The skill lies in knowing when medical management has failed and surgery has something to offer. Surgery with resection of necrotic bowel may indeed be life-saving, but large segments of bowel may need to be removed, leaving the children with diarrhoea and malabsorption at follow-up. No single infectious agent has been implicated and many aetiologies have been suggested. The major theory is that the cause is linked with feeding an immature ischaemic bowel too quickly. Although it is not a condition seen outside hospitals, it is an important cause of neonatal mortality and morbidity and one of which family doctors should be aware.

Haemorrhagic disease of the newborn (see Chapter 3) may present as isolated rectal bleeding, though in severe cases there are other bleeding points as this is a general coagulopathy.

Outside the newborn period (GP Overview 6.5)

Anal fissure. It would be unusual for there to be a large bleed from an anal fissure. The bleeding would be at the time of passing a stool and not in between. Visual inspection will lead to the diagnosis. Treating the associated constipation leads to cure.

Anal stenosis needs to be considered in chronic cases.

Gastroenteritis presents with mucous and bloody streaking of a diarrhoeal stool.

Intussusception. Outside the newborn, the important differential diagnosis of acute bleeding is bacterial infection or intussusception. The bleeding of an intussusception is associated with mucus production and the passing per rectum of what is described as redcurrant jelly. The symptoms are of intermittent acute abdominal pain with screaming and pallor followed by a period of quietness. Although there may be classical signs of an intussusception with a sausage shaped mass palpable centrally and emptiness of the right iliac fossa, a classical history makes investigation mandatory. In this situation, particularly when the history is short, an experienced radiologist may make the diagnosis and reduce the intussusception with a gastrograffin or air enema. When the history is longer, and the intussusception is irreducible, surgery is necessary (see Chapter 15, p. 323).

Inflammatory bowel disease. Ulcerative colitis may present with acute rectal bleeding although

one would only seriously consider this as the diagnosis if the symptoms became recurrent. The condition can occur in the toddler age group.

Meckel's diverticulum is very rare and is a diagnosis of exclusion. The embryological remnant of gastric mucosa in the midgut can painlessly bleed. The bleeding point may be demonstrated by radioisotope scanning of the abdomen in which a bleeding focus is shown in the ileum. Treatment consists of surgical excision.

Persistent rectal bleeding

It is important to reassure parents that, although the source of the bleeding must be sought, the malignancies which give rise to these symptoms in adults are not found in children. If there is significant rectal bleeding on more than two occasions, unless the cause is an anal fissure, a lower bowel endoscopy is always essential.

Causes (GP Overview 6.5)

The diagnosis of an anal fissure should present no problem providing a good history is taken and a careful examination is made. Assuming that there is no anal stenosis, in which case dilatation is necessary, the treatment consists of curing the constipation with adequate doses of lactulose.

Rectal polyps are uncommon but are a significant cause of bleeding. The presence of a rectal polyp should lead to a colonoscopy in case there are polyps higher up.

Cow's milk allergy (CMA) is a rare cause of rectal bleeding. Cow's milk intolerance more often causes protracted diarrhoea. This type, which is associated with gastrointestinal blood loss, is linked with a low serum copper and albumin and iron deficiency.

Inflammatory bowel disease. Any child from the age of 3 upwards with persistent rectal bleeding and ill health could have Crohn's disease or ulcerative colitis. The symptoms overlap, and the final diagnosis may not always be clear despite extensive investigations.

Ulcerative colitis. This presents as bloody diarrhoea, classically in the teenager but occasionally are the extra-gastrointestinal manifestations. Investigations include full blood count, liver function, orosomucoids and acute phase reactants such as CRP or ESR. A low serum albumin, raised CRP and anaemia are common. Barium enema shows superficial ulceration and loss of haustrations. The rectum is always affected. The bowel is continuously affected, in contrast to the patchy pathology of Crohn's disease.

Remission is induced with prednisolone 2 mg/kg/day for 4–6 weeks. Maintenance of the remission is achieved with sulphasalazine in a dose of 30–50 mg/kg/day. Most children have long remissions on this regime. Surgery is indicated for 2 weeks of failed medical treatment, massive haemorrhage or toxic megacolon; it may also be necessary for chronically relapsing ulcerative colitis. There is an increased risk of malignancy of 4% between 10 and 20 years from the onset of the disease.

Crohn's disease. The history, symptoms and signs may be indistinguishable from ulcerative colitis, hence the classical presentation is abdominal pain and rectal bleeding. These symptoms may not be so severe as in ulcerative colitis. Crohn's disease has a habit of being more difficult to diagnose, the presentation often being growth failure, general ill health and even behavioural changes. It is common for the families of children with Crohn's disease to complain of a 1-–2-year delay in making the diagnosis.

Investigations include:

1. full blood count and ESR or plasma viscosity
2. a biochemical profile looking at plasma proteins and liver function
3. serum CRP and orosomucoids
4. barium follow-through looking for stricture formation (Crohn's)
5. lower bowel endoscopy.

Crohn's disease is more common in northern Europeans with an incidence of 4:100 000. Any part of the gastrointestinal tract may be affected: 50% of the cases are ileocaecal. The general manifestations include clubbing, perianal fissure, oral ulceration, uveitis and a general arthritis. Barium follow-through studies show dilated small bowel proximal to narrowed segments.

in children as young as 3 years old. Unlike Crohn's disease, the symptoms are primarily gastrointestinal. Asymmetric joint involvement in the lower limbs, erythema nodosum and renal stones

The treatment of Crohn's disease is not significantly different to that of ulcerative colitis with the use of systemic steroids and sulphasalazine in the same doses. Recent work has focused on the success of elemental diets to induce remission; the involvement of a paediatric dietician is obligatory. These diets are very unpalatable. If sulphasalazine fails, metronidazole should be tried. Nutrition requires supplementation with folic acid, zinc and magnesium. In very severe cases, total parental nutrition is advised. Surgery is indicated for failure of medical management.

Both ulcerative colitis and Crohn's disease are so unusual and difficult to manage that only paediatric gastroenterologists should supervise the follow-up. Prognosis is very variable with complete cure or chronic relapse.

FOOD INTOLERANCE

Allergy to food and, in particular, to cow's milk may mean different things to doctors and certainly to parents. It is therefore helpful to distinguish allergy from intolerance. A classic example of food allergy is the anaphylactic reaction to peanut in which, because of a massive release of histamine, a child can have a life-threatening type I allergic reaction. There are many other foods which give rise to mild or severe urticaria in sensitive individuals but few which cause anaphylaxis. Usually, the connection with the food is more vague, and intolerance is a better term. Cow's milk can certainly cause anaphylaxis but usually the problems are:

- vomiting
- diarrhoea
- failure to thrive because of an enteropathy
- anaemia and blood loss
- constipation
- eczema.

Cow's milk allergy (CMA)

In atopic individuals with a family history of CMA, allergy to cow's milk may be primary with a severe reaction on first or second exposure. Typically, there is severe vomiting and diarrhoea each time an attempt is made to introduce formula feeds to a breast fed baby. No investigations are necessary and alternative milks should be used when breast milk is no longer available or appropriate. For convenience, all the milk companies manufacture a soya milk. There are theoretical reasons for using a modified cow's milk preparation such as Pregestemil (Mead Johnson) or Pepti Junior (Cow and Gate) as soya can be antigenic and babies with severe CMA may develop soya allergy. In practice, soya milks are easily available and cheap.

Secondary CMA/intolerance following an attack of acute gastroenteritis is more common. This manifests as diarrhoea each time cow's milk is reintroduced. If the diarrhoea recurs early in the reintroduction and is associated with vomiting, this is likely to be true cow's milk allergy (a reaction to cow's milk protein). If the diarrhoea occurs only when full strength feeds are reintroduced, it may be lactose intolerance. Nowadays, the distinction is academic as early management is the same for both conditions. All the substitute milks, whether soya or casein hydrolysate based, are free from cow's milk protein and lactose. It is common practice to use the hydrolysed casein milks such as Pregestemil when the symptoms are gastrointestinal. Opinions differ about how long the infant should stay free from cow's milk. If it is a secondary intolerance based on unconvincing evidence, a cautious cow's milk challenge can be done at home after a month. If the evidence is convincing or the allergy was primary, such challenges may be risky and should be performed in hospital. A small amount of cow's milk is offered under close supervision; over 24 hours the amount is slowly increased. RAST tests, measuring milk antibodies, and skin tests to assess immediate hypersensitivity are only helpful if the history is unclear. In addition an eosinophilia in the peripheral blood and a high IgE are supportive findings. Even then there are many false positives, particularly in atopic individuals. As in the case of coeliac disease, a true enteropathy develops in longstanding CMA. The histology is similar but the pathology more patchy.

The relationship between cow's milk and eczema is more controversial and the link with infant colic even more tenuous. Investigations play no role and the history is paramount.

Gluten intolerance in the form of coeliac disease is a permanent condition, but 20 years ago, when it was common to give gluten-containing foods early in weaning, a severe temporary gluten intolerance was common. This entailed rechallenging later in childhood any baby diagnosed as intolerant to gluten under the age of 12 months. Nowadays, it is advised that gluten be offered at a later age and the associated reduction of the temporary gluten intolerance gives the impression that coeliac disease is less common.

LIVER DISEASE IN CHILDHOOD

Liver disease in children is very rare. The average family doctor is unlikely to come across a child with liver problems apart from cases of hepatitis A. Nevertheless, it is important to understand what can be done for children with liver disease now that transplantation offers a real alternative to death in early childhood. The most important message is that persistent jaundice in babies needs investigation.

Neonatal hepatitis or biliary atresia
(see also p. 56)

Physiological jaundice is common in the newborn; when babies go home within the first 24 hours, GPs will come across jaundiced babies. What is meant by persistent jaundice? If, after 2 weeks of life, obvious jaundice persists, the situation needs careful assessment. If the baby is healthy, particularly if it is breast fed, and the stool retains the yellow, mustard or even green normal colour, investigations are not urgent. There should be no bile in the urine. In doubtful cases, liver function tests can be performed to measure the conjugated component of the jaundice.

A baby with liver problems will switch from the healthy yellow colour of physiological jaundice to the greener bile-stained yellow of an

---

> **Box 6.7** Causes of neonatal hepatitis
>
> - Metabolic, e.g. galactosaemia, tyrosinosis or other amino acid problem
> - Congenital viral infection—toxoplasmosis, rubella, CMV, herpes, hepatitis B (TORCH)
> - α_1-antitrypsin deficiency
> - Cystic fibrosis
> - Idiopathic

obstructive pattern. These babies are usually not thriving, in contrast to the healthy breast fed baby where persistent jaundice is not so unusual. If liver function is abnormal, the baby has either neonatal hepatitis or biliary atresia or, more rarely, a choledochal cyst obstructing the flow of bile. The causes of neonatal hepatitis are listed in Box 6.7. The challenge is to differentiate these causes from biliary atresia before 6 weeks of age. This is because the only treatment available for biliary atresia at this age is a portogastroenterostomy—a surgical procedure named after the Japanese surgeon Kasai. The Kasai procedure is palliative but buys several years of valuable growth until liver transplantation is possible. Ascending cholangitis is a common postoperative complication caused by organisms from the bowel getting into the biliary system.

Investigations which should be performed in babies with abnormal liver function are listed in Box 6.8. The liver can be imaged with CT scanning or, more usually, by ultrasound looking

---

> **Box 6.8** Investigations in babies with abnormal liver function
>
> **Blood**
> - Amino acids
> - α_1-antitrypsin and phenotype
> - Galactose-1-uridyl transferase levels
> - Viral titres:
>   —hepatitis B
>   —herpes
>   —toxoplasmosis
>   —cytomegalovirus (CMV)
>   —rubella
>
> **Urine**
> - Amino acids
> - CMV isolation
> - Reducing substances

for a gallbladder and the presence of adequate bile canaliculi within the liver. Bile flow can be assessed by nuclear medicine scanning with an isotope called HIDA which is given intravenously, taken up by the liver and excreted into the bile. The uptake of HIDA into the bile is stimulated by the administration of phenobarbitone to the baby 3 days before the test.

Despite all these tests, the diagnosis is not always clear; liver biopsy and even laparotomy may be necessary to exclude biliary atresia.

When the diagnosis has been made, there follows a long period of supportive care. Whatever the aetiology of the liver disease, the aim of follow-up is to ensure adequate nutrition and growth. This may involve overnight nasogastric tube feeding to give the necessary high calorie diet. Supplementation with vitamins A, D, E and K is important. Cholestyramine is necessary to bind bile acids and prevent diarrhoea. Liver transplantation is feasible from one year if the infant is well grown, but is better performed later.

If the diagnosis is neonatal hepatitis, the prognosis depends on the cause. Specific conditions will respond to treatment. Galactosaemia is treated with a lactose free diet. The children should remain lactose and galactose free at least into their teens. The outlook is good but IQ and fertility are suboptimal on long-term follow-up. The jaundice which is linked with cystic fibrosis is not so much a neonatal hepatitis but is more associated with a sluggish enterohepatic circulation. The disorders of amino acid metabolism are mainly treated with specific diets. The treatment of tyrosinosis is vastly improved since the use of NTBC. Liver disease associated with α_1-antitrypsin deficiency carries a worse prognosis and may rapidly lead to cirrhosis which can only be treated with transplantation.

The rare liver enzyme deficiencies may or may not be associated with liver dysfunction. Gilbert's disease, caused by deficiency of gluceronyl transferase, is mild and familial. The jaundice may only be clinically obvious at times of stress such as infection. Crigler–Najjar syndrome is more severe, the levels of unconjugated bilirubin being high enough to endanger the child's develop-

ment. These children have even been treated with home phototherapy.

Liver problems in the older child

Not all liver problems present as jaundice, and not all causes of hepatomegaly imply liver dysfunction. Apparent hepatomegaly is often observer error. In a compliant child or a child with soft abdominal musculature, it is easy to palpate the liver two fingers' breadth below the costal margin. It may be possible to tip the spleen. It is more the texture of the liver that is important. Causes of hepatomegaly are listed in Box 6.9.

Acute hepatitis

Hepatitis A (HAV)

Hepatitis A virus (HAV) is an RNA virus spread by faecal–oral transmission. In developed countries the incidence is falling. Blood product transmission is very rare as is vertical transmission (mother to fetus). The incubation period is between 2 and 6 weeks. Children usually have a mild illness with anorexia, nausea and vomiting; many cases are asymptomatic or without jaundice (anicteric). The illness normally lasts from 2–4 weeks and the characteristically elevated serum transaminases (AST/ALT) return to normal levels after this time.

Rarely cholestatic hepatitis occurs; fulminant hepatitis is extremely rare. Confirmation of the diagnosis depends on serological tests for IgM anti-HAV (antibody to hepatitis A virus). No

---

Box 6.9 Causes of hepatomegaly

- Haemolytic anaemia such as sickle cell disease or thalassaemia
- Leukaemia or other malignancy
- Storage disorders such as glycogen storage or Gaucher's disease
- Hepatitis—acute or chronic
- Wilson's disease
- Reye's syndrome
- Portal hypertension, perhaps linked with hepatic vein thrombosis in the neonatal period

specific treatment is required apart from bed rest; dietary restrictions are not necessary. Hospital admission is not required unless the hepatitis is severe. Contacts can be given HNIG (human normal immunoglobulin) as prophylaxis.

Hepatitis B (HBV)

Hepatitis B virus (HBV) is a DNA virus with a worldwide prevalence. In the Far East 80% of children have been infected by the time they reach adolescence. The incubation period is long—between 45 and 160 days. The routes of transmission include:

- perinatal transmission from carrier mothers (? breast feeding also)
- exposure to blood (blood transfusions, needle stick injuries)
- family contacts.

Perinatally acquired infection is generally asymptomatic with no obvious jaundice but elevation of ALT and S. bilirubin occurs. The risk of becoming a carrier following infection is very high (90%) in this group. Older children also have a mild, often asymptomatic illness with non-specific symptoms of anorexia, nausea and malaise. The risk of developing carrier status in this group is 10%.

Fulminant hepatitis is very rare (1%) but chronic hepatitis may develop and lead eventually to cirrhosis and primary hepatocellular carcinoma. The diagnosis depends on positive serological tests for HBV antigens and IgM antibodies to the core antigen (anti HBc). There is no specific treatment available.

Prevention of hepatitis B. All pregnant women should be screened for their hepatitis B status. Babies born to mothers who are HBsAg positive should begin a course of hepatitis B vaccination within 24 hours of birth. Second and third doses are given at 1 month and 6 months of age. If the serology of the mother suggests a higher risk to the infant (e.g. mother is 'e' antigen positive), then the infant should receive also hepatitis B specific immunoglobulin.

Immunisation of at risk individuals. Those at risk of being exposed to hepatitis B, in particular those caring for children, include the following groups:

- household contacts of hepatitis B carriers
- health care workers who have direct contact with blood
- staff/clients of residential accommodation for people with severe learning disabilities
- children with chronic renal failure
- haemodialysis/haemophiliac patients and children receiving repeat blood transfusions; relations involved giving these products.

Hepatitis C RNA virus (non-A, non-B hepatitis)

Hepatitis C virus (HCV) has a worldwide prevalence. Most cases occur either in intravenous drug users or those who received blood transfusions before screening for HCV began (1991). Transmission is via blood transfusions and pre- and perinatal exposure. Needle stick injury can also cause transmission (risk 3–10%).

The incubation period is 6–8 weeks. Most cases are asymptomatic or mild and go on to the carrier state with chronic persistent or chronic active hepatitis; 20–30% of cases develop cirrhosis, and hepatocellular carcinoma is a later complication.

Diagnosis. Serological tests are available for antibodies to hepatitis C (anti-HVC) and interferon treatment is being evaluated.

Hepatitis D (delta hepatitis)

Hepatitis delta virus (HDV) is a defective RNA virus which requires hepatitis B virus for replication. It occurs as a co-infection with hepatitis B virus or as a superinfection in HBsAg positive patients. Chronic infection leads to cirrhosis in 50–70% of cases.

Hepatitis E

Hepatitis E virus is an RNA virus. It causes outbreaks of hepatitis in developing countries. Transmission is via food or water, although person to person spread via the faecal–oral route does occur.

Diagnosis relies on the detection of IgM or IgG

antibodies using ELISA. No specific treatment or vaccine is available.

Infectious mononucleosis

This infection may cause hepatitis in about 40% of cases and is usually asymptomatic. Rarely fulminant hepatitis occurs.

Cytomegalovirus

Cytomegalovirus infection may also cause hepatitis.

Chronic active hepatitis

This condition presents in all ages but in children it is seen mainly in the teenage years. The symptoms are chronic malaise and ill health. Hepatomegaly and mild jaundice are present clinically and liver function is abnormal. Autoantibodies confirm the auto-immune nature of the disease which may lead to cirrhosis. In girls, there is a link with systemic lupus erythematosus. The diagnosis is confirmed on liver biopsy. Treatment is with prednisolone, 2 mg/kg for one month; each relapse should be treated promptly.

Wilson's disease

Wilson's disease is caused by abnormal copper metabolism. There is increased hepatic copper content and a raised serum copper. Serum caeruloplasmin is low. The presentation may be neurological or hepatic. Occasionally, the condition may be detected by routine eye screening; cases of Wilson's disease have hallmark brown rings in Descemet's membrane in the cornea—Kayser–Fleischer rings. Untreated, the condition is progressive and fatal; however treatment with the chelating agent penicillamine is effective.

Reye's syndrome

Occasionally, a child presents with deepening coma, hypoglycaemia and deranged liver function. This condition seems to follow a viral or gastroenteritis type of illness. The early cases were often related to aspirin; the possible development of Reye's syndrome is the reason why aspirin should not be given to children. The child may not be jaundiced but the pathognomonic laboratory finding is a very high ammonia level. Death is due to cerebral oedema. Although there is no specific therapy, the children can make a full recovery with supportive care; they are best managed in units where intracranial pressure monitoring can be performed.

INFANT FEEDING AND NUTRITION

Breast or bottle

Breast

It is the duty of all health professionals concerned with infant nutrition to encourage and facilitate breast feeding. In countries where there is a significant infant mortality from gastroenteritis, bottle feeding should be strongly discouraged. In the UK, if maternity services have done their best to make breast feeding the first choice and despite this a mother elects to bottle feed, that woman should not be made to feel a second class citizen. If, despite a clear message that breast milk is natural, safer than bottle feeding and that breast feeding promotes bonding, the mother elects to bottle feed, that is her right. The final argument in favour of breast feeding is the recent work showing that babies who are breast fed have a higher IQ at the age of 2. The problem is that bottle feeding is easy for mothers, easy for babies and easy for midwives; an obvious display of formula milks in the maternity unit or the health centre is counterproductive to what we are trying to achieve.

In countries like Africa or India where breast feeding has never been questioned, when there is no choice and the family support is guaranteed, early practical difficulties can be overcome. These difficulties should not be underestimated, and in the UK the health service fails mothers with problems (Box 6.10) by knowing what to do in theory but not putting it into practice.

Although maternity units have lactation sisters, practical tips are to be obtained from organisations such as the National Childbirth Trust

Box 6.10 Causes of failure to breast feed

- A small baby with an inadequate suck
- A high Caesarean section rate causing mothers to be separated from their babies in the first hours which are crucial to bonding
- Lack of privacy in postnatal wards
- Poor technique and practical problems such as sore nipples

Box 6.12 Disadvantages of breast feeding

- Unknown quantity
- Breast milk jaundice
- Infection with CMV/hepatitis/HIV
- Risk of poor weight gain/rickets
- Drugs, e.g. anti-thyroid/anti-metabolites
- Psychological—guilt re failure to establish

(NCT). The main difficulties arise in the first few days. Mothers should be encouraged to put the baby to the breast on demand—that means whenever the baby cries. If the position of the nipple in the mouth is correct, this will not lead to soreness. When the flow of milk has been induced by frequent contact between mother and baby, breast feeding can be said to be established. When there are specific problems which can overwhelm a busy lactation sister, the voluntary organisations play a useful role.

The advantages and disadvantages of breast feeding are listed in Boxes 6.11 and 6.12.

Box 6.11 Advantages of breast feeding

Nutritional
- Whey/casein ratio 60/40, curd easily digestible
- Long chain fatty acids polyunsaturated
- ? IQ factor
- Lower Na^+ load
- Contains lactoferrin (inhibits pathogenic *E. coli* and promotes lactobacilli in gut)
- Enhances structural changes in gut in response to feeding (gut hormones, e.g. insulin, enteroglucagon and motilin)
- Contains cyclic AMP and GMP important for regulation processes of maturation

Anti-infective
- Secretory IgA

Humoral
- Lactoferrin
- Interferon
- Lysozyme

Cellular
- Macrophages
- Lymphocytes

Bonding
- Facilitated

Ease
- Preheated, sterile, prepared

Bottle

All the formula milks are excellent and very similar. They are as near as the manufacturers can get to breast milk in chemical composition. Even the breast milk 'intelligence factor' has now been added. If it is true that breast milk has a specific component which optimises brain nutrition in pregnancy and the first few months of life, that component is now thought to be the long chain polyunsaturated fatty acids (LCPs) which are different in cow's milk to human milk. It is therefore not surprising that the latest 'humanisation' of formula feeds is focused on the type and amounts of these fatty acids. When the baby matures, he has the ability to manufacture LCPs from other fat sources.

All milk companies market a step-up milk for babies who are 'not satisfied'. There is no scientific justification for these milks which contain more casein. More controversial are the even stronger milks which are aimed at the 6–12-month infant with special nutritional needs. These are called follow-on milks and have not yet found their place. If a baby is not thriving and weaning is not progressing, or has ongoing respiratory problems which hamper growth it would be reasonable to use a follow-on formula.

There are no specific difficulties with bottle feeding. Babies with a cleft palate may require a special teat but most cope with standard feeding. There is the potential that a demanding baby will be overfed, leading to obesity.

Basic principles of dietetics

Although doctors may have access to dieticians, it is important to know how much food a baby or infant should take in order to achieve satisfactory growth. A newborn baby takes on average

150 ml/kg per day. Babies feed ad libitum which means they are offered milk only when they are hungry rather than on a rigid 4-hourly regimen. Breast milk and formula milks contain a balanced amount of protein, carbohydrate and fat: 150 ml/kg gives approximately 110 kcal/kg/day (Table 6.3).

As the baby gets older and takes solid food, the fluid intake will diminish and it will not all be milk. By the time the baby is 12 months, he will take only 80 ml/kg/day.

Dietary supplements

If a bottle fed baby does not thrive, the intake can at least be accurately measured. If this is equal to or more than 150 ml/kg per day, it is not a nutritional problem; other factors then enter the diagnosis such as milk intolerance, increased demand such as in severe eczema, or chronic illness as found in the premature baby with chronic lung disease. In the situation where growth is poor because of increased demand or inability to feed due to breathlessness, it is helpful to understand the role of dietary supplements. For the newborn there are two sources of dietary supplements—carbohydrate and fat.

Carbohydrate supplements

Sugar or glucose is likely to cause diarrhoea or over-sweeten the milk. Glucose polymers provide 4 kcal/g without sweetening the milk and only increase the osmotic load presented to the bowel by a small amount. If the calorie content of milk is approximately 70 kcal per 1000 ml, addition of 2–4 g of a glucose polymer increases the intake by 8–16 kcal per 1000 ml. These supplements are easily given and available on prescription; an example is Maxijul.

Table 6.3 Content of milk

Food	Energy
1 g protein	4 kcal
1 g carbohydrate	4 kcal
1 g fat	9 kcal

Fat supplements

The family doctor is unlikely to initiate supplementary fat feeding: these babies require investigation and the skills of the paediatric dietician. The proportion of fat to carbohydrate as a fuel is important. Fat is an energy rich supplement, 1 g providing 9 kcal; too much fat however can cause ketosis which leads to vomiting. The supplement Calogen is a mixture of fatty acids. For convenience, a combined glucose polymer/fat supplement can be used (Duocal).

Vitamin and mineral supplements

Breast fed babies up to the age of 6 months do not need added vitamins if the health and nutrition of the mother is good. After 6 months, they need vitamins A and D. Formula fed infants do not need vitamin supplements before 6 months. After 6 months, if their intake of milk is small or they are being given ordinary cow's milk, they should also be given vitamins A and D. After the age of one year there are no routine recommendations, but so many children eat very badly in the 'terrible twos' that a supplement containing vitamins A, C and D as a minimum should be given every day.

The following minerals are important and deficiency may cause symptoms: calcium, phosphorus, magnesium, sodium, potassium, chloride, zinc, copper, selenium and iodine. Calcium is found mainly in milk, so children on milk exclusion diets for cow's milk intolerance will require supplemental calcium.

Iron deficiency – see page 278.

Vitamin D deficiency. Rickets is uncommon these days though it is still seen in infants who are not weaned by the age of 18 months. It is less common in the white population and more common in Asian or black children. Breast milk is adequate as the sole source of vitamin D for 6 months. After that, deficiency will depend on the nutrition of the mother and the amount of sunshine to which the infant is exposed. There are no symptoms except those associated with other deficiencies such as iron. The infant may therefore be lethargic. The signs are bowing of the legs, splaying of the wrists and ankles, and

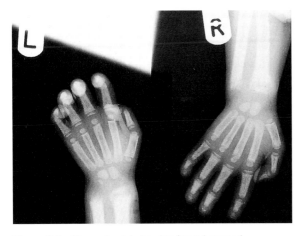

Figure 6.2 X-ray of wrist showing frayed cupped epiphyses ('champagne glass') appearance in rickets.

cupping and fraying of metaphyses (Figure 6.2). Additional signs include craniotabes, frontal bossing, 'rickety rosary', hypotonia and seizures. Diagnosis is confirmed by X-ray, a raised alkaline phosphatase in the blood and a low blood level of vitamin D_3 (25-hydroxycalciferol). The condition can be prevented by weaning onto cow's milk, fortified cereals and bread, fish and vegetables. Treatment is with vitamin D supplements. Unfortunately, the only liquid preparation available is 1,25-dihydroxycholecalciferol (alphacalcidol), 500 ng/day. It works well but is primarily aimed at treating rickets with a renal cause when the kidneys cannot convert 25-hydroxy vitamin D to the 1,25-dihydroxy vitamin D stage. The prognosis is excellent, with full recovery of the bones within 6 months.

Weaning

Weaning is the introduction of foods alternative to milk which provide the full range of nutrients appropriate for the infant's age. It is a gradual process, beginning at approximately 4 months and reaching completion by the age of 2 years. One would expect that a 2-year-old would have three meals a day; whilst milk might provide some nutrition, most would come from solid food. Sadly, in the UK, this is not the case. The reasons for food refusal and poor diets are com-

plex, but many infants persist in their reliance on milk well into infancy giving rise to iron deficiency, constipation and possibly behavioural disorders. The model mother begins with non-wheat cereal, pureed fruit such as banana or apple, and pureed vegetables such as carrot or mashed potato. In contrast the more typical mother buys commercial instant 'wet' tins or jars, having neither the time nor the inclination to prepare pureed versions of family food. In the hurried and inexperienced environment of modern family life, tolerance, understanding and patience are lacking and mothers give way to demands for milk feeds and the junk food which is readily accepted by the toddlers. There is no easy solution; we cannot turn back the clock, and today's children have to fit in with the pace of society and the inexperience of the modern family. Nevertheless, an understanding of the cause of food refusal and inadequate diets helps health professionals understand the problems even if they cannot provide an instant solution. Progress can only be made by health visitors providing practical advice in the home and a firm consistent approach by all members of the family.

Obesity

The hospital paediatrician has no role to play apart from differentiating pathological causes of obesity from simple or constitutional causes. Trying to slim fat children is a waste of time. Children who have simple obesity are relatively tall for their age and parental height. Their bone ages are marginally advanced. Children with syndromes such as Prader–Willi or growth hormone deficiency are short and the parents are not necessarily fat.

Fat children need understanding, sympathy and love. Unfortunately, either the obesity gene runs in the family or everyone eats too much at home. As a result, there is little incentive to take exercise or seriously cut down on intake because the whole family has to get involved. If the children are teased, and are then reprimanded in the obesity clinic, life becomes intolerable for them. If any health professional—whether in general practice, the community or the hospital—has the energy to run an obesity clinic, its aims should be simple. Weight reduction is unrealistic—not gaining weight should be the goal. A dietician should be involved but there is a limited number of times that the same message can be given. The only hope is that some rapport may be established between the child and the doctor so that the child has an incentive to please and the doctor has the enthusiasm to motivate.

At the end of the day, even if weight gain continues unabated or the family default from the clinic, all that matters is that the child was understood; there is no need to feel that we have failed.

FURTHER READING

Tripp J, Candy D 1992 Manual of paediatric gastroenterology and nutrition. Heinemann, Oxford

7

Genetic disease and congenital disorders in primary care

Michael Modell

Genetics is becoming more and more relevant to the practice of paediatrics, both in hospital and in the community.

About 10% of the population carry (are heterozygotes for) one of the common inherited disorders. Though carriers can be very common, individual inherited diseases are rare in most ethnic groups (for example, cystic fibrosis affects about 1 in 2000 infants), but collectively these disorders affect many people and have a disproportionate impact on the family and the medical services because they tend to be chronic and severe. In addition a genetic disorder in one family member often means that relatives and future children are at risk. It is increasingly possible to detect and advise carriers of inherited diseases, both in the general population and within affected families, and to detect and advise individuals with a genetic predisposition to premature onset of coronary heart disease or some forms of cancer.

GENES

Most of our physical characteristics are dictated by genes contained in the 23 pairs of chromosomes. For each characteristic, there is one gene from the individual's mother and one from the father. Each chromosome contains a single long strand of DNA. This is made of two paired chains of nucleotides, associated with binding proteins. Each nucleotide of DNA (Figure 7.1) is composed of one of four possible nitrogenous bases—adenine (A), guanine (G), cytosine (C), or

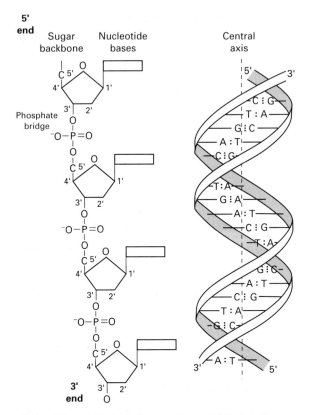

Figure 7.1 Right, the helical structure of DNA. Left, the chemical structure of DNA.

thymine (T)—plus a sugar (deoxyribose) and a phosphate ion. The phosphate ion forms a bridge between the sugar molecules from which the bases protrude. Two strands are joined face to face along their length by hydrogen bonds in such a way as to lead them to form a spiral—the double helix. Each base can pair only with one other base: A with T and C with G. DNA duplicates before cells divide, the two strands separate, and each is used as a template by the enzyme DNA polymerase to make a new complementary strand. Genes are the sections of the DNA molecule where one strand carries the code for a specific protein, three nucleotide bases coding for one amino acid. These coding sequences only comprise about 2% of all the DNA. Each nucleated cell contains the complete genetic code for the organism, probably 50 000–100 000 genes.

In order to direct the synthesis of a protein, the coding sequences of the relevant gene are copied to produce the single stranded messenger RNA (mRNA). This then moves out of the nucleus into the cytoplasm and binds to ribosomes which contain the machinery for protein synthesis. The smaller transfer RNA (tRNA) brings the appropriate amino acids to this complex, and this is followed by production of the corresponding protein.

Mutations and congenital abnormalities

Mutations are alterations in the structure or arrangement of DNA or chromosomes. Those that arise in somatic cells affect only the person in whom they occur. Somatic mutations occur frequently, most are corrected spontaneously, and a few eventually lead to cancer or some other disease. Mutations in germ cells (ova and sperm) can be passed on to succeeding generations. Mutations within genes can interfere with production of the relevant proteins, with the result that a protein is not made at all, is manufactured in too small a quantity, or malfunctions.

Congenital abnormalities (malformations) are more common than inherited diseases, though some (about 10%) are inherited in a Mendelian fashion. Major malformations affect about 2% of newborn infants. Many more have minor or moderate abnormalities such as birthmarks or anomalies of the fingers or toes. Some abnormalities will only be diagnosed later in infancy, as when a renal abnormality is discovered following a urinary tract infection, or when a cardiac problem is diagnosed because a murmur is heard at the 6-week check-up. Only a minority of congenital abnormalities are the result of environmental factors such as infections, drugs or maternal disease. If genetic disease and congenital abnormalities are taken together, it has been estimated that about half can be either prevented or effectively treated (Table 7.1).

Mendelian inheritance

Classical patterns of inheritance are illustrated in Figure 7.3. If two or more relatives have the

Table 7.1 Prevention of congenital abnormalities (or their effects). Source: Modell et al 1996, by permission of Oxford University Press.

Preventive measure	Examples
Avoiding abnormalities by pre-conception care	Malformations in diabetes Fetal alcohol syndrome Congenital rubella Spina bifida (folic acid)
Early detection by screening in pregnancy including ultrasound, followed by prenatal diagnosis and selective abortion	Haemoglobin disorders Cystic fibrosis Down's syndrome Many structural abnormalities (for example, heart)
Medical treatment following neonatal screening	Phenylketonuria Congenital hypothyroidism
Early paediatric surgery following ultrasound in pregnancy or clinical examination of the newborn	Some heart or renal abnormalities Undescended testes; hypospadias Inguinal hernia

same disease, especially if they come from more than one generation, this suggests that the condition is dominant or X-linked. People with a recessively inherited disease seldom have a family history unless they belong to a society in which consanguineous marriage is common. The condition may of course recur in a sibling.

RECESSIVELY INHERITED CONDITIONS

We all carry one or more genes for a recessively inherited disorder, but these disorders can become apparent only when an individual inherits two genes for the same condition from both parents. On average, 25% of the offspring of carrier couples will have the disorder, 50% will be healthy carriers, and 25% will not have the mutant gene at all. Some recessively inherited diseases are common because carriers are more likely to survive than non-carriers and therefore have an evolutionary advantage; for example, between 3 and 25% of many Asian and African populations carry a haemoglobin disorders (sickle cell or thalassaemia) because carriers have increased resistance to malaria, their red blood cells being inhospitable to the malaria parasite.

In rare instances there may be problems for carriers; thalassaemia carriers for example have small hypochromic red blood cells and often a somewhat low haemoglobin, so they are often

mistakenly thought to be iron deficient and are at risk of iatrogenic iron overload.

SOME EXAMPLES OF SINGLE GENE DISORDERS
Cystic fibrosis (CF)

Cystic fibrosis is the most common serious autosomal recessive condition of Causasians, affecting 1 in 2000–3000 in various populations. The CFTR (cystic fibrosis transmembrane conductance regulator) gene on chromosome 7 encodes a protein containing 1480 amino acids which is involved in transmembrane ion transport. At least 350 CF mutations have been identified, but the major one, found in about 70% of cases, is a deletion of three base pairs coding for phenylalanine.

Clinical features – see page 134.

The haemoglobin (Hb) disorders

Adult haemoglobin (HbA) is composed of two α and two β globin chains coded for by genes on chromosomes 11 and 16 as shown in Figure 7.2.

The more common major haemoglobin disorders such as sickle cell disorders (SCD) and homozygous β thalassaemia (thalassaemia major) are caused by β chain abnormalities. However,

Chromosome 11 The beta globin gene cluster

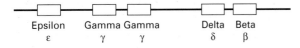

| Epsilon | Gamma | Gamma | | Delta | Beta |
| ε | γ | γ | | δ | β |

Chromosome 16 The alpha gene cluster

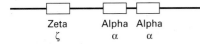

| Zeta | Alpha | Alpha |
| ζ | α | α |

Figure 7.2 The alpha and beta globin gene clusters. *Notes:* Between and even within the genes there are long sequences of DNA that do not code for proteins. The epsilon gene on chromosome 11 and the zeta gene on chromosome 16 are involved in making very early embryonic haemoglobins.

400 or more variants of haemoglobin have so far been identified which are the result of single amino acid substitutions in one of the globin chains. The clinically important **abnormal haemoglobins** (HbS, HbC, HbE, HbD) are caused by different point mutations in the coding sequences of the β globin gene that cause structural and charge changes in the haemoglobin molecule. In sickle haemoglobin (HbS) the amino acid valine is substituted for glutamic acid at position 6 of the β globin chain. The thalassaemias are caused by reduced or absent production of one of the globin chains of haemoglobin. The haemoglobin that is produced has a normal structure. Over 100 different mutations have been shown to cause β thalassaemia, and the clinical severity of the disease depends to some extent on the underlying mutation. Normally there are two functioning α genes on each chromosome 16. In α⁺ thalassaemia one is deleted, but the condition is nearly always harmless, since even in homozygous α⁺ thalassaemia plenty of α globin is still made and there is only a slight reduction in haemoglobin level. This condition is common in people of Indian or African origin. By contrast, in α⁰ thalassaemia both α genes are deleted from the same chromosome, and this mutation involves a serious genetic risk. Carriers are healthy, but homozygous α⁰ thalassaemia causes stillbirth or neonatal death. This form of thalassaemia occurs in South East Asians and Cypriots.

Sickle cell disorders (SCD)

Sickle cell disorders affect approximately 5000 people of African–Caribbean and occasionally Asian origin in the UK. HbS undergoes polymerisation in the deoxygenated state, causing red blood cells to become crescent-shaped (sickle). Sickled cells can cause blockage of small blood vessels in various tissues including bone and spleen. The deformed red blood cells are destroyed and removed from the circulation, leading to chronic haemolytic anaemia with a raised reticulocyte count. The children are normal at birth and the symptoms of sickle cell disease usually appear after 6 months of age as the concentration of fetal haemoglobin (HbF) falls to be replaced by HbSS rather than HbAA. Affected children have a baseline haemoglobin concentration of between 7 and 11 g/dl, may be slightly jaundiced, and have a palpable spleen. By later childhood the spleen usually becomes impalpable because of repeated infarction. Folic acid requirements are increased due to chronic haemolysis, and supplements should be given.

β Thalassaemia

The thalassaemias are caused by reduced or absent production of one of the globin chains of haemoglobin. The most common form, homozygous β thalassaemia (thalassaemia major), is caused by underproduction of β globin chains. A pale languid child, usually of Mediterranean, Middle Eastern, Asian or African ancestry, presents in the first year of life (Hb concentration 4–7 g/100 ml) with an enlarged liver and spleen.

Carrier detection

Carriers of Hb disorders can be easily identified by conventional blood tests using a 5 ml sample of blood sent to the laboratory with a request for a 'haemoglobinopathy screen'. β thalassaemia trait results in microcytosis (MCH 19–27 pg, normal range 27–32 pg) with a raised HbA_2 (> 3.5%). The main differential diagnosis is iron deficiency, when the HbA_2 is normal and the serum ferritin reduced. The sickle cell mutation

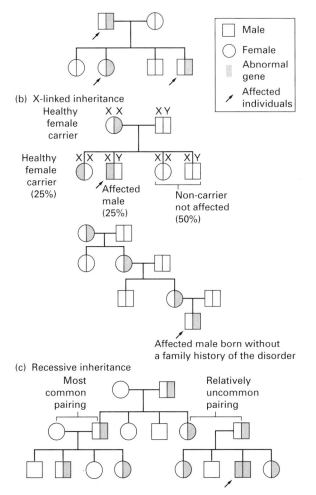

(a) Dominant inheritance

Male
Female
Abnormal gene
Affected individuals

(b) X-linked inheritance

Healthy female carrier   X X   X Y

Healthy female carrier (25%)   X|X   X|Y   X|X   X|Y
Affected male (25%)   Non-carrier not affected (50%)

Affected male born without a family history of the disorder

(c) Recessive inheritance

Most common pairing   Relatively uncommon pairing

Figure 7.3 Classical patterns of Mendelian inheritance. Carrier (heterozygote) status is shown by shaded half-symbols throughout. The arrows indicate individuals who have, or may develop, the disease.

causes a charge change which makes it easy to separate HbS by electrophoresis.

Adolescence

Adolescence is likely to be a particularly difficult time for young people with longstanding severe chronic diseases such as cystic fibrosis and the haemoglobin disorders. There may be problems with compliance with treatment (the most common cause of death in young adults with

thalassaemia). In some conditions (thalassaemia, cystic fibrosis, occasionally sickle cell disease) delayed puberty and infertility can cause enormous stress. Early hormone replacement therapy is important, both to accelerate puberty and to lessen the likelihood of osteoporosis. In young adults referral to a reproductive endocrinologist is often indicated, as various methods of assisted reproduction may need to be considered.

Support associations are a vital source of information and social support. Many families are helped by sharing their problems with others who have had similar experiences, though they may need to be warned that at branch meetings they may meet individuals with particularly severe disease. The associations also often support research, and campaign for extra resources.

X-LINKED DISORDERS

In females, mutant genes carried on the X chromosome usually have a recessive mode of inheritance. However, because half of a female's X chromosomes are randomly inactivated, there may be a mild biochemical abnormality. The frequency of clinical manifestations in females varies from less than 10% in haemophilia to 30% in the fragile X syndrome. Males have only one X chromosome, so the genes on it are 'dominant'; thus it is males who usually suffer from X-linked disorders. Carrier females are usually related to a known affected male, but there may be no affected relatives, because either the woman carries a new mutation or has inherited the abnormal gene in the female line, without a known affected male. Reliable identification of carriers is usually possible using DNA methods. This means that prenatal diagnosis is often feasible, and that 50% of sisters of the index case can be shown not to be carriers and can be reassured.

X-linked diseases include haemophilia from factor VIII deficiency, affecting about 1 in 5000 to 10 000 males, and Duchenne muscular dystrophy (DMD). Children with DMD present with delay in walking or falls, characteristically using their arms to 'climb up' their legs. The gene responsible, and its protein product dystrophin, have been identified. DMD has an incidence of about 1 in 3500 males and results in increasing muscular weakness, hypertrophy of muscles such as those of the calves, a usually fairly mild mental impairment and death from respiratory failure around the age of 20. Diagnosis involves DNA studies and measurement of the serum creatine kinase (50–100 times normal).

Fragile X syndrome

The fragile X syndrome probably accounts for 5–10% of undiagnosed cases of boys with severe learning difficulties. It is called fragile X because, in affected individuals, there appears to be a 'fragile' area (it does not take up stain and so looks as if it could break) near the tip of the long arm of the X chromosome.

The pattern of inheritance has puzzled geneticists for some time, as clinically normal males sometimes transmit the full disease to a grandson, and about a third of female carriers are intellectually impaired. The explanation lies in the type of mutation causing the disorder. Fragile X syndrome is the most common example of an inherited disorder, being caused by a multiplication of a normal set of trinucleotide (CGG) repeats within the fragile X mental retardation (FMRI) gene. The full mutation results in hundreds of copies of a normal CGG sequence (Huntington's disease and a number of other inherited disorders affecting the CNS are caused by similar mutations). Interestingly, the full mutation may be inherited by the offspring of an individual who has already got a moderate increase (pre-mutation) of the CGG sequence but is clinically normal. This apparently happens only if the mutation is passed on from a female (rather than a male) carrier of the pre-mutation.

It is now possible, by DNA studies, to identify carriers of this syndrome; the family doctor may consider discussing this test with a woman who has a close relative with severe undiagnosed learning difficulty.

AUTOSOMAL DOMINANT INHERITANCE

Dominantly inherited diseases become apparent when only one of a pair of chromosomes carries the mutation. The children of a person with a dominant disorder have a 50% chance of inheriting the same gene and so developing the disease, though sometimes the gene is not fully expressed. In some affected children the condition arises from a new mutation in the sperm or ovum. The recurrence risk within the family is usually low, because this mutation has not been incorporated into the parent's genetic makeup. New mutations are more common with older parents, especially older fathers. There are, broadly speaking, two groups of dominant disorders—sporadic and familial.

Sporadic disorders. Some disorders, such as severe forms of osteogenesis imperfecta, are not inherited because they cause death in infancy or prevent reproduction. New cases arise from new mutations. Until recently this also applied to about 80% of cases of achondroplasia. Improved obstetric management (Caesarean sections because of a narrow pelvis) has increased the proportion of familial cases.

Familial disorders. These conditions usually cause disease only after reproduction has started, and so are likely to be handed on to offspring. Examples include Huntington's disease (about 1 in 3000 births) and adult polycystic disease of the kidney (1 in 1250).

Familial hypercholesterolaemia (FH)

Dominantly inherited FH often results in very premature death from coronary artery disease, especially in males. It is treatable in the pre-symptomatic phase by means of dietary and lifestyle advice and lipid-lowering drugs such as the statins, that result in a 40% reduction in low density lipoprotein (LDL) cholesterol. FH is usually caused by a mutation in the LDL receptor gene which leads to an increased plasma concentration of this, the major cholesterol transport lipoprotein. The diagnosis is based on a combination of hypercholesterolaemia (often present in childhood) and clinical features such as arcus senilis and tendon xanthomas; these often do not appear until the third decade. There may be a family history of a raised serum cholesterol and/or premature coronary artery disease.

The most cost effective method of case finding appears to be to contact close relatives of index cases. The British Paediatric Association Ethics Advisory Committee (1994) accepted the recommendation that predictive genetic testing is appropriate in childhood if there is effective medical intervention that can be offered. Predictive testing however raises ethical issues, such as the risk of damaging a healthy 'self image', the difficulty in obtaining informed consent for testing from children, and recommending a lifetime of medication and a special diet; the latter is not restricted to genetic disease and would also apply to a child or adolescent who was discovered to have diabetes. Diagnosis is not so urgent for FH, however, so testing should be done at a time when a fully informed family feels able to cope with the consequences.

Neurofibromatosis type 1

This autosomal dominant disorder affects 1 in 3000 people. A third to a half of cases result from new mutations, others are likely to have a positive family history. See page 219.

CHROMOSOMAL ABNORMALITIES

The number and structure of an individual's chromosomes can be examined by growing available cells (e.g. blood lymphocytes, amniotic fluid, skin fibroblasts) until they are actively dividing. Chromosomes in the metaphase of mitosis are then fixed and stained using methods that produce the characteristic banding appearance (*karyotyping*). The 22 pairs of autosomes and two sex chromosomes can be distinguished by their size, the position of the centromere (which divides the chromosome into two arms), and characteristic banding patterns.

About 10% of diagnosed pregnancies have a chromosomally abnormal conceptus. Nine tenths of these die in utero, accounting for over half of first trimester spontaneous abortions. The incidence of abortion and the chance of the birth of

a child with a chromosomal disorder increase with maternal age (Figure 7.4).

There are four different types of chromosomal disorders. The most common is *aneuploidy*, resulting in a fetus in which one or more chromosomes are present in too many or too few copies. It is not surprising that this has a catastrophic effect when one considers the large number of genes in one chromosome. Only the fetus with a less severe abnormality is likely to survive past the first trimester of pregnancy. A fetus with three copies of the small chromosome 21 may be viable, for example, and will have Down's syndrome (see below). In *deletion* a piece of the chromosome breaks off; in *translocation* this piece is transferred to another chromosome. Translocations can be either balanced (correct number

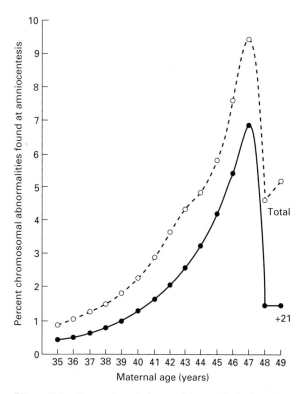

Figure 7.4 Chromosomal abnormalities—data for fetuses at amniocentesis. The incidence at birth is about 30% lower, because of late miscarriage of chromosomally abnormal fetuses. The apparent fall in incidence of fetuses with trisomy 21 (solid line) after maternal age 46 may be an artefact due to small sample size or the result of an increased rate of early miscarriage of chromosomally abnormal fetuses.

of gene copies, but in a different order), or unbalanced (too many or too few genes). Occasionally one arm of a chromosome is lost, and the other one duplicated. Finally, in *mosaicism* one set of body cells has one chromosomal composition, and the other a different one (e.g. Turner mosaic 45X and the normal 46XX). Most chromosomal disorders are the result of new mutation and have a low risk of recurrence. Disorders arising from unbalanced translocations are exceptions: these are inherited from a healthy parent with a balanced translocation.

Down's syndrome

Most children with Down's syndrome are identified at or soon after birth by their characteristic physical appearance, including eyes that slant up, often with prominent epicanthic folds, loose skin on the nape of a short neck, flat occiput, a narrow palate, flat bridge of the nose, short, broad hands and malformed ears. Other features include an increased gap between the first and second toes, incurved fifth finger and Brushfield spots of the iris. There is decreased muscle tone in neonates and infants with Down's syndrome. Trisomy 21 is found in about 75–80% of infants suspected to have Down's syndrome. 40% of affected babies have a congenital heart defect, and gastrointestinal malformations such as duodenal atresia also occur in about 5% of cases. The incidence of acute leukaemia in these children is 10–20 times normal. There is also an increased frequency of hypothyroidism.

It is only possible to give the parents of a Down's baby a range of likely achievements. The intelligence quotient (IQ) is very variable and tends to fall further behind with age. Thus the mean IQ at the age of one year is about 70, falling to 45 at age 3–5 years and 30 six years later. A few Down's individuals have only a moderate learning difficulty, some are profoundly handicapped, and most are in the middle. The median age for speaking in three word sentences is 4 years, compared to 2 years for normal infants. Intellectual attainment is influenced by genetic (intelligence of parents) and environmental (institutional care compared with living at home)

factors. These children often have additional problems such as defects of sight and hearing which may, unless corrected, aggravate their handicap. Males are almost always infertile, but there have been a number of instances of women with Down's syndrome bearing children. Life expectancy has improved significantly in recent decades, and individuals without congenital heart disease may live to the age of 60 years or more. The principal causes of death are infection, heart disease and malignancy. Finally, many Down's individuals develop Alzheimer's dementia at a relatively early age. This has been confirmed by autopsy examinations of the brains of individuals who have lived to more than 40 years of age.

Number of sex chromosomes

A disorder of sex chromosome number is present in about 0.25% of live births. Congenital malformations are usually less frequent and less severe than in autosomal aneuploidies. The IQ may be somewhat below average. The most common are Turner's syndrome (XO, 1 in 3000 female births, but mosaicism is common) and Klinefelter's syndrome (XXY, 1 in 1000 male births). An XO chromosomal make-up is common at conception, accounting for 1–2% of pregnancies. The vast majority of these fetuses abort spontaneously.

MULTIFACTORIAL DISORDERS

Many of the common chronic diseases of adult life cluster in families much more frequently than would be expected than by chance alone. It is likely that conditions such as asthma, diabetes, glaucoma, idiopathic epilepsy, hypertension, manic depression and schizophrenia are the result of the interaction of several genes (polygenic effects) or of genetic and environmental factors (multifactorial effects). The same applies to congenital malformations such as congenital dislocation of the hip, cleft lip and palate, pyloric stenosis, neural tube defect and club foot. Many normal characteristics such as height, blood pressure, intelligence and hair colour are inherited in the same way. The features of this type of inheritance include:

- An empirical 2–10% rate of recurrence in siblings and offspring of an affected person (higher for adult onset mental disorders).
- The more severe the case, the more likely is a positive family history and recurrence in a subsequent pregnancy.
- There is an increased likelihood of recurrence in other relatives, if more than one close relative is affected.
- The risk is highest amongst close relatives of an affected person.
- Some of these conditions are more common in one sex than the other, and children of affected individuals of the less frequently affected sex are more at risk. For example, pyloric stenosis is five times more common in boys than in girls, and a female index patient has a four times greater risk of producing an affected child than a male index patient.

It is often possible to give parents a more exact risk of recurrence by taking account of other information. Some diseases for example are associated with particular HLA types (e.g. ankylosing spondylitis, insulin-dependent diabetes, rheumatoid arthritis and thyrotoxicosis). Offspring of an affected parent who carry the relevant HLA antigen are much more likely to develop the disease in question than those without the antigen.

MITOCHONDRIAL DISORDERS

Cells contain several hundred mitochondria, with their own circular DNA coding for a number of enzymes involved in cell metabolism. Mitochondria are inherited from the mother only, as there are many in oocytes, but sperm leave their cytoplasm outside the ovum after fertilisation. A number of rare diseases exist that are caused by alterations in mitochondrial DNA. They affect both sexes, but are transmitted only by the mother.

GENOME IMPRINTING

This means that certain physical characteristics

(phenotype) of an individual are expressed differently depending on whether a particular gene, or group of genes, was inherited from the father or the mother. In rare cases two copies of part or all of a chromosome originate from one parent and none from the other, perhaps because one chromosome is lost from a trisomy in utero. This is known as uniparental disomy. Examples are the Prader–Willi syndrome (congenital hypotonia and slow development, with hypogonadism, small hands and feet and characteristic facial features), and the Angelman syndrome (fat, hyperactive, happy children with a large mouth and red cheeks and unusual fits). Both result from a deletion of the same part of the proximal long arm of chromosome 15. The transmission of the Prader–Willi syndrome is always paternal, and that of the Angelman syndrome maternal.

GENETIC SCREENING AND PRENATAL DIAGNOSIS

The objective of most current genetic screening programmes is to detect carriers and carrier couples at risk of producing a child with mainly recessively inherited disorders. They are then offered the possibility of prenatal diagnosis. The alternative to screening is to identify couples by waiting until an affected child is born. That seems a pity; most Western European families are small, and genetic advice after an affected birth will deny most couples at risk reproductive choice. A preventive approach is still justified for many of these disorders (not so obviously for sickle cell disease, because of its unpredictable nature), though the prognosis is improving. Most of these disorders often shorten life and the treatment is harrowing.

Until recently, individuals affected by genetic disease and carriers have been biochemically identified by direct analysis of the product of the relevant gene such as haemoglobin (haemoglobin disorders) or by failure of the enzymic step that the product catalyses (phenylketonuria). It is now possible to study abnormal genes directly by analysing DNA from any tissue. Analysis is usually by the polymerase chain reaction (PCR). This is a simple, cheap method of amplifying the target DNA (if present) a million times or more within a few hours. PCR is so sensitive that it can be used to amplify DNA sequences from a single cell, starting with only two copies of the gene in question. In some cases when the relevant mutation is unknown, segments of DNA adjacent to the abnormal gene can be identified; in this case family studies are an essential part of the diagnostic process. With a fatal inherited disease, even if the exact mutation has not yet been identified, it may be of critical importance to subsequent pregnancies in family members to collect a lithium heparin blood sample from an affected patient before death for storage and later DNA analysis. DNA methods have made it possible to make a genetic diagnosis using prenatal diagnosis in the first trimester of pregnancy by chorionic villus sampling (CVS). This is possible for all conditions where the DNA basis is known, and has thus widened the options available for couples at risk. It also greatly reinforces the importance of *early* identification of genetic risk—before, or in very early pregnancy. Fetal cells from CVS divide more rapidly than those obtained from amniocentesis, allowing diagnosis of a chromosomal abnormality after only a few days, rather than waiting two or three weeks.

At the moment most screening is done in antenatal clinics. This is efficient, in that it uses an existing system for collecting specimens and it targets the group (pregnant women) most immediately at risk. However it has a number of disadvantages, the most important being that carrier couples are almost inevitably diagnosed too late for early prenatal diagnosis, and often too late for diagnosis at all in the presenting pregnancy. The ideal would be to detect these couples in primary care, ideally before reproduction, or at least in the first couple of months of pregnancy when they first present to their GP or community midwife. They then have the full range of reproductive options including 'taking the risk', not having children, or opting for early instead of mid-trimester prenatal diagnosis (so

perhaps avoiding a harrowing termination at 20 weeks of pregnancy).

As with all screening programmes, carrier testing should be offered at an appropriate time, the approach should be acceptable to the population at risk, full information should be provided, participation should be voluntary, and distribution of the service equitable. Carrier screening has been well established for many years for thalassaemia, sickle cell and Tay–Sachs disease. The quality of screening programmes for haemoglobin disorders has been shown to be very variable in different parts of the United Kingdom. Many couples at risk for sickle cell disorders are missed, but about 80% of those identified in the first trimester accept the offer of prenatal diagnosis. This falls to 40% for those identified later in pregnancy. Around 85% of couples at risk of producing a child with cystic fibrosis could be identified by examining DNA from a mouth wash for the most common mutations. Several national pilot screening programmes have demonstrated that screening for CF is acceptable to individuals, but at present screening is only carried out in a few antenatal clinics and rarely in primary care.

PREGNANCY SCREENING TECHNIQUES

Ultrasound

A gestational sac can be visualized by 5–8 weeks, and the fetal heart beat from about 7 weeks onwards. If there has been vaginal bleeding in early pregnancy then ultrasound examination is helpful in confirming whether a viable conceptus is still present. The other main indications for ultrasound are:

- detection of multiple pregnancies
- to aid the diagnosis of an ectopic pregnancy
- calculation of gestational age
- to guide procedures such as chorionic villus sampling and amniocentesis
- monitoring of intrauterine growth
- the detection of a low-lying placenta or of fetal malformation in high risk pregnancies

- as a screening procedure to detect congenital abnormalities in the low risk population.

A word of warning. The accuracy of the 'routine' 19-week fetal anomaly scan depends on the quality of the ultrasound machine and the expertise of the operator. Probably only about half of major congenital abnormalities are detected in non-tertiary referral units. The other danger is of making an incorrect diagnosis of abnormality, thus causing considerable parental distress.

Blood testing

Serum alphafetoprotein (AFP) estimation

The level of AFP in maternal serum is raised in some fetal malformations that disrupt the continuity of the fetal skin. The most common causes of a raised AFP are underestimation of the gestational age and multiple pregnancies. A maternal serum AFP of more than about 2.5 MoMs (multiples of the median) includes all pregnancies where the fetus has anencephaly and most where it has spina bifida, in addition to non-viable pregnancies and growth-retarded fetuses. Careful ultrasound is replacing amniocentesis as the next step in ascertaining whether or not there is a neural tube defect.

Diagnosis of chromosomal abnormalities

Definitive diagnosis of a chromosomal abnormality in a fetus is by cytogenetic studies following chorionic villus sampling or amniocentesis. It is only possible to detect about 35% of all Down's syndrome pregnancies, using age alone (35 years and over) as the criterion for offering prenatal diagnosis. However, if maternal serum concentrations of human chorionic gonadotrophin, unconjugated oestriol and AFP (the 'triple test') are measured at 16–17 weeks of pregnancy and interpreted in relation to maternal age, it is possible to calculate more accurately the risk of carrying a Down's syndrome fetus. Amniocentesis is usually offered to women with a risk greater than 1 in 250, but even this approach will not detect 40% of fetuses with a chromosomal

abnormality. It is possible to diagnose a Down's syndrome fetus in the first trimester of pregnancy by ultrasound examination (increased thickness of the nape of the neck) and by the measurement of another placental product, the pregnancy associated plasma protein A (PAPP-A).

Chorionic villus sampling (Figure 7.5)

The chorionic villi are of embryonic origin and can be used to study its chromosomes, DNA and certain enzymes. The risk of CVS to the pregnancy is only a little higher that that of amniocentesis, provided the procedure is carried out in an expert centre. Very early CVS might be associated with an increased risk of the birth of a child with limb abnormalities, so CVS should be only done at or after 10 weeks' gestation.

Amniocentesis (Figure 7.6)

Amniotic fluid is collected at about 16 weeks after the last menstrual period; it also contains fetal cells which can be cultured and examined

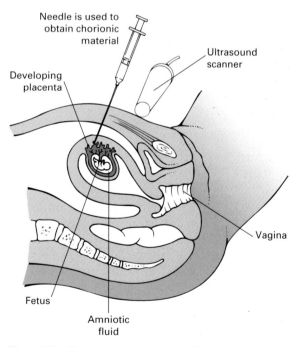

Figure 7.5   Transabdominal chorionic villus sampling.

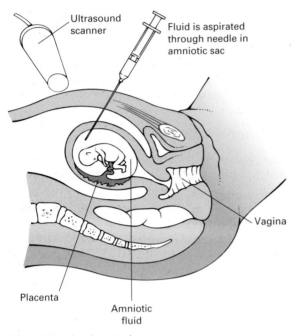

Ultrasound scanner

Fluid is aspirated through needle in amniotic sac

Vagina

Placenta

Amniotic fluid

Figure 7.6 Amniocentesis.

for chromosomal or DNA abnormalities. It takes up to a couple of weeks of culturing the cells to get enough mitoses for reliable karyotyping. There appears to be an increased fetal loss of about 0.5–1% with this procedure. There is possibly a slightly increased risk of breathing difficulties immediately after delivery and of correctable orthopaedic deformities such as club foot. At present the main indications are:

- increased risk of a child with certain single genetic defects
- increased risk of a child with chromosomal abnormalities
- a failed or doubtful CVS.

Both CVS and amniocentesis are invasive; potentially more exciting is the possibility of extracting fetal DNA from small numbers of cells of fetal origin which can be isolated from the maternal circulation. This approach is still very experimental.

PRE-IMPLANTATION DIAGNOSIS

Prenatal diagnosis is very upsetting to a couple at genetic risk, because it may lead on to termination of a wanted pregnancy. Pre-implantation diagnosis is gradually becoming an option in some cases, for example haemoglobin disorders, Duchenne muscular dystrophy and cystic fibrosis. Using techniques developed for in vitro fertilisation, eggs from the female are mixed with sperm from her partner. A fertilised ovum is then grown to the eight cell stage, a single cell is removed, and its DNA is amplified by PCR to see whether or not it is affected by the disease. If the cell appears to be healthy the rest of the embryo is implanted into the mother's uterus. CVS is still advised to confirm that all is well after pre-implantation diagnosis.

REPRODUCTIVE INFORMATION AND ADVICE

The paediatric responsibilities of family doctors begin before the children are born. The objective of providing reproductive information (if possible for couples rather than just women) is to increase the chance of the birth of a healthy baby. Ideally, this information should be provided *before* pregnancy, rather than in the first trimester, to minimise risk factors at the time of conception.

The following areas should be covered:

The need for referral to an obstetrician or reproductive endocrinologist because of a bad obstetric history or infertility.

Implications of advancing maternal age. The general risk of miscarriage increases with advancing maternal age. It is about 10% for recognised pregnancies in women aged 20–35, about 20% in women aged 35–40, and at least 30% for women over 40. As far as chromosomal abnormalities are concerned, the risk of Down's syndrome (normally 1 in 1000 births at age 30) increases to about 1 in 400 at 35, and 1 in 100 at 40 years of age.

Are the couple related? Consanguineous marriage is favoured by many (mainly Muslim) communities, because of its social advantages. It may however increase the risk of a recessively inherited disease, particularly if there is a family history.

Implications of a family history of possible genetic disease. A carefully constructed family tree, using the symbols shown in Figure 7.7, is the key to identifying many people at genetic risk who would benefit from referral to a clinical geneticist or other specialist. There may be a history in the close family, or more distant relatives, of:

- identified genetic disease
- unexplained intrauterine deaths, stillbirths or neonatal deaths; these are sometimes due to chromosomal abnormalities or inherited metabolic diseases
- unusually deep or prolonged neonatal jaundice, caused for example by X-linked glucose-6-phosphate dehydrogenase deficiency, carried by about 7% of the world's population (WHO 1989)
- death in infancy; this can be caused by

numerous genetic conditions of slightly later onset, such as sickle cell disease or metabolic disorders
- unexplained failure to thrive, repeated respiratory infections (cystic fibrosis) or specific symptoms such as a bleeding tendency in a male (haemophilia)
- severe learning difficulty (fragile X syndrome), sensorineural deafness, or blindness.

Need for genetic screening tests because of ethnic background (see above).

Rubella immunisation status and other infections. The average number of annual births of babies with congenital rubella has fallen from 48 in the early 1970s to 4 in 1991–5. This figure rose to 12 in 1996, following a decline in the uptake of the measles, mumps and rubella vaccine. It is important to remember that refugees and other immigrants may be susceptible to rubella. Reassuringly, there is no evidence that rubella vaccine inadvertently given during the first trimester of pregnancy is teratogenic. *Toxoplasma gondii* is a protozoan intracellular parasite found in many animals, but sexual reproduction and spore production occur only in the intestine of the cat. It is thought to be transmitted to humans (and other animals) through contact with cat faeces, or by eating undercooked meat. Congenital toxoplasmosis occurs in about 10% of children of mothers who were infected in pregnancy and can cause miscarriage, neonatal disease and severe ocular problems. The risk of toxoplasmosis may be reduced if pregnant women cook meat carefully and wash their hands after handling raw meat. Those with pet cats should also cook the cat's meat well and wear gloves when cleaning up cat litter. Pregnant women seem to be particularly susceptible to listeriosis (caused by *Listeria monocytogenes*, a small Gram-positive bacillus, which in the non-pregnant usually causes only a mild influenza-like illness). Infection in pregnancy may lead to miscarriage, stillbirth or severe neonatal infection. To prevent infection, pregnant women are advised to avoid foods that may be contaminated with listeria. These include undercooked poultry and cooked chilled meals, pâté and soft cheese.

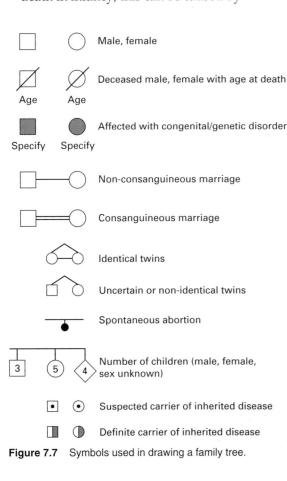

Figure 7.7 Symbols used in drawing a family tree.

Smoking and alcohol. The risks of smoking (miscarriage, bleeding in pregnancy and premature birth, with an increase in prenatal morbidity) rise in proportion to the number of cigarettes smoked. It is also a modifiable major risk factor for cot death. Stopping smoking in early pregnancy can reduce the risk to the fetus and newborn baby.

It is difficult to separate environmental factors from the effect of alcohol when presented with a child who is somewhat slow physically and mentally and whose parents drink heavily. The deleterious effects of alcohol are likely to depend on the amount drunk. Many social drinkers will have healthy children, and the fetal alcohol syndrome (FAS) represents the most severe damage. The features include learning difficulties, poor growth, and various congenital abnormalities which may involve the face, limbs, heart and nervous system.

Folic acid supplementation before conception, and vitamins in pregnancy. Since the Medical Research Council study showed that 4 mg/day of peri-conceptional folic acid significantly reduced the risk of recurrence of a neural tube defect, all women have been recommended to take 0.4 mg folic acid daily, starting from when they begin trying to conceive until the twelfth week of pregnancy. This is twice the average dietary intake. The richest sources of folic acid are green leafy vegetables (lightly cooked), jacket potatoes, yeast and beef extracts, and cereals and cereal products fortified with folic acid.

Not all vitamins are good news in pregnancy: excessive intake (more than 10 000 iu/day) of *Vitamin A* or related compounds in the first two months of pregnancy appears to double the normal risk of congenital abnormality. Liver normally contains a relatively large amount of vitamin A and it has been suggested that pregnant women should not take tablets containing vitamin A, or eat more than 50 g of liver a week or 100 g of liver sausage or pâté.

Maternal disease, e.g. diabetes or epilepsy. There is a threefold increase (to about 6%) in the incidence of congenital malformations in the children of mothers with frank insulin dependent diabetes, the risk being highest for mothers with diabetic vascular complications. The risk falls to around the normal 2% if the diabetes is well controlled around conception and in early pregnancy.

Anticonvulsants are associated with an increased risk of congenital abnormalities. Reassessment by a specialist may be indicated if a woman taking this medication is contemplating pregnancy. The aim is to minimise the number of different anticonvulsant drugs taken around conception. Women taking carbamazepine and/or valproate have an increased risk of a child with a neural tube defect, and should be advised to take additional folic acid daily before conception.

Drugs. It is always wise to check the comprehensive, regularly updated table of the effects of drugs taken in different stages of pregnancy and lactation included in the British National Formulary. Fortunately, relatively few drugs in common use appear to cause congenital malformations, the most important exceptions being anticonvulsants, lithium, warfarin and cytotoxic agents.

ASPECTS OF GENETIC COUNSELLING

The aim of genetic counselling is to provide people with objective, accurate, understandable information, or to advise them where they can obtain such information. Couples or individuals should then be encouraged to make up their own minds, with the doctor supporting them in any decision they make. The 'right' choice differs for each person depending on individual circumstances and social and cultural background.

Counselling in primary care is most likely to be given to adults who are concerned that they may have inherited a specific illness affecting a blood relative, prior to screening for carriers of a recessive disorder, to newly identified carriers (Box 7.1), to women (or couples) before antenatal tests, and after the offer of prenatal diagnosis. Patients often find it helpful to be given clearly written leaflets containing the relevant information at the first consultation. They can then return

---

> **Box 7.1** Issues to raise with parents before and after a screening test for a recessively inherited disease. Source: Modell et al 1996.
>
> *Counselling before a test*
> - You may be a carrier
> - Brief description of the condition
> - Implications for child bearing
> - Limitations of test (e.g. 85% of CF mutations only are identified; does not test for other conditions)
>
> *Counselling carriers* (leaflets may be available)
> - Carriers are healthy
> - More information about the disease
> - Desirability of testing partners and relatives
> - Reproductive risks

at a later date if they have further questions. These leaflets can usually be obtained from the appropriate organisation or generated from 'patient education' software packages. The careful family history is a most important tool for identification of genetic risk.

THE ROLE OF THE CLINICAL GENETICIST

A couple whose baby has been born with a probable genetic disorder (apart from the common recessively inherited diseases) will usually need referral to a specialist genetic clinic. There may be diagnostic uncertainty, and patterns of inheritance in apparently similar conditions often vary. Referral for genetic assessment is also suggested for a child with more than one significant congenital abnormality (excluding skin blemishes and over-riding toes), especially if there are additional causes for concern such as an odd facies, slow development or a history of similar problems in other members of the family. The study of children with structural defects is called *dysmorphology*.

Reaching a diagnosis requires a careful and detailed family history, a full examination and appropriate investigations including chromosome and DNA studies. Specific patterns of abnormalities are called *syndromes*, and computerised databases contain details of thousands of rare syndromes. These may be caused by single gene defects or chromosomal abnormalities. Clinical geneticists, specialist nurses and (in some areas) genetic associates work closely together. Counselling for specific genetic diseases has to cover many areas, such as:

- What is the inheritance, and is the condition likely to be equally severe in future affected children?
- What are the implications for the family in terms of treatment and likely outcome?
- Does the diagnosis explain all the child's problems (for example, in the older child, deafness or a learning difficulty)?
- Should the child be referred to another specialist (e.g. neurologist, community paediatrician)?
- Is carrier detection or prenatal diagnosis possible?

THE NEW GENETICS
Genetic engineering

In 'genetic engineering' the DNA code of living organisms is altered. One of the applications of this new technology is the engineering of bacteria to manufacture proteins such as insulin, growth hormone, factor VIII and hepatitis B vaccine, used in the treatment and prevention of various diseases.

Gene therapy

The objective of gene therapy, another example of genetic engineering, is to cure genetic diseases—either by introducing a functioning gene when one is absent, or by replacing a defective gene with a normal one. Somatic cells only are targeted, thus ensuring that the altered genetic make-up is not passed on to children (germ cell gene therapy would cause many ethical problems, its safety is uncertain, and affected future generations would have no say in their inheritance). The main initial candidates for gene therapy are recessively inherited disorders. However there are a number of problems:

- There must be a full understanding of the genetic defect and how it causes the disease.
- There must be a safe and effective way of inserting the new gene. Many vectors are viruses

such as retroviruses and adenoviruses, which can be integrated with the host's DNA after removal of many of the viral genes. However, delivery systems now include other viruses and non-viral vehicles such as liposomes. In some instances the gene and its regulatory sequences are inserted via a self-replicating artificial chromosome.

- The gene has to be inserted into an appropriate target cell—a stem cell rather than one that is no longer going to divide and multiply. A disease such as thalassaemia that is potentially curable by bone marrow transplant could theoretically be treated by inserting the healthy globin gene into bone marrow cells.
- The transformed cell must be able to function and compete with cells with the mutate genes.

- The vector may have toxic or mutagenic effects (perhaps because it is a potentially pathogenic virus). It may also have to be repeatedly administered.

In cystic fibrosis the cloned gene has been inserted into adenoviral vectors and administered by spray to the nasal mucous membrane. Even if the problem in the lungs is rectified, however, patients will still be susceptible to other complications such as diabetes or cirrhosis.

Possible candidates for gene therapy include not only single gene conditions but also cancer (alteration of cells to enhance the immune response, or the response to chemotherapy or to induce 'cell suicide') and AIDS (producing an increased resistance to HIV infection).

FURTHER READING

Harper P S 1993 Practical genetic counselling, 4th edn. Wright, Bristol

Jones K L 1996 Smith's recognizable patterns of human malformations, 5th edn. W B Saunders, Philadelphia

Lever A M L, Goodfellow P (eds) 1995 Gene therapy. British Medical Bulletin, Churchill Livingstone, Vol 51

Modell M, Mughal Z, Boyd R 1996 Paediatric problems in general practice, 3rd edn. Oxford University Press, Oxford

Modell B, Modell M 1992 Towards a healthy baby—congenital disorders and the new genetics in primary care, Oxford University Press, Oxford

Mueller R F, Young I D 1995 Emery's Elements of medical genetics, 9th edn. Churchill Livingstone, Edinburgh

Scriver C R, Beaudet A L, Sly W S, Valle D (eds) 1995 The metabolic and molecular basis of inherited disease, 7th edn. McGraw-Hill, New York

Weatherall D J 1991 The new genetics and clinical practice, 3rd edn. Oxford University Press (for the Nuffield Provincial Hospitals Trust), Oxford

Internet addresses

Genetics
http://www.vh.org/Providers/Textbooks/ClinicalGenetics/Contents.html

Congenital disorders
http://www.uab.edu/pedinfo/DiseasesCongenital.html

CHAPTER CONTENTS

8

Child and adolescent mental health

David Cottrell

INTRODUCTION AND DEFINITION

Emotional and behavioural problems are common in childhood and adolescence and can cover a wide range of presentations, from the toddler with sleeping difficulties to the depressed, withdrawn, and possibly suicidal teenager. Generating one definition for a child[†] psychiatric disorder given this range of problems is difficult but essential for purposes of research, communication and service planning.

One commonly accepted definition is that a child has a psychiatric disorder if:

- behaviour, thoughts or feelings differ quantitatively from the norm, and
- as a result of this difference, the child is either suffering significantly or development is being significantly impaired.

Development here could refer to motor, social, emotional, language or cognitive development. Quantitative differences are stressed because the behaviours, thoughts and feelings referred to are broadly similar to those experienced by all children, but to a greater or lesser degree; for example, children with psychiatric problems feel more tearful, they have more temper tantrums, they go to school less. When deciding what constitutes the 'norm', children must be compared with others of similar developmental age.

[†]For convenience, the word 'child' will be used to refer to children and adolescents. Where problems arise specifically in relation to either childhood or adolescence, this will be made clear in the text.

Behaviour must also be persistent; transient 'symptoms', for example after minor stressful events, are so common as to be considered normal in most situations. This is different from adult mental health where disorder is often judged to exist because of the presence of qualitative differences in thoughts, feelings or behaviour, for example the presence of hallucinations. Some children do of course show qualitative differences from the norm; examples include teenagers with psychosis and younger children with pervasive developmental disorders. These problems are relatively rare. For the most part, child mental health disorders concern children whose 'symptoms' may seem similar to those of many other children. This can lead to confusion and the kind of unhelpful statements that are sometimes heard suggesting that children with quite significant mental health problems are 'just naughty'.

EPIDEMIOLOGY

Using this broad definition it is possible to make some estimates of the prevalence of child mental health problems. There have been a number of good, population based studies over the last twenty years with broadly similar findings (see Table 8.1). These suggest prevalence rates of 5–10% in rural areas, rising to 10–20% in more socio-economically deprived inner city areas. The lifetime risk for having had at least one psychiatric disorder in childhood has been estimated as being as high as 50%. Children seen in general practice and in paediatric outpatient clinics have rates of psychiatric disorder higher than 20% and in some studies as high as 40%. Most of these children present with physical symptoms and the majority are not recognised by the general practitioner or the paediatrician as having a psychiatric disorder. Nevertheless, in one study, behaviour problems were the third most common reason for children to be presented to their general practitioner. Population based studies show that only about 10% of children with problems are in touch with mental health services, and that these do not necessarily have the most severe problems.

General practitioners and community paediatricians see many children with psychiatric disorders. Given that many of these problems are treatable, especially if identified early, it is crucial that those who come into contact with children consider the possibility of psychiatric disorder as a routine part of assessment, whatever the presenting difficulties.

ASSESSMENT

Assessment in child psychiatry is a complex procedure. The aetiology is multifactorial; in most children, a number of factors in the child's family and environment come together to create the clinical picture. Problems presenting in a similar way may have widely differing patterns of causation, and there is therefore no substitute for carrying out a detailed assessment of all of the possible domains which may contribute to a child developing problems.

A cumulative stress model is helpful when considering assessment. Imagine a set of kitchen scales: as more and more causative factors are loaded onto one side of the scales, the balance tips over and at this stage the child becomes symptomatic. Protective factors in the child's environment may counter this swing despite the presence of adverse factors. Assessment is therefore concerned with identifying as many possible

Table 8.1 Prevalence of child psychiatric disorder

Age	Prevalence %	Comments
3 years	7	Moderate to severe behaviour problems
	15	Mild behaviour problems
10–11 years	7	Rural (Isle of Wight), 1970
10–11 years	14	Urban (London), 1970
14–15	21	Rural (Isle of Wight), 1970
4–16 years	18	Canada, large population sample, mixed urban & rural, 1987
7–12 years	23	General practice

Box 8.1   Common aetiological factors

Individual
- Genetic influences
- Gender
- Intelligence
- Temperament
- Physical characteristics (chronic illness, sensory deficit)

Family
- Parental mental illness
- Discord and disruption
- Large family size
- Inconsistency and lack of supervision
- Lack of warmth
- Lack of secure attachments

Environment
- Socio-economic deprivation
- Poor housing
- Lack of safe play space
- Overcrowding
- Poverty
- School ethos

---

causes and protective factors as possible. Even relatively 'small' causative factors may tip the balance, and so it is crucial to examine all areas of the child's life. A common mistake is to assume that the problem is understood because a few obvious precipitants have been identified. This approach may miss other factors, the removal of which may tip the scales back and allow the child to proceed along a more normal development path. This is particularly important as some of the most obvious causes, which are therefore easiest to identify, are also the most difficult to change. Some of the more important aetiological factors are summarised in Box 8.1 and discussed below. Many of these are strongly associated with psychiatric problems in childhood. However, the association is usually with problems in general rather than with any specific diagnosis.

Individual influences

There are a number of innate characteristics of children that may predispose to difficulties but these interact with environmental influences from a very early age to produce a particular pattern of development. Later observed differences are therefore a product of this interaction

between nature and nurture, and arguments about the primacy of one or the other are unhelpful. Specific genetic influences on psychiatric disorder in childhood are the subject of much current research but are rarely the single most important contribution. Genetic research usually provides the most powerful evidence we have for the crucial role of environmental factors.

Gender is important: boys have significantly more problems, particularly for conduct disorders, but gender differences vary according to specific diagnoses. Intelligence is also related to overall levels of disorder with an inverse relationship between IQ and prevalence rates of psychiatric disorder. Children with a 'difficult' temperament (operationally defined as biological irregularity, predominantly negative mood, slow adaptability to new situations, and intense emotional reactions) are also at greater risk of developing later psychiatric disorders. Children with chronic illness or disability (up to 20% of the total child population according to the definition used) have a 2–3 times higher risk of developing psychiatric disorders than the healthy child population. This risk is even greater if the central nervous system is involved as part of the child's illness or disability.

Family influences

As would be expected, families have been shown to have a major influence on the presence of psychiatric disorder in children. Rather than any one particular factor, it is the presence of a combination of any of the factors listed below that seems to be most damaging:

- parental mental illness, particularly maternal depression
- family disruption and marital discord
- large, disorganised families
- inconsistent parents who do not set clear rules and who do not monitor and supervise children effectively
- paternal criminality
- lack of warmth in family relationships.

Many studies have looked at the impact on children of different family structures, for example single fathers, multi-family communes, etc. There is little evidence that the family structure itself is associated with problems. Children of single parents do have more emotional and behavioural problems but this is largely accounted for by the greater socio-economic hardships experienced by such families. What seems to be important is the quality of emotional relationships within the family. The quality of the child's attachment relationship to his or her carers is crucial. Secure early attachments have lasting positive effects on the child's later development and capacity to form relationships with others. Children who have not had the opportunity to form secure attachments are at greater risk of social and emotional difficulties which persist into adolescence and adult life.

Environmental influences

Whilst the family is the major environmental influence on children, as they grow up and spend more time outside the home wider environmental influences also have a direct effect on the child as well as an indirect effect via their parents. The evidence is less conclusive about these factors but there is no doubt that rates of disorder increase in socio-economically deprived urban areas because of poor housing, lack of safe play space, overcrowding and poverty. School is clearly another major influence. Schools drawing from the same catchment area can have markedly different rates of achievement, absenteeism and behaviour problems, suggesting that the way in which the school is managed can have a significant impact on the presence of problems in the child.

Conclusions

When carrying out an assessment it is necessary to consider all of the factors described above. As well as thinking about which individual, family and wider environmental influences are involved, it is important to consider how these factors have influenced the child. Some are predisposing and make the child more likely to have difficulties in the first place, some are precipitants, and some are perpetuants in that they maintain the problem and keep it going. Given the need to consider all possible causes, it may be helpful during assessment to consider the grid shown in Figure 8.1. There may not always be relevant aetiological factors operating in each box of the grid but the possibility should always be considered. The last line of the grid concerns the presence of protective factors such as the presence of a warm confiding relationship with an adult. These too should be considered. When a full assessment has been carried out, treatment then consists of developing an intervention package which will remove as many of the causative factors as possible and create the possibility of protective factors where they are absent.

INTERVIEWING

The task of the assessment interview (or interviews) is to gather as much information as possible about potential causative factors, as outlined above. This task is complicated by the fact that it is adult carers, not the children themselves, who usually present asking for help. Children may not agree with parental interpretations of

	Individual factors	Family factors	Environmental factors
Predisposing factor	Hearing deficit		
Precipitating factors		Birth of sibling	
Perpetuating factors		Inconsistent parental response	Poor housing and overcrowding
Protective factors			

Figure 8.1 The assessment grid. An illustration of possible aetiological factors operating in a preschool child with a behaviour problem.

events and indeed may not even accept that there is a problem at all. Parents may be very worried that they are to be blamed for any problems. However, most treatment interventions involve the parent having to do something different. The art of such an assessment is to form a partnership with parents such that they are convinced of the need to do things differently with their child without feeling at the same time blamed for their child's problems. General practitioners, with their unique knowledge and experience of families, are often well placed to carry out such an assessment and to facilitate appropriate referral. Nevertheless, more time may be needed than is often available for a 'typical' general practice or paediatric consultation. It may be necessary to see all of the family, and sufficient space must be available with toys and play materials appropriate for the child. Whilst seeing the family together allows for observation of family relationships it is also important to see the child and the parents separately.

TREATMENT

As indicated in the assessment section, treatment packages are usually individually tailored for the child and family, with the intention of modifying the specific aetiological factors identified. All health professionals should be able to carry out a basic assessment and implement simple treatment interventions for mental health problems. More complex problems may require referral to a specialist mental health team. Making a referral to a mental health team is an important skill in its own right. There is still a stigma attached to these services, and many parents worry that a referral means that they are being accused of inadequate parenting. It is important to remember that, although it is the child who may be symptomatic, it is the parent(s) who need to be engaged in treatment as, if they do not support the process, the child will never get the treatment that is needed.

Making a referral

It is vital that referrers know about the service

that they are referring into and convey accurate information about the kinds of things that will happen, for example waiting times, length of assessment interview, and who will be invited. Most mental health teams invite the whole family for first assessments; these can often take up to 90 minutes. Often two or more staff may be involved in initial interviews. Details about the kinds of questions asked are widely available and the reader is referred to the references at the end of this chapter. If the family feel that the referrer knows about the service and approves of it then they are more likely to attend.

Services in the UK are patchily distributed but most areas have a dedicated mental health service for children, adolescents and families. At the minimum this is likely to include a multidisciplinary team comprising psychiatrist, psychologist, nurse, and social worker. Teams may have a child psychotherapist, or other staff, for example occupational therapists, who have had some additional training in individual therapeutic work with children. In many areas the service will prefer to receive referrals to the team as a whole and will then allocate cases according to their assessment of which team member can offer help most appropriately. Not all referrals will necessarily see a doctor. In some areas there is also a specialist child psychology service which may, or may not, be contributing staff to work within the multidisciplinary mental health team. It is important to know precisely how services are configured in your own area if you are to obtain the best help for your patients.

Mental health services are predominantly outpatient in nature. Some districts run day units for more disturbed children but most have to refer out of district to specialist regional units if admission is required. Mental health teams should offer a range of different psychological treatments, as outlined below, and may also offer consultation to the referrer concerning management as an alternative to taking on direct work with the child and family.

The referrer must give a clear message about the nature of the referral and why the child is being referred. It is not unusual for mental health teams to meet parents who had not known they were going to see a psychiatrist or a psychologist until they received the appointment letter. The referrer's assessment and formulation should be explained to the family. Euphemisms like 'a colleague who is expert in these matters' should be avoided. Tell the family they are going to a mental health service and why. Do not pressure parents into attending. Psychological treatments require the co-operation of parents and will not work unless families are willing to work. Suggest a mental health referral, but if the family are clearly against it do not forcefully persuade them to attend; instead suggest reviewing the situation and try discussing referral on a later occasion. Referral letters should contain brief information about the presenting problem, the referrer's assessment of likely aetiological factors, including any relevant past history, and a brief description of the family members.

Psychological treatments

Treatment packages are often eclectic in nature, with elements of a variety of different therapies offered to families. Sometimes a combination of therapies is used as when parents are offered marital work and the child is offered some individual counselling. Listed below are brief descriptions of the kinds of treatments which should be available in all child mental health services.

Behavioural treatments

These are based on learning theories and involve the manipulation of environmental antecedents and consequences of behaviours. Learning theory provides a rationale for thinking about everyday behavioural management of children and leads to an emphasis on clear and consistent rules, careful monitoring of the child, and the implementation of clear sanctions if rules are breached, along with the use of positive reinforcement for desired behaviour. Used properly, behavioural treatment should start with a period of baseline observation before proceeding to a detailed and individual formulation, and the development

of an individual treatment programme which is regularly reviewed. It should not consist of the blanket distribution of star charts to all children with behavioural problems without consideration of the specific issues leading to that child's presentation.

The use of positive reinforcement and extinction (ignoring unwanted behaviour) is very effective for the management of many common behaviour problems especially in pre-school children, for example sleeping and feeding difficulties and temper tantrums, and should probably be the treatment of first choice for these difficulties. It is also widely used as part of a package of interventions for older children and teenagers with disruptive behaviour problems. More complex behavioural techniques also exist for the management of other problems. Response prevention (the active prevention of ritualised responses to obsessional thoughts, for example stopping a child from repetitive hand washing in response to obsessional thoughts about contamination) is probably the treatment of first choice for obsessive compulsive disorders. Some form of graded desensitisation is recommended for phobic disorders.

Cognitive treatments

Cognitive treatments were initially developed in adults, but are being successfully transferred to work with younger people. They have arisen from behavioural and social learning theories and are based on the notion that children may have specific deficits or distortions in their thinking which will lead them to misunderstand or misinterpret their own behaviour and that of others. Cognitive techniques have been used successfully in helping children with attention deficit and conduct disorders to solve problems more effectively, thus improving their ability to interact with others and to deal with classroom demands. They have been used with children as young as 5 or 6 years but are used mostly with older children and teenagers. They are often used in conjunction with behavioural techniques, with specific cognitive strategies being used more commonly as the child gets older.

Cognitive methods are probably the treatment of first choice for the management of depression. Specific techniques involve helping the child to identify accurately different feelings and their immediate antecedents and consequences, exploring the child's causal beliefs about his own and others behaviour, and rehearsing specific strategies for countering distorted cognitions. Patients are seen individually and often for a fixed number of weekly appointments—usually about 8. There is some evidence that, in depression, one-off 'booster' or intermittent follow-up sessions may help to prevent relapse.

Family treatments

Family systemic therapy has changed the way that most child mental health teams operate in the last 10–15 years and is now probably the most common type of intervention used. The basic premise is that children cannot be understood, or helped, outside the context in which they are living. The problems of the child are seen as a manifestation of interactional difficulties within the family group, and treatment is directed at that group not the individual child. A series of family group meetings is held in which the therapist assists the family in exploring their effect on each other and in constructing a new and more helpful set of beliefs and expectations about the members of the family. The process is so complex, with so many people in the room at once, that family therapists often work with colleagues observing the session through a 'one-way' screen or on closed circuit television. Family therapy has been used with almost all presenting problems. It tends to be used most when there are obvious family interactional difficulties, but can be helpful even when they seem absent. There is growing evidence of its efficacy and it is probably the treatment of first choice for some conditions, such as anorexia nervosa. Similar techniques are also used to work with couples who are experiencing difficulties in their relationship; indeed therapy that starts by looking at the interactional effects of the family on the child often ends by exploring the parental relationship in particular.

Psychodynamic treatments

These are a range of therapies that have in common a regular contact with the child, usually weekly for one hour, in a regular place, to explore the child's inner world and experiences. Therapists are usually non-directive and work with the child's feelings, including those about the therapist that arise in the session; these may represent a repetition of feelings in earlier relationships (transference). Therapists use a variety of media for facilitating communication, play being central in younger children. Different schools of therapy may also use art, music, or drama as the main medium of communication.

Most centres would probably try to work first with parents or families to help adult carers better meet the needs of children. If this is not possible, not sufficient, or has failed then individual work with the child may be the most appropriate treatment. It is a scarce and expensive resource and is often used with children who have been victims of trauma, particularly abuse.

Group treatments

These tend to be used less frequently, perhaps because of the practical difficulties in getting people together, but can be very helpful in certain situations. Their orientation can vary from educational to psychodynamic. Parents' groups which emphasise understanding behaviour problems and learning specific techniques for dealing with them have been shown to be very effective in conduct disorders. Group work can also be effective for social skills training in children and adolescents, with the group itself providing an opportunity for young people to practise social interaction. Groups for younger children in primary schools have been shown to be effective in reducing emotional and behavioural problems. Groups can also help victims of trauma and abuse make sense of their experiences.

Pharmacological treatments

These are used much less than in adult mental health. There is clear evidence that stimulants such as methylphenidate are effective in reducing restlessness and distractibility in children who meet the criteria for hyperkinetic disorder. In children in whom stimulants are not successful, other drugs such as tricyclic antidepressants or clonidine may be effective but should probably only be used by an experienced child psychiatrist.

There is no good evidence that antidepressants are effective in children and adolescents. However, it must be remembered that lack of evidence of effectiveness is not the same as evidence of ineffectiveness. There are strong links between depression in adolescence and that occurring in adulthood, when antidepressants are effective. For this reason, antidepressants are sometimes used in practice but should probably be reserved for older teenagers with more severe forms of depression and in whom other treatments have failed.

Antidepressants (clomipramine and specific serotonin re-uptake inhibitors) have also been shown to be effective in obsessive compulsive disorders.

Tricyclic antidepressants were used in the past for the treatment of enuresis. They are not as effective as behavioural treatments, have high relapse rates, and have a high rate of side-effects. If a pharmacological treatment is indicated then vasopressin analogues are more appropriate.

Major tranquillisers are used in adolescents as part of the management of psychotic symptoms in much the same way as they are in adult psychosis. Low dose haloperidol is also used for the treatment of tic disorders.

There are few indications, if any, for the use of minor tranquillisers in children or adolescents. If they are used, for example to help re-establish a normal sleep pattern or to help sleep after an acute trauma, their use should be strictly time limited.

Consultation

The goal of consultation is to help other professionals to manage problems more effectively. It is collaborative in nature, and aims explicitly to increase the skills and knowledge of the consultee. It is becoming increasingly used by child mental health teams as a way of dealing cost effectively with an increasing referral load. It is not, however, a second best option to direct therapeutic work with the child. If cases are selected for consultation correctly, the process of consultation will empower referrers and enable them to provide for the needs of the referred child or family. In addition, the knowledge derived from the consultation should be of use in other cases, increasing the quality of work generally carried out by the consultee.

Consultation may be to individuals or to groups and, although it usually starts by being based on particular cases, often proceeds to look at organisational aspects of the consultee's work setting. It may be reactive and 'one-off', for example following a specific referral, or proactive, for example regular consultation to a children's home or to a paediatric team.

Residential and day treatments

These treatment settings allow for the assessment and management of more complex and/or more severe psychiatric problems. There is an increasing trend not to admit younger children to residential units but instead to use day units. Adolescents with complex problems may be helped by day units but some, with serious depression, eating disorders, obsessive compulsive disorders or psychosis, are likely to need admission during the acute phase of their illness. These units usually have teaching staff and education on site and allow for more intensive treatment, over longer periods of time, and in a group setting. The milieu of the unit itself, with a regime of warmth and consistency, is an important part of the therapeutic package. There are also more opportunities for group work.

SPECIFIC CLINICAL SYNDROMES

Classification in child mental health is not an exact science: new operational criteria and new diagnostic groupings appear in successive generations of both the International Classification of Diseases (ICD) and the American Diagnostic and Statistical Manual (DSM). This section will describe briefly some of the more common syndromes, outlining their presentation and what is known about their aetiology and management.

Conduct and behavioural problems

Conduct disorder refers to children presenting with severe, persistent, and repetitive antisocial behaviour (see Box 8.2).

It is the most common disorder in children and adolescents: epidemiological studies suggest rates as high as 4–8% in children up to 10–11 years of age and 10–15% in adolescents. It is much more common in boys, and children tend to come from families with disadvantaged backgrounds with family histories of mental illness, aggression and criminality. Parents are more likely to use coercive methods of discipline, and high levels of inconsistency are coupled with a lack of parental supervision. As children get older there is a strong likelihood of delinquency.

Oppositional defiant disorder refers to younger children (under 10 years) with persistent behaviour problems in the home but who have not displayed significant antisocial or delinquent behaviour.

Management of conduct problems is difficult and needs to be collaborative, involving family, school and perhaps social or probation services where there are significant antisocial problems outside the home. Behavioural techniques to promote consistency, good supervision, and reinforcement of positive behaviour are probably the most common strategies. These may be coupled with sessions for the child, either individually or in a group, to enhance social skills and problem solving abilities. Parent training groups have become popular recently and there is emerging evidence that these may represent a cost effective means of addressing conduct problems. Children with conduct disorders are often failing at school and any attempts at treatment must pay attention to academic work as well as behaviour management in school. Remedial education is likely to be needed.

In pre-school children, the most common conduct problems are eating and sleeping difficulties and temper tantrums. Assessment of these problems often reveals patterns of behaviour in which children's difficulties are being reinforced by parents who, after a struggle, give in to the child's demands. A child's ability to acquire control over his or her eating, sleeping and behaviour depends on both that child's individual temperament and developmental status, and the parent's capacity to adapt to this. Factors which interfere with this adaptation commonly include poor social conditions (overcrowding, poor housing, lack of safe play space) and parental mental health problems and/or marital difficulties. These common pre-school problems often co-exist and may reflect difficulties in the wider parent–child relationship. As they are common in primary care and paediatric settings, and as early intervention can be very effective, they will be discussed in more detail. Most of these problems can and should be managed in the primary care setting, following the kind of family oriented assessment described above. Only those children whose problems prove intractable should be considered for referral to more specialist services.

Eating problems

Problems with feeding are common in toddlers: 10–20% of mothers report difficulties with faddiness, slowness and food refusal. Assessment must consider three areas:

1. why the child might not want to eat (snacks between meals, development of autonomy and desire to self feed, distractibility and

---

Box 8.2 Symptoms of conduct disorder
• Fighting and aggressiveness
• Persistent disobedience
• Severe temper tantrums
• Bullying
• Cruelty
• Destructiveness
• Stealing
• Lying
• Firesetting
• Truancy
• Running away

playfulness, child's own likes and dislikes, misery)

2. why feeding may be over-important to the parent (lack of knowledge about normal variations, rigidity of diet or of discipline, feeding as a way of showing love, unrealistic fears and anxieties)

3. what methods are being used to make the child eat.

Management needs to address parental anxiety and re-establish sensible eating patterns by suggesting that attractive and varied food be provided in small, manageable portions and avoiding excessive display of concern about feeding. Children should be praised (this can include giving snacks or treats after meals) for eating properly but not given snacks, including sweets and milk, between meals. Tonics and other medications are generally unhelpful.

Sleeping problems

It is normal and very common for infants and small children to wake during the night. By the age of 3 years, most children will sleep through the night. Sleep disturbance usually consists of either difficulty in settling to sleep, frequent waking, or sometimes both. Assessment can be helped by asking parents to keep a sleep diary covering:

- the time the child is put to bed
- the consistency of bedtime routines
- the time the child falls asleep
- the time of any night-time waking
- the amount and timing of sleep during the day
- the amount of activity during the day.

As usual, questions about what has been tried so far and whether there is parental agreement about how to deal with the problem are crucial. The sleep diary often reveals an obvious cause for the problem and may suggest a common-sense solution. It is often sufficient to establish a specific bedtime and a settling routine such as bath, drink and a story. If this fails, the use of star charts to positively reinforce an improved

sleep pattern may be helpful. Some authorities recommend letting the child cry without paying attention. This is very difficult for both the parent and the child, but effective. Alternatively, a programme of gradually establishing a routine by firmly setting small, incremental, manageable goals may be more acceptable. Medication is rarely of any help in dealing with sleeping difficulties.

Nightmares. Nightmares are frightening dreams which may cause the child to cry out or wake up. They occur in 'rapid eye movement' sleep and are common, not indicative of mental health problems and best treated by reassurance. The content of the dream can often be recalled. If the dream is repetitive in content, consider referral to a child mental health team as this may indicate underlying anxieties. Management should in the first instance ensure that any stressors are alleviated and that the child is safe. Encouraging children to talk about dream content, act out the dream in play, or draw pictures of it can be very helpful. Suggesting that the child then constructs new and happier endings for the dream, which in turn can be drawn, discussed, or acted out, can help to change the frightening content of the dreams.

Night terrors. These occur in stage IV sleep (the deep sleep that precedes rapid eye movement sleep). The child cries out (usually about 2 hours after going off to sleep) and is found sitting up with open eyes, looking terrified, but not responsive to questions. The child may appear hallucinated, fending off something with the hands and may talk incoherently. Waking the child is difficult and after a few minutes he or she may settle to sleep without ever really waking. In the morning there is no recall for the episode. Night terrors are not the same as nightmares and are not indicative of mental health problems although they may be precipitated or exacerbated by stress. They often run in families. The best management approach is reassurance; alternatively, the child may be woken up before the night terror is expected to occur, hence disrupting the pattern of sleep. Sleep walking is another stage IV phenomenon, not dissimilar to night terrors. It too is best treated by reassurance, with appropriate attention to safety, for example locking windows and doors.

Temper tantrums

This is a common problem during the pre-school years but there is remarkably little research on the subject. Tantrums are the child's normal response to discipline, and they usually start at around 18 months of age before gradually disappearing. If they do not go, it is usually because of an interaction between the parents' inconsistent or unclear communication about rules, including inadequate or excessive control, and the child's poor understanding of demands or inability to communicate his or her wishes. Diary keeping is a helpful part of assessment; parents are asked to keep an 'ABC' chart detailing antecedents, behaviour and consequences of tempers. Assessment should also consider the parents' own experiences as children, their attitude to discipline generally, and their anxieties and fears about possible harm to the child if tempers are allowed to run their course (such as epileptic fits or heart attack). This is often an issue when children are seen as being 'special', perhaps because of early health problems, perinatal complications or chronic illness. Parental anxiety or depression and marital disharmony will also contribute to unresolved tantrums.

For parents to deal successfully with temper tantrums it is necessary for them to agree on a management strategy in order to avoid the child playing one against the other. Straightforward advice about clear rules, ignoring unwanted behaviour, and praising desired behaviour should always be considered first. If this does not work, attention needs to be paid to the other factors listed above which may interfere with parental ability to carry out this simple advice. Problems that persist may need referral to specialist mental health teams.

Hyperkinetic disorders

ICD 10 uses the term 'hyperkinetic disorders' but the terms 'attention deficit disorder' (ADD) or 'attention-deficit/hyperactivity disorder' (ADHD) are probably more commonly used, especially by parents.

Clinical features

The clinical features of hyperkinetic disorder are impaired attention and overactivity with impulsive, distractible and disruptive behaviour which is most evident in structured, organised situations that require concentration and self control, for example the classroom. It is more common in boys and is associated with specific learning difficulties (dyslexia) and with motor clumsiness (dyspraxia). Symptoms nearly always start in the pre-school years but, because of the wide range of normal behaviour in that age group, caution should be exercised in making the diagnosis before the age of 5 years. For the diagnosis to be made, the main features should be present in more than one setting.

The core hyperkinetic syndrome as described above is present in 1–2% of the population. The American diagnosis of ADHD, which can be made in children with situation-specific difficulties, is more common: quoted prevalence rates are as high as 5–10%. Specific cognitive impairments are associated more commonly with pervasive than with situational difficulties. Associated conduct problems are common but not necessary for the diagnosis to be made.

Management

Assessment must include a careful developmental history as well as an account of all the symptoms in all settings. Management usually involves a careful explanation of the problems and behavioural advice for parents and teachers. These children are often failing at school and have low self-esteem and poor peer relationships. Steps must be taken within the school to address these difficulties. For children with clear hyperkinetic disorder, stimulant medication (methylphenidate or dexamphetamine) is likely to be the treatment of choice and is of proven efficacy. Methylphenidate—starting at a dose of 5 mg twice daily and building up to as much as 30 mg twice daily—is the usual starting point for drug treatment. Side-effects (abdominal pain, sleep problems, loss of appetite and growth retardation) do occur but are dose related and often fade once the dose is established. It is often necessary to juggle with the dosage (times and amounts) before the most appropriate regimen is found. Once established, medication may have to be continued for some years but should be reviewed regularly. Some children will not need to continue medication; this can only be established by a trial without drugs.

Cognitive behavioural treatments for individual children and social skills training may be of help in some cases. Dietary manipulation may also be of benefit in a few cases. There is clear evidence that in some children with hyperkinetic disorders reactions to particular foodstuffs play an important role. Unfortunately no particular food has been implicated; the relevant dietary ingredient must be identified for each child, and this is sometimes a long and difficult process.

The prognosis is not always good but is better in the absence of conduct disorder or other associated problems, when the child is of normal intelligence, and when the family are supportive and co-operative with treatment. Poorer outcomes include ongoing schooling and behaviour problems, delinquency, educational failure, and difficulties with employment and relationships in adult life.

Emotional disorders

Children suffer from the same kinds of emotional disorders (for example anxiety, depression and obsessions) as adults but their presentation is heavily influenced by age. As with adults, they may present with a mixture of symptoms from different emotional disorders. The diagnosis is complicated by the difficulty, especially for younger children, of describing inner experiences to outsiders.

Depression

Depression can occur in pre-pubertal children, although it becomes more common with increasing age. It does not always present with persistent depressed mood; instead children may have sudden episodes of unexplained sadness and weepiness coupled with social withdrawal, anger and irritability, physical symptoms and a falling off in school work. The child may not enjoy normal activities as much as usual, if at all, but often has periods of relative normality. As the child gets older, biological features such as loss of appetite, diurnal variations in sleep and mood, and loss of energy may be more prominent, as will sustained lowering of mood.

Co-morbidity is common, especially with conduct disorder in adolescents. Family histories of depression are common and are often helpful in making a diagnosis.

Recent evidence suggests that individual cognitive behavioural treatment for the depressed child is effective and is probably the treatment of choice. This should take place against the usual backdrop of support and advice for parents and teachers. Attention should also be paid to alleviating any stressors in the child's environment identified in the assessment. Despite proven effectiveness in adults there is, as yet, no evidence for using antidepressant medication in children and teenagers with depression. Given that antidepressants are effective in adults, however, most child psychiatrists would consider their use in older teenagers where the pattern of presentation is similar to that in adults and when other treatments have failed. Although suicide is rare in adolescence, any treatment plan must include advice to parents about monitoring for the possibility of self harm.

Suicide and self harm

Completed suicide is fortunately very rare in children under the age of 14 but the incidence rises with age. Boys outnumber girls, and in older adolescents it is the third most common cause of death.

Attempts at self harm (most usually overdoses) are far more common, occurring in 1% of the population aged 12–15. In this group girls outnumber boys. 15–25% will repeat their attempt within a year and 1–2% are likely to eventually succeed in their attempts.

Children who self harm are more likely to be socially isolated, to have chronic physical health problems, and to come from families with parental marital difficulties, communication problems and inconsistent discipline. Common precipitants are relationship disputes, either with peers or with family. Depression in the adolescent, a past or current history of psychiatric illness in the family, and current child abuse should be seen as high risk factors in young people who do self harm.

Although violent means of attempting self harm, for example attempted stabbing and hangings, do indicate high risk, the reverse is not true. Medically insignificant overdoses may mask serious suicidal intent; all children who self harm should therefore be admitted to a paediatric ward and assessed by a member of a child mental health team before discharge. Assessment in the accident and emergency department is not usually helpful as the assessment needs to involve the family as well as the young person and may require information from school and other agencies—this takes time to organise. Drop-out rates are high, but often useful therapeutic work can be carried out in the crisis situation on the ward in the immediate aftermath of the attempt.

Anxiety disorders

Separation anxiety. All toddlers are expected to show some degree of anxiety about separation from carers to whom they are attached. For a few, this can become a serious problem: anxiety becomes so severe, or persists for so long after it would be expected to decline, that it interferes with the child's normal social functioning and development. Many situations that involve separation from an attachment figure also involve exposure to other potential stresses. It is important to ascertain that the child's anxiety is not related to a fear of these other stresses, i.e. it is a phobia, rather than the fear of separation. In practice, in young children, this can be more difficult than it might seem.

Fears and phobias. Specific fears and phobias are common in children and show a developmental progression. Fears of animals and of the dark are so common in pre-school children as to be considered normal. As the child gets older and encounters new situations, other fears—of school and of social situations—arise. In adolescents, anxiety related problems similar to those found in adults (agoraphobia, panic disorder, generalised anxiety disorder) emerge.

Obsessive compulsive disorder. Obsessions are persistent, intrusive, repetitive thoughts. Often they are accompanied by ritualised behaviours (compulsions) performed by the person to reduce the anxiety generated by their obsessive thoughts. This is a relatively rare presentation in children but can be a very disabling condition if left untreated. There is often a positive family history. Some obsessional thoughts and rituals occur normally in children and usually emerge at around 6–7 years. In most children these fade with time and this normal aspect of development only occasionally becomes a clinically significant problem.

School refusal and truancy. This is not strictly speaking a diagnostic category but is still a common presentation. School refusers can be distinguished from truants by the anxiety that school attendance causes. In some cases this anxiety can be masked by physical symptoms but usually emerges if attendance is insisted upon. School refusers are also more likely to be girls, to have a good record of academic attainment, and to have other emotional symptoms when compared with truants. Truants tend to come from large disorganised and chaotic families, have a history of other conduct and antisocial behaviours, and present in the final years of schooling. School refusal peaks at 5 years (starting school) and at 11 years (secondary transfer) (see Table 8.2). General management principles are described below but the involvement of educational staff (teachers, educational social workers and educational psychologists) in the management of school refusal is essential.

Post-traumatic stress disorder. This is being increasingly recognised in children and young people. Mild anxiety symptoms and/or developmental regression, for example the re-emergence of bedwetting, are common following minor upsets and should be managed in primary care.

Table 8.2 Contrasting features of school refusal and truancy

School refusal	Truancy
Girls = boys	Boys > girls
Good academic record	Poor academic record
Other emotional symptoms present, especially anxiety	Other conduct problems present
Peaks at 5 and 11 years	Most common in final years of compulsory schooling
	Large, disorganised families
Physical symptoms common	Physical symptoms rare

Reassurance and sensible behavioural management advice are often sufficient.

Where symptoms are severe and persistent, specialist help is needed. Symptoms in these cases are not dissimilar to those in adults, with recurrent and intrusive memories of the traumatic event, together with more generalised anxiety and fearfulness. Sleep disturbance is common. The exact presentation, as so often in children, depends on the child's developmental level. Children are often encouraged by adults not to think about upsetting thoughts or events. The management of post-traumatic stress should be the opposite of this advice, with the child and family being encouraged to tell and re-tell the 'story' of the traumatising event in an effort to make sense of it. Disturbing dreams can also be retold in this way. It may help to get children to draw pictures of disturbing events, or even act them out in play, if verbal accounts are difficult for them.

Assessment of anxiety disorders

The exact aetiology of anxiety disorders is not always certain although specific triggers and precipitants can often be identified. Genetic factors play a small but significant role, especially in obsessional problems. Behaviours designed to alleviate symptoms, but which in fact maintain them, can commonly be discerned if a careful history is taken of how children and families are dealing with the symptoms. Parents understandably wish to protect their children from distress and therefore may select strategies for dealing with anxiety problems which involve avoidance of the anxiety provoking trigger, be this separation, school, obsessional thought or whatever. This may reduce short-term anxiety but is likely to increase the chances of similar symptoms returning. The pattern can escalate and self-perpetuating vicious circles develop very quickly.

Assessment must therefore include clarification of the exact nature of the anxiety and its precipitants. Information must be sought concerning the coping mechanisms that the child is using and also the explanations and coping strategies of the family. Attention must also be paid to other potential stresses in the environment of both the child and other family members.

Management of anxiety disorders

Treatment aims to promote understanding of the vicious cycle of self-maintenance that can escalate anxiety related symptoms. This often involves some degree of education about anxiety and its physical, emotional, cognitive and behavioural components. Careful history taking of precipitants and coping mechanisms may be aided by getting families to keep diaries of key events. In younger children, therapy focuses on encouraging parents to ensure that the child is not exposed to unnecessary stress but at the same time is not allowed to avoid stressful situations altogether. Brief focused counselling together with sensible behavioural advice may be sufficient. This can be carried out in primary care or in paediatric settings. As with other problems, referral to specialist mental health teams should only take place if problems are particularly severe or persistent, or if simple treatment strategies have not proved successful.

With separation problems relating to nursery attendance there is good evidence that a swift separation is the treatment of choice, but many parents need a lot of preparation for this. Arranging for them to go to the school office and have a cup of coffee prior to looking into the classroom before leaving is often very helpful. Young children find the moment of separation itself the most difficult and usually cope well very soon afterwards if it is not drawn out. Parents, however, carry away an image of a distraught child which they think about all day and which may make it harder for them to separate the following day.

In older children, graded exposure to the source of anxiety may be needed, perhaps supplemented by training in relaxation and diaphragmatic breathing to combat physical symptoms of anxiety and give the child something to do in the midst of an anxiety attack. As the child gets older, individual and group treatments may contribute to the management package but involvement of parents (and teachers in school refusal) is still crucial. Formal family therapy may be needed in some instances when simple advice is not sufficient, in order to involve parents in management plans. In obsessional difficulties it is not uncommon to find that, although it is the child who has the obsessional thoughts, the whole family are engaged in carrying out the consequent compulsive behaviour. A combination of behavioural techniques (response prevention) and family work is nearly always needed.

Medication is less useful in anxiety disorders. Minor tranquillisers do not have a place in ongoing treatment but may, occasionally, be used in acute crises on a strictly time limited basis. There is some' evidence to support the use of some antidepressants (specific serotonin re-uptake inhibitors) in obsessive compulsive disorders but these are not usually seen as a first choice treatment. They can be valuable when family and behavioural treatments have failed.

Developmental disorders

Developmental delay is associated with an increased risk of child psychiatric disorder. This section covers not delay, but specific disorders which are seen as being linked to developmental problems.

Enuresis

This can be diurnal or, more commonly, nocturnal. It is helpful to distinguish between children with primary enuresis (who have never been dry) and those with secondary enuresis. It is a common condition: 5% of children still wet the bed at 7 years. Enuresis is more common in boys and strongly associated with a positive family history. Other factors associated with enuresis include social disadvantage, large families,

---

GP Overview 8.1 Enuresis

- Primary—never dry at night, usually dry in daytime
- Secondary—previous nocturnal continence then relapse

Incidence
- 15% of 5-year-olds
- 3% of 10-year-olds
- 1% of 14-year-olds

Causes
- Delayed maturation
- Emotional/psychological
- Urinary tract infection
- Familial
- Polyuria (hypercalcaemia, diabetes mellitus/insipidus, chronic renal failure)
- Urological (incontinence rather than enuresis)
  —ectopic ureter
  —meatal stenosis
  —posterior urethral valves

History
- Recent changes to routine, e.g. school, house move, new sibling
- Check for UTI symptoms
- Check FH enuresis
- Consider spinal/urological causes

Examination
- Check for renal enlargement/tenderness
- Check spine/scrotum

GP tests
- Dipstick urine for sugar, protein, blood
- MSU for culture
- consider renal function, serum Ca^{++}

Management
- Full explanation of problem to child/parents
- Star chart
- > 6 years old, alarm buzzer
- Short-term treatment with DDAVP (tricyclics should be avoided because of cardiac side-effects)

recent life events, and low intelligence. Only about 20% of children who wet the bed have a concurrent psychiatric disorder. There is an association with urinary tract infections, which should always be looked for, but successful treatment of the infection does not guarantee dryness.

Genetic, family and environmental factors all seem to play a part and should be assessed, together with questions about sleeping arrangements (who sleeps where) and location of the toilet. Assessment should include examination of the abdomen, back and lower limbs in addition to mental state.

In the first instance, management should consist of sensible advice about consistent, regular bedtime routines with praise for dryness and no punishment for wet nights. Both excess fluids and excess fluid restriction before bed should be avoided. This is often successful on its own but can be reinforced by getting families to use formal 'star charts' to help maintain a consistent pattern. Star charts reinforce existing behaviour; they will therefore not be effective if the child is wet every night and there are no dry nights to reinforce.

If star charts fail, a pad and alarm system should be used in addition to charts and praise for dryness. Management of enuresis should be undertaken by the primary care team, and more than 90% of children should be dry with this graded approach using advice, charts and alarms. Local practice varies but in many districts resistant cases are then taken up by community paediatric services. In some families the child may continue to wet because of more serious family difficulties. These children may need referral to a specialist child mental health service. Medication with vasopressin analogues can be used to treat enuresis but is associated with high relapse rates when discontinued. Nevertheless, use of these drugs may be useful as a short-term holding operation (for example a school trip) or where parental intolerance of the child and/or the problem makes compliance with other strategies unlikely.

Soiling

50% of children achieve faecal continence by 18–24 months, and by 4 years almost all will have achieved bowel control. Soiling is thus a relatively rare event, present in perhaps 1–2% of 7-year-olds and more common in boys. It is associated with enuresis. Primary soiling difficulties may be due to difficulties in learning, either because of inherent developmental problems (where retention is uncommon) or because of training difficulties. The latter may occur in chaotic and inconsistent families or in those with bizarre ideas about toilet training. Disagreements about potting may become a battleground for autonomy between the child and parent. Physical causes include painful anal conditions, such as fissure, which may lead to retention and overflow. Soiling presenting in toddlers is only very rarely caused by Hirschsprung's disease. Secondary soiling in older children who have already achieved continence is often part of a range of 'protest' behaviours. Such children often have stressful, chaotic life circumstances.

Assessment must include a full and detailed account of toilet training as well as the parents' current attempts to deal with the problem. It is essential to find out, and use, the family's language for faeces and defaecation.

As with enuresis, management of soiling should be carried out in primary care with only resistant cases being referred on. It should always involve explanation to the child and parents of the possible mechanisms involved, particularly if there is evidence of retention and overflow. If retention is present it must be treated first, with laxatives initially but, if necessary, other more vigorous treatments. The family then need help in 'retraining' the child's bowels. This usually involves a regular potting routine where the child sits on the pot for a few minutes only at regular intervals (4–5 times daily or more may be necessary) and is rewarded for so doing. It is important that sitting on the pot and 'trying' is rewarded, not cleanliness, as rewarding the latter may encourage further retention. Star charts may help reinforce this programme. Parents may need help in avoiding provoking anxiety in the child, and this may lead to family therapy in those families with more serious difficulties.

Tic disorders

Tics are involuntary, rapid, recurrent, non-rhythmic motor movements or vocal productions. Their aetiology is uncertain but, like most developmental problems, they are more common in boys than girls. A family history is often present. Simple, transient tics are common: 10–20% of the population may be affected at some time. The onset is usually in middle childhood or early adolescence, may be precipitated by stressful life events, and starts with simple movements involving only one muscle or muscle group. In most children the tic resolves spontaneously. In a few cases the tics persist and may go on to involve multiple muscle groups and vocal productions (coughs, grunts or words). At its most severe, combined motor and vocal tics (known as Tourette's syndrome) can be a very distressing and disabling condition. Simple, transient tics should be dealt with by reassurance and ignored. In complex tics, treatment can be difficult and prognosis poor. Specialist mental health assessment is recommended. Low dose haloperidol is probably the treatment of choice but, as the condition is exacerbated by stress, psychological treatments and attention to stress reduction in the environment may also be of benefit.

Pervasive developmental disorders

These conditions are characterised by difficulties in three broad areas:

1. qualitative abnormalities in reciprocal social interactions with others
2. abnormalities in patterns of communication
3. a restricted and repetitive range of interests and activities.

Infantile autism

Children with autism have severe and persistent difficulties in all three domains listed above. It is fortunately a rare condition (about 4 per 10 000), and more common in boys than girls. Associated learning difficulties are common. Affected children are often emotionally unresponsive from a very early age. They do not seek out gestures of affection and do not respond to them. They may avoid eye contact and do not develop the normal pattern of attachment with separation anxiety seen in ordinary toddlers. Although the exact pattern of presentation varies from child to child, the central problem is a failure to understand social interactions and an inability to respond appropriately in social contexts.

Language problems are widespread and most children do not develop early non-verbal means of communication such as pointing or gesturing to indicate need. Almost half of autistic children will not develop any useful speech at all. The rest have great difficulties in using speech socially and to convey meaning. There is an associated inability to engage in creative and fantasy play.

Autistic children usually have a restricted range of interests and may engage in endless repetitive play. They may become very attached to routines and to particular inanimate objects.

Asperger's syndrome

These children have similar problems to those with autism in relation to reciprocal social interactions and restricted interests, but have relatively normal cognitive and language development. Asperger's syndrome is more common in boys and there is a marked association with clumsiness. Despite their normal language skills, affected children may still have major communication difficulties because of their lack of understanding of social interactions. Presentation may be later than in autism and some children are not identified until middle childhood.

There is some debate about whether Asperger's syndrome is a separate condition to autism or just represents a milder variant. In practice, there is so much variation within each condition that many children do not seem to fall neatly into either category.

Management of pervasive developmental disorders

There is no cure for these conditions. Management strategies are geared towards helping affected children and their families cope with the child's difficulties and promote maximal developmental progress. Early identification is crucial; assessment should be multidisciplinary (usually involving paediatricians, psychiatrists, psychologists and speech therapists) and lead to careful consideration of appropriate schooling. Autistic children do best in special schools, or special units within mainstream schools, where their particular needs can be met. Children with Asperger's may do well in mainstream school initially but often find the social demands of school increasingly difficult as they progress through the school system. Transfer to high school is often very difficult.

The diagnosis of a pervasive developmental disorder is usually devastating for parents. They need reassurance that their behaviour has not caused the child's condition and a considerable amount of social and emotional support, although not necessarily formal counselling or therapy. National and local support groups may have a key role, in addition to primary care staff. Parents also need advice and guidance on the appropriate behavioural management of the child to avoid repetitive rituals becoming too restrictive. Behavioural treatments are more effective if carried out in the child's home as autistic children have great difficulty generalising their behaviour to new settings.

Disorders of social functioning

The importance of secure early attachments to carers has long been recognised as central to a child's subsequent development. Research is beginning to show that insecure early attachments are associated with inadequate care and predict later social, emotional and behavioural difficulties. Increased recognition of specific patterns of behaviour associated with poor caregiving which do not 'fit' with existing diagnostic categories have recently led to the inclusion of two new diagnostic categories in ICD 10.

Reactive attachment disorder

The key feature is a persistently abnormal pattern of relationships with a caregiver, developing before the age of 5 years and characterised by

---

Box 8.3 Symptoms of reactive attachment disorder

- Fearfulness
- Hypervigilance
- Resistance to being comforted
- Ambivalent responses to caregivers (a mixture of approach and avoidance)
- Looking away when being held
- Withdrawal
- Misery
- Aggression towards self and others

---

contradictory social responses, most often seen at times of parting and reunion—see Box 8.3.

Such behaviours persist across different social settings yet respond to major changes in the child's social environment, for example placement in a more appropriate home. These children can be distinguished from those with pervasive developmental problems primarily by their responsiveness to major environmental change. Also, they do have the capacity for reciprocal interaction and do not show qualitative impairments in language (although they may have language delay). This condition is nearly always found in relation to significant child abuse.

Disinhibited attachment disorder

This refers to a persistent pattern of abnormal social functioning that is resistant to environmental change. Typically children show clinging and non-selectively focused attachment behaviour at 2 years but by 4 years are attention-seeking and indiscriminately friendly. Attention-seeking behaviour and difficulties in peer relationships persist into later childhood. This syndrome is most commonly seen when children have had a persistent lack of opportunity to develop selective attachments. This is most likely to happen if children have been reared in institutions or when they have been subject to frequent changes in caregiver and have had multiple early family placements.

Eating disorders

These are distinct from early feeding problems although recent research suggests a link between the two. Anorexia nervosa and bulimia nervosa both arise in adolescence and involve characteristic disturbances of body image. Obesity can present at any age.

Anorexia nervosa

The key psychological feature of anorexia nervosa is a dread of fatness with a distortion of body image such that, even if emaciated, the patient may not see herself as thin. This in turn leads to self induced weight loss. The typical clinical and endocrine features are listed in Box 8.4.

Typically the condition starts with dieting. Teasing about weight or shape may precipitate this. High calorie foods such as carbohydrates are usually avoided and this may continue for some time before concerns are raised, by which time dieting may be out of control. Patients are often very preoccupied with their diet, sometimes to the exclusion of all other interests.

The condition occurs in about 1% of adolescents and most commonly becomes a problem at around the age of 17. It does occur in boys (the female:male ratio is about 10:1) in whom the clinical picture is remarkably similar. In those cases where presentation is pre-pubertal, there is an association with early feeding and behavioural difficulties. The aetiology is complex and multifactorial. Suggested theories include a fear of becoming physically and emotionally mature, and anorexia as the only means of gaining some autonomy in families where this would otherwise be impossible. The onset of puberty is clearly an important factor, as are family communication patterns and societal pressures to conform to ideals of thinness. There are increasing reports of higher rates of sexual abuse in childhood in adults with anorexia nervosa.

Management must include a structured programme to increase weight alongside psychotherapeutic approaches for the child and family. In severe cases this has to take place in an inpatient setting. Cognitive behavioural approaches are being increasingly used to supplement other therapies. There is some evidence that family therapy may be more effective than individual psychodynamic therapies in younger adolescents. The prognosis is not always good. About two thirds will attain normal weight but only about half of patients will resume menstruation or regain normal eating patterns. The mortality is about 5%.

Bulimia nervosa

Bulimia is 2–3 times more common than anorexia in teenagers and occurs predominantly in girls. There is a persistent preoccupation with food, a dread of fatness, and a cyclical pattern of disturbed eating with bouts of overeating followed by bouts of self induced vomiting, purgative abuse, and use of diuretics or appetite suppressants. There may then follow a period of severe dieting leading to further craving and bingeing. The significant weight loss seen in anorexia nervosa is absent but there may be serious electrolyte disturbances secondary to laxative abuse and vomiting.

Bulimic symptoms may occur as part of the picture of anorexia nervosa or may follow a period of anorexia nervosa as normal weight is regained. It is, however, a syndrome in its own right. The theories of its aetiology are similar to those of anorexia.

There is most evidence for the effectiveness of cognitive behavioural treatments in bulimia.

Box 8.4 Changes associated with anorexia nervosa

Clinical
- Avoidance of 'fattening' foods
- Self-induced vomiting and/or purging
- Excessive exercise
- Use of appetite suppressants, diuretics or laxatives
- Body weight maintained at least 15% below that expected
- Depression
- Irritability
- Obsessionality
- Insomnia
- Low self-esteem

Endocrine
- Amenorrhoea
- Elevated growth hormone
- Elevated cortisol
- Altered thyroid hormone
- Altered insulin levels

Management usually involves educational input about healthy eating and the effects of starvation on bingeing, with diary keeping and self monitoring of eating behaviours. This leads in turn to identification and modification of dysfunctional thoughts and beliefs that perpetuate the disturbed eating pattern.

Obesity

This is an increasingly common problem in children and adolescents and may lead to hurtful teasing and to relative social isolation. As in adults it is not an easy problem to manage. Sensible advice about diet, exercise, and the longer-term implications of obesity should be given and reinforced using simple behavioural techniques, but this is often insufficient to bring about anything but short-lived change. Lasting reduction in weight needs lifestyle changes not short-term diets, and experience suggests that it is difficult to modify a child's eating and exercise patterns unless the rest of the family are willing to co-operate as well.

Gender identity disorder

This is very rare and occurs when a child has persistent and intense distress about his or her assigned gender, together with a desire to be of the other gender. It is usually present from pre-school years; affected children display a marked preference for, and preoccupation with, the activities stereotypically associated with the other gender. Typically boys will want to play with girls rather than other boys, will avoid rough and tumble play and will choose to play with female dolls. Children are often not distressed by their own feelings about gender, but may be very distressed by the reactions of others to this. Boys in particular can be subjected to severe teasing and bullying at school. Follow-up studies indicate that, of boys who demonstrate this kind of behaviour, most will go on to develop a homosexual or bisexual orientation.

Management is controversial: some argue that this is not a condition that should be treated. There is no evidence that psychotherapy can change eventual sexual orientation although behavioural techniques may modify gender role behaviour in childhood. Support and counselling may be necessary to help children deal with the reactions of others and to help parents deal with their own feelings about their child's development.

Substance misuse

Substance misuse in young people is a cause of much societal and family concern, with regular media reports of children dying as a result of drug use. There seems little doubt that substance abuse is increasing in young people although actual figures are hard to come by. The most commonly abused substances are alcohol, tobacco, solvents and cannabis—all of which may be used in early adolescence. Doctors will come across young people in middle to late adolescence who use opiates, stimulants, ecstasy and hallucinogens.

Most drug use in adolescence is 'recreational' in that drugs are used in group settings as part of a social experience. Peer pressure and a desire to be accepted in the group may play a key role in initiating drug use. In these circumstances drug use may be intermittent but regular and with little in the way of either physical or psychological dependence.

Although the long-term physical effects of regular substance misuse may be serious, with alcohol and tobacco being particularly dangerous, many of the substances used are not particularly dangerous in the short term in their own right. Risks arise more from the effects of intoxication or from the means of administration. Thus young people may get into dangerous situations when intoxicated, the risks of traffic accident being high if drugs are taken in public places. The use of inhaled aerosols may precipitate respiratory and/or cardiac arrest, and the use of polythene bags in association with other solvents may lead to suffocation. Injection of any drug carries serious risks of infection.

In primary care settings it is important always to be aware of the possibility of substance misuse contributing to the clinical presentation and to enquire in the history about this in as 'non-judgemental' a way as possible. Recreational substance misuse does not usually concern mental health services, who usually only become involved when substance misuse has become a core feature of the young person's behavioural repertoire. Referral to specialist services should always be considered when there is risk of physical damage or when withdrawal symptoms are evident, and when there is significant social dysfunction. Solitary substance misuse outside the group or social setting should be a cause for concern as this may mask other psychiatric problems, for example depression.

Substance misuse leading to widespread social dysfunction is often part of a wider pattern of disorder. Commonly, young people who have been referred have had conduct problems for many years and, as they have grown older, substance misuse has been incorporated as part of this picture. Having dealt with any physical withdrawal, management usually involves dealing with these other problems in the ways outlined in other sections of this chapter rather than focusing specifically on the substance misuse.

Psychosis

Psychosis very rarely occurs before puberty but the risks increase as children proceed through adolescence. Many adults with schizophrenia or with bipolar affective disorder can trace their first episodes of illness back to adolescence.

Schizophrenia

The core symptoms of schizophrenia are the same in young people as in adults—see Box 8.5. Acute and florid presentations are relatively easy to diagnose. If the onset is gradual with thought disorder, social withdrawal and deteriorating school performance it may not always be easy to recognise the condition for what it is; careful, specialist assessment is needed.

Acute transient schizophreniform episodes do occur, and typically present with a rapidly changing and variable state of acute onset, including typical features of acute schizophrenia but with high levels of affective symptoms and

---

Box 8.5 Symptoms of schizophrenia
• Auditory hallucinations in the third person • Thought insertion • Thought withdrawal • Thought broadcasting • Thought echo • Delusions of control • Delusions of influence • Delusions of passivity • Other persistent and culturally inappropriate delusions • Formal thought disorder • Catatonia

associated with acute stress. Such transient psychoses can resolve completely within 2–3 months, but early prediction of which young people will follow this path rather than go on to develop more persistent symptoms is not yet possible.

Treatment should be with neuroleptic medication as in adults. Families need support and education about the child's needs, as do school staff. Work to reduce expressed emotion in the family may reduce relapse. The prognosis is better if the onset is acute and with a substantial affective component.

Bipolar affective disorder (manic depressive psychosis)

Bipolar disorders can have their onset in adolescence. Like schizophrenia, the core symptoms are the same as in adults but the presentation is influenced by the child's developmental stage, making diagnosis difficult in younger adolescents. Depression has already been covered. Mania usually has an acute onset with heightened mood, activity and mood congruent delusions. Treatment is similar to that in adults. The acute manic phase needs to be managed with neuroleptic medication. There is a high likelihood of further episodes if the initial one is manic; lithium therefore needs to be considered as prophylactic medication.

Children with physical symptoms

From the mental health perspective, children with physical symptoms may be referred because of chronic or acute illnesses with which they are having problems coping, or because of concerns that psychological difficulties are either exacerbating or causing physical symptoms. The numbers of children involved are large. Chronic illness or disability affects up to one fifth of the child population, depending upon exact definitions.

All services for children with physical health problems have to consider how the associated social and psychological problems of children and their families will be met. Failure to do this not only leads to a lower quality of care for the child and family as a whole but may even make the physical problems worse.

Chronic illness

As observed earlier, children with chronic illness are more likely to have psychiatric disorders. Parents are also profoundly affected by the illness of their children and are more likely to have psychological problems, as are the siblings of the affected child. Marital problems are more common, but parents are not more likely to divorce. Children with poorly controlled chronic illness are likely to come from dysfunctional families with more conflict, disorganisation and poor supervision. Communication is often poor and there is a relative lack of warmth. Having a child with a chronic illness also has adverse effects on the family's economic situation, with reduced earning opportunities for parents and increased costs of caring for the ill child. It is not clear whether these family associations are causes or effects of the chronic illness. Most children with chronic illness and their families cope very well. What is clear is that for some families with a chronically ill child, a pattern is set up where psychological problems in the child and family adversely affect the child's physical health and compliance with treatment which, in turn, adversely affects the mental health of the family.

Specific physical diagnoses do not predict specific psychiatric disorders. However, characteristics of the chronic illness such as duration, severity, chronicity, visibility (high visibility pre-dicts fewer problems), and interference with normal functioning do predict likelihood of psychological problems.

Physical symptoms with no organic cause (somatoform disorders)

At the 'milder' end of the spectrum, symptoms of pain are very common. Recurrent abdominal pain (RAP), defined as three or more episodes in 6 months, severe enough to lead to absence from school or interference in normal functioning, occurs in 25% of 6-year-olds. Most RAP does not have an organic cause; this is not true for other painful symptoms such as headache but these too can be exacerbated by psychological factors. Children with recurrent painful symptoms are often from families with a history of painful symptoms, leading to suggestions that this is one way in which some families communicate distress.

More severe problems include the classic 'conversion' disorders which are fortunately relatively rare, occurring in 1–2% of referrals to child mental health teams. Common presentations are disturbances of gait, other disorders of motor function, pseudoseizures, and disturbances of sensation and vision. Such problems are rare under the age of 5 years. A family background of emotional over-involvement and poor communication is common. Episodes often start with a period of genuine physical illness and there is often a 'model' for the patient to copy—someone known to the family who has a similar symptom. Theories about the 'sick role' and 'illness behaviour' suggest that symptoms may be maintained by the child getting some advantage or 'secondary gain' from the symptoms. However, it is not thought that these symptoms are under conscious control. Often, despite the seriousness of the physical symptoms, there is no major underlying family or child psychopathology. Also to be included in this category are the chronic fatigue syndromes. The aetiology of these presentations is still unclear but their management has much in common with that described below for non-organic disorders.

Management

Management of all children with physical symptoms, whatever the cause, is best carried out as part of an ongoing collaborative relationship between the paediatric, child mental health and primary care teams. If children and families can see that mental health staff are part of the team this can facilitate referrals, if and when they are needed, and make joint assessment easier. Regular meetings between staff from these teams to discuss potential problems (psychosocial ward rounds) facilitate communication within staff groups as well as between staff and families. Some mental health professionals are specialising in this area of work, and the terms 'liaison psychiatry' and 'health psychology' are being used increasingly to describe this work. In chronic illness the main burden of communicating the diagnosis to children and families and providing support rightly falls on paediatric staff. However, referrals to the mental health team are appropriate for those families who find coping with the child's illness too difficult or for those children who develop specific psychological problems. There is also a role for mental health teams in supporting children through difficult and painful procedures.

Treatment of non-organic disorders also involves close collaboration. Physical investigation must be thorough and seen to be thorough by the family. Most treatment plans stress recognition of the symptoms irrespective of cause, coupled with a gradual rehabilitation of the child back into a normal routine. Symptoms are managed with as little secondary gain as is possible and 'well' behaviour encouraged and rewarded. Specific child or parental anxieties must be explored (it is not possible to reassure someone effectively until it is known what that person is worried about) and any underlying stresses removed, where possible. In cases of hysterical motor disturbance physiotherapy is a helpful adjunct and provides the child with an 'escape with honour' from the symptoms.

CONCLUSION

Child and adolescent mental health problems are common in the population and more common still in primary care and paediatric settings. Their aetiology is complex and multifactorial, and requires careful assessment, but these problems are treatable. It is essential that general practitioners and paediatricians have a basic grasp of the principles of assessment and can apply simple management techniques. A knowledge of local child and adolescent mental health services is also required, along with the ability to refer families in a way that encourages attendance. This is more likely to happen if paediatricians and general practitioners are already working closely with their local child mental health team.

FURTHER READING

Black D, Cottrell D (eds) 1993 Seminars in child and adolescent psychiatry. Royal College of Psychiatrists/Gaskell, London
Eiser C 1990 Chronic childhood illness. Cambridge University Press, Cambridge
Rutter M, Taylor E, Hersov L (eds) 1994 Child and adolescent psychiatry: modern approaches, 3rd edn. Blackwell, Oxford

9

Neurology

Martin Bellman

Nerve cells in the central nervous system (CNS) do not regenerate, therefore their protection and preservation is particularly important. In general, children with suspected neurological disease should be referred to an experienced paediatrician for assessment unless it is absolutely clear that they have a minor time-limited problem (Box 9.1).

CONVULSIONS (Figure 9.1)

A convulsion (seizure) may occur for many reasons. It is a symptom which must be assessed carefully in order to establish the underlying diagnosis. It is important to distinguish between epileptic and non-epileptic convulsions. The crucial piece of evidence is an accurate eye-witness account and this should always be sought and documented as quickly as possible.

Non-epileptic convulsions

Febrile convulsion (FC)

Febrile convulsions occur in up to 5% of children

Box 9.1   Symptoms that require paediatric referral

Urgent (same day)
- Significant decrease of conscious level
- Prolonged first convulsion (> 10 minutes)
- Paralysis
- Ataxia

Non-urgent (within 2 weeks)
- Recurrent brief convulsions
- Severe/prolonged headaches
- Regression of developmental skills

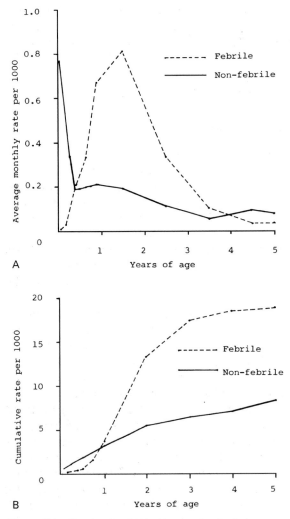

Figure 9.1 Graphs showing incidence rates for first convulsion. A: Average monthly rates by age at first convulsion. B: Cumulative rates by age at first convulsion.

tepid (not cold) sponging, reducing the ambient temperature and giving drinks.

Infants aged less than 12 months should be referred urgently to hospital in case of meningitis. The only indication for lumbar puncture is to exclude meningitis if there is clinical doubt.

Hospital referral is not necessary if:

- the child is neurologically normal
- age > 1 year
- the fever has subsided
- there is a definite cause for fever
- the parents can cope.

Drugs. Prophylactic anticonvulsant medication should not be given universally after an FC. If FCs are recurrent there is a risk of a complex or prolonged seizure; parents can be given diazepam for rectal administration if the FC lasts longer than 5 minutes. Some paediatricians prescribe continuous sodium valproate if prolonged FCs recur.

The prognosis is good except in the following circumstances:

- prolonged convulsion (> 30 minutes)
- complex convulsion (focal or multiple)
- positive family history (first degree relative) of epilepsy
- age < 1 year.

In these children the risk of subsequent FCs is increased. If two or more factors are present, the risk for epilepsy is approximately 10%. Mesial temporal sclerosis may occur after prolonged FCs and cause subsequent temporal lobe epilepsy.

In the vast majority of cases, parents can be reassured that there is no long-term sequel to a febrile convulsion. It is an extremely frightening experience for them, however, and many think the child is dying during the first convulsion, hence they require sympathy and time.

Reflex anoxic seizures

These are brief tonic-clonic convulsions which rarely occur after breath-holding attacks because of brain hypoxia/ischaemia during a temporary cardiac arrest. This occurs because of excessive vagal tone, which can be mimicked for diagnostic

aged 6 months to 5 years as an idiosyncratic response to fever. The majority are brief (< 5 minutes) generalised tonic-clonic seizures which may rarely recur within 24 hours during the same febrile episode. In the long term, approximately 33% of children will have another FC. There is a familial tendency, with a high concordance (80%) in monozygotic twins.

Management. In all cases, parents should be advised to reduce fever with paracetamol and cool the child by removing excess clothing, gentle purposes by ocular compression under EEG and ECG control. Treatment with atropine may be successful. Reflex anoxic seizures are always benign; firm reassurance, with behavioural advice to try to avoid the precipitating breath-holding attacks, is indicated. Whilst parents should be advised on the value of distracting a child who is 'brewing up' for a breath-holding attack, a policy of placating the child at all costs is more likely to damage social development than is the occasional seizure!

Differential diagnosis

Several paroxysmal events can mimic epileptic convulsions and should be excluded (Box 9.2).

Epileptic convulsions (Box 9.3)

Epilepsy is a recurring tendency to have con-

Box 9.2   Possible non-epileptic diagnosis of 'convulsive' episodes

- Tics
- Syncope
- Breath-holding attacks
- Cardiogenic collapse
- Vertigo
- Daydreams
- Gratification/behavioural phenomena
- Sandifer syndrome (sudden head movements due to gastro-oesophageal reflux in children with cerebral palsy)

Box 9.3   Simplified classification of childhood epileptic seizures

Partial (focal)
- Simple—elementary symptoms (motor, sensory)
- Complex—psychomotor
- Partial progressing to secondary generalisation

Generalised
- Absence:
    —typical (petit mal)
    —atypical
- Myoclonic including infantile spasms
- Tonic-clonic (grand mal)
- Atonic

Mixed
Unclassified

---

vulsions because of a neurological or metabolic abnormality. It is not an appropriate diagnosis for a single seizure. Epilepsy is relatively common and affects approximately 1 in 200 of the adult population. It is entirely compatible with a normal lifestyle.

Generalised epilepsies

Abnormal cerebral discharges arise from both hemispheres, and symptoms are bilateral.

Tonic-clonic/generalised (grand mal) epilepsy. Approximately 80% of epilepsy is of the major tonic-clonic type. Symmetrical jerking affects the arms, legs and face (in any order or simultaneously) during the characteristic clonic phase. It usually subsides after a few minutes and the child sleeps for several hours. On waking, the child often feels generally unwell for up to 24 hours. Rarely in children there are residual neurological abnormalities, e.g. slurred speech, poor balance, limb paralysis or paraesthesia (Todd's paralysis), which resolve over the next 2–5 days.

The diagnosis is made on a reliable history, and an EEG is not usually necessary.

Treatment. Drugs should only be prescribed when the diagnosis has been confirmed, i.e. usually after the second or subsequent convulsion. The first line drugs are sodium valproate and carbamazepine. Phenobarbitone and phenytoin are no longer in the first line category because of their side-effects. Monotherapy is preferred; each drug is titrated against fit control and side-effects up to the maximum level. If control is not achieved with one drug, another can be added. Second line drugs are phenytoin, phenobarbitone, topiramate, vigabatrin, lamotrigine and gabapentin. They can be tried alone or in combination. It may not be possible to eliminate seizures completely, and in some children it is better to accept a few convulsions rather than excessive adverse effects. This strategy must be clearly negotiated with child and parents. Drug therapy for epilepsy is developing rapidly and new generation drugs are being produced which are highly effective and have few side-effects.

Absence (petit mal) epilepsy. This accounts for approximately 2% of cases of epilepsy and is most common in girls aged 5–12 years. It is often missed by parents and is first noticed by teachers or other professionals observing the child's behaviour. During attacks, the child does not lose consciousness; the eyes stare, then drift, and the eyelids flicker. The attacks are brief, lasting 5–15 seconds (rarely up to 30 seconds), but during that period the child is unaware of his or her surroundings. If the attacks are frequent, learning at school is compromised. The diagnosis is made by the characteristic description and the EEG which shows regular, 3 per second, spike and wave abnormalities. Clinical attacks can sometimes be precipitated by hyperventilation (for at least 2 minutes) which can be done as a diagnostic test.

Treatment. Sodium valproate or ethosuximide is usually very effective and well tolerated.

Prognosis. Typical absence attacks usually cease in adolescence but major epilepsy develops in up to 50% of cases.

Myoclonic convulsions. A myoclonic jerk is a sudden involuntary contraction of muscle without loss of consciousness (isolated myoclonic spasms on falling asleep are a normal phenomenon).

Myoclonic epilepsy of childhood. This affects children from the age of about 3½ years and is often preceded by tonic-clonic seizures. There is no warning and the spasm may be violent, causing the child to fall suddenly without any saving reaction. If the child is standing or sitting at a table, serious injury may result. There is no post-ictal phase and the child carries on (unless injured). Spasms may occur as startle attacks in response to noise, touch or flashing lights. The EEG is abnormal, showing atypical spikes and waves, sometimes with photosensitivity.

There may be no underlying cause but some cases have degenerative brain disease and show other progressive neurological symptoms. Idiopathic cases are generally benign and respond well to treatment with sodium valproate. Refractory seizures may require second line drugs such as nitrazepam, clonazepam, vigabatrin or lamotrigine.

Lennox–Gastaut syndrome (petit mal variant). This is usually associated with severe learning difficulties and brain disorders. The attacks consist of head drops or nods, absences and myoclonic spasms, alone or in combination, and may be very frequent. The EEG shows diffuse slow spike waves. Treatment is difficult and requires trials of lamotrigine, benzodiazepines and steroids. A ketogenic diet can be tried as a last resort.

Infantile spasms (salaam attacks). The incidence is approximately 1 per 5000 children aged between 3 and 18 months. 70% of cases present in the first 6 months of life. Attacks are momentary; typically the trunk flexes and the arms extend or flex at the elbow. The child may simultaneously cry out, grimace or laugh. The attacks often occur in repetitive runs for about 1 minute and may happen many times a day. The most frequent diagnostic confusion is with infantile colic. Cases should be referred for urgent paediatric assessment as early treatment may ameliorate the generally very poor prognosis. Many children show developmental regression; when this is combined with the classical EEG picture of hypsarrhythmia, the triad is known as West's syndrome.

Treatment should be started as early as possible with ACTH injections for 6 weeks or vigabatrin, followed by benzodiazepines or sodium valproate.

Approximately half the cases have no identifiable cause and the child was previously normal (cryptogenic). In these cases the prognosis is relatively good and about 50% recover. In the other half, a neurological abnormality can be demonstrated on the history or investigation (symptomatic). In this group the prognosis is poor: approximately 75% will have learning difficulties and 10% die. Persistent epilepsy (grand mal and Lennox–Gastaut syndrome) is a frequent sequel.

Status epilepticus is a convulsion or series of convulsions persisting for longer than 30 minutes without recovery of consciousness in between. This situation requires emergency treatment as continuation can cause increasing cerebral oedema, intracranial pressure and thus hypoxia leading to neuronal death. First aid is to remove sources of potential danger (e.g. fire), secure the airway and administer oxygen. The only medication suitable for use in primary care is rectal diazepam liquid. This is absorbed rapidly and is effective in 80% of cases. It can safely be given by parents or other carers. If rectal diazepam is not available, the child must be urgently transferred to hospital where the drug of choice is intravenous diazepam. Resuscitation facilities must be available as cardiac and respiratory depression and arrest may occur. In approximately 10% of cases, status epilepticus cannot be controlled by rectal or intravenous diazepam; alternative drugs are rectal or intramuscular paraldehyde, intravenous phenytoin, and intravenous infusion of chlormethiazole or lignocaine. If these are unsuccessful by 60–90 minutes, then general anaesthesia with thiopentone and muscle paralysis can be used. In status epilepticus the brain's metabolic rate is very high and nutritional requirements must be maintained in order to prevent irreversible neuronal damage.

Partial epilepsies

Temporal lobe epilepsy (TLE) (partial complex seizures/psychomotor epilepsy). This is the most common form of epilepsy in children (approximately 20% of all cases). The average age of onset is 5–6 years, and attacks may continue into adult life.

Clinical features. A wide variety of sensations may occur including hallucinations of smell, taste, sound or vision, strange emotional feelings—'déjà vu' and 'jamais vu'—and sensations of sickness and vertigo. These attacks are often frightening and TLE is in the differential diagnosis for children with unexplained behaviour disturbances and nightmares. Motor automatisms occur such as repetitive movements which can be semi-purposive, e.g. dressing, lip smacking or hand washing.

The EEG shows abnormal discharges in one or other temporal region. Brain imaging may show a focal abnormality, including mesial temporal sclerosis, following prolonged febrile convulsions.

Treatment. Carbamazepine is the first line drug of choice and lamotrigine the second. Surgical removal of a defined focus can be successful.

Prognosis. Roughly one third recover comple-

tely during childhood, a third continue having epilepsy (TLE and grand mal) but are mentally normal, and a third have learning difficulties. Poor prognostic factors are onset before 2 years of age, low IQ and frequent seizures (more than one a day).

Partial seizures with elementary symptoms. In simple partial seizures consciousness is not lost. If the motor cortex is involved there is unilateral jerking in the appropriate part of the body. In Jacksonian fits there is a 'march', usually starting in the thumb or fingers and extending up the arm to the rest of the body on that side. When the epileptic focus is in the sensory cortex, abnormal sensations of temperature change, numbness or paraesthesiae are felt. There are many other possible sites: in the occipital lobe they cause visual phenomena and in the hippocampus laughing (gelastic) attacks.

Treatment. Carbamazepine is the first choice, followed by phenytoin or sodium valproate.

Partial seizures with secondary generalisation. Focal epilepsy may spread to surrounding areas of the brain to culminate in a generalised grand mal seizure. Treatment is with sodium valproate or carbamazepine, alone or in combination.

Benign focal (Rolandic) epilepsy is relatively common (approximately 10% of cases of epilepsy), starting at the age of 7–10 years and occurring more frequently in boys than girls. Seizures occur mainly during sleep and consist of focal limb jerking and sometimes adversive turning of the head and eyes. Abnormal sensations, especially of the tongue and mouth, may be felt. Consciousness is not lost and the child is aware of surroundings but cannot respond. The EEG shows spikes in temporal and central areas.

A positive family history is common. The prognosis is excellent with 75% recovering within 5 years and 100% before adulthood.

Partial (minor) status epilepticus (epilepsia partialis continua). This consists of continuing minor jerking of a limb, the face or tongue, often associated with slurred speech, dribbling and disorientation. The physical signs may be subtle and the child may present with lack of responsiveness. The prognosis is poor and treatment as for major status epilepticus may be needed

Table 9.1 Adverse effects of anti-epileptic drugs

Drug	Indication	Side-effect
Carbamazepine	Generalised/partial epilepsy	Dizziness, ataxia, diplopia, rash
Sodium valproate	Generalised/partial/myoclonic epilepsy	Anorexia, hair loss, weight gain, tremor, rarely liver failure
Phenobarbitone	Generalised/partial epilepsy in infancy	Behaviour change (aggression, hyperactivity), sleep disturbance
Phenytoin	Generalised/partial epilepsy (rarely used now)	Ataxia, gum hypertrophy, hirsutism, acne, nystagmus
Nitrazepam	Myoclonic epilepsy, infantile spasms	Sedation, ataxia
Clonazepam/Clobazam	Myoclonic epilepsy (second line in all epilepsies)	Behaviour change, weakness, hyper-salivation
Ethosuximide	Absence/myoclonic epilepsy	Vomiting, headache
Lamotrigine	Lennox–Gastaut syndrome (second line in all epilepsies)	Flu-like illness. Raises levels of valproate and carbamazepine. Transient rash
Vigabatrin	Generalised/partial epilepsy, infantile spasms	Confusion, irritability, dizziness. Rarely visual field defect

to gain control. A defined cerebral focus can be treated surgically; hemispherectomy may be indicated.

Anti-epileptic drugs (AEDs)

All AEDs have side-effects which limit the dosage (Table 9.1). The aim is to achieve the best seizure control with the lowest dose, and compromise is often necessary. Monotherapy is always preferable as it minimises the risks of adverse effects and interactions. Most AEDs inhibit CNS activity, so drowsiness and mental slowing are almost universal side-effects, as are nausea and skin rash.

HEADACHE

Headaches occur in children more frequently than is often thought. A positive family history is common, not just in migraine.

Medical assessment

History

Features of the headache. Characteristics such as good relief from analgesics suggest benign headaches, whereas headache on waking or sneezing may be caused by a brain tumour.

Past history. Neurological illness, including head injury.

GP Overview 9.1   Headache

Common causes
- Febrile illness
- Sinusitis
- Migraine
- Tension/stress
- Meningitis/encephalitis

Others to consider include:
- Torticollis
- Head injury
- Cerebral tumour/abscess/cyst
- Benign intracranial hypertension
- Subarachnoid haemorrhage
- Intracerebral haemorrhage
- Severe hypertension
- Dental pain
- Temporo-mandibular joint pain

History—look for symptoms of raised intracranial pressure
- Duration, site, time of day, associated symptoms, ?vomiting, frequency
- Any precipitating factors, e.g. migraine with food/ drink
- Explore emotional/family aspects if tension/stress possible
- Check for meningitis/purpuric rash

Management
- Acute febrile illness—temperature control and antibiotics if appropriate
- Meningitis suspected—hospital admission
- Migraine/tension/stress
  —use of headache diary and explanation
  —dietary exclusion, e.g. chocolate, cheese, tartrazine
  —simple analgesics
  —possible prophylactic treatment, e.g. pizotifen

Family history. Migraine.

Social history. School progress, worries about self, family or friends.

Examination

- Neurological, including optic fundi
- Ears, nose and throat
- Teeth
- BP
- General (abdomen and chest).

A thorough history and examination, with negative results and confirmation that there is no sinister underlying medical condition, is a potent therapeutic tool.

Tension headache

This occurs most commonly in children of school age who have emotional stress concerning their academic progress or personal relationships. The headache is often diffuse, midline or band-like rather than unilateral. It often occurs in regular association with a stressful situation such as school.

It may be severe and not relieved by simple analgesics. A school report is essential with particular enquiry about bullying, especially if there is associated school refusal.

Treatment

Treatment is by reassurance after a normal examination and discussion of potential stress factors. The child should be reviewed after about one month by the GP, school doctor or school nurse. If the problem persists or serious emotional factors are uncovered, referral can be made to a child and family mental health team.

Migraine

This affects approximately 5% of children; about 75% have a positive family history. Classically, it presents as a unilateral, throbbing severe headache. It may start behind the eye and radiate outwards.

Associated symptoms

- Dizziness
- Nausea and vomiting
- Visual phenomena—blurring, flashing lights, stars, scotomata, photophobia
- Abdominal pain
- Hemiplegia—this is very frightening and may alternate between one side and the other (fortunately rare in children)
- Ataxia, vertigo and visual abnormalities occur in basilar artery migraine which is also rare in children.

Treatment

Symptomatic. Many children find relief by resting (lying down) in a quiet dark room.
Drugs:

- Simple analgesics (preferably soluble) should be tried first up to a maximal dose.
- Prophylactic medication, e.g. pizotifen or propranolol, if the attacks are very troublesome and frequent. These drugs are not worthwhile if the frequency is less than once a week.
- Symptomatic—5HT agonists, e.g. naratriptan are more often effective than ergotamine. A useful feature of these drugs is that their successful use is diagnostic of migraine. However, both must be used cautiously in children and should not be prescribed for children under 12 years old without the support of a specialist.

Diet. Some children are allergic to substances such as chocolate, eggs, cow's milk, gluten, cheese and food additives. If the history suggests an association, an exclusion diet can be tried with the help of a dietician.

HEAD INJURY

Head injuries, mostly due to road traffic accidents, are the most common cause of death in children after the first year of life in developed countries; sadly, developing countries are catching up in this respect.

The proportionate size of the head decreases throughout the first 16 years of life so the head of a young child is particularly at risk. In a fall, it is often the first part of the body to hit the ground.

Assessment

History

- Distance fallen
- Previous relevant conditions, e.g. epilepsy, cerebral palsy, bleeding disorder
- Nature of surface fallen onto
- Neurological state immediately afterwards, especially loss of consciousness, seizures, vomiting, ataxia
- How accident happened.

Examination

- Examine the head for swelling, bruises, lacerations, depressed fracture, anterior fontanelle in infants. Measure head circumference.
- Look in ears and nose for bleeding or CSF leak (check any clear fluid with Clinistix to detect glucose in CSF).

Urgent admission to hospital should be arranged in the following circumstances:

- suspected skull fracture
- impaired conscious level
- focal neurological abnormality
- seizures
- persistent vomiting
- social concern regarding ability of carers to observe child accurately
- suspicion of non-accidental injury.

If none of the above applies, the child can go home and the carers must be instructed how to observe the child for signs of raised intracranial pressure. This involves waking the child at 2-hourly intervals over the following 12 hours.

Management of severe head injury

This can be a first aid emergency; the priority is to clear the airway and give cardio-pulmonary resuscitation (CPR) if necessary. A paramedical ambulance team should be called if possible. If equipment is available, an intravenous line should be set up to treat surgical shock. The spine and any fractured limbs should be stabilised before transport to hospital. In the accident and emergency department the child must be attended by a senior trauma specialist or paediatrician.

Supportive treatment may include:

- plasma and blood transfusion
- ventilation—possibly hyperventilation to reduce pCO_2 and lower intracranial pressure
- anti-epileptic medication—phenobarbitone or phenytoin
- antibiotics if skull fracture is present
- monitoring of intracranial pressure clinically or by pressure transducer.

Skull X-ray or, preferably, CT/MRI head scan should be performed if fractures and/or intracranial bleeding is suspected. A neurosurgical opinion should be obtained if there is clinical deterioration, whether or not a skull fracture is present.

Prognosis

Children often make a remarkable recovery after serious head injury. The most important prognostic factors are the duration of loss of consciousness and amnesia. The long-term risk of epilepsy is approximately 6%; in 50% of cases this presents within 12 months of the injury.

Intracranial haemorrhage

Subdural haemorrhage

Bleeding occurs when the fragile cortical veins between the arachnoid and pia mater are torn by direct damage or from a shearing force. Subdural haemorrhage occurs at any age and in neonates is due to birth trauma. In older children it can be caused by head injury, accidental or non-accidental; the latter often occurs from shaking, and retinal haemorrhages must be sought.

Chronic subdural haemorrhage (effusion/collection) occurs when haemorrhages have not been treated. It causes persistent raised intracranial pressure because the fluid collections are not completely reabsorbed. They are important sequelae of non-accidental injury or bacterial meningitis and present with irritability, failure to thrive, developmental delay and focal neurological abnormalities. If available, a CT or MRI scan is performed; if it is positive a neurosurgeon should be consulted about possible drainage.

In infants a diagnostic/therapeutic subdural tap can be performed by carefully inserting a needle through the unfused lateral sutures 1–2 cm either side of the midline at the anterior fontanelle.

Extradural haemorrhage

This is rare in children and occurs because of tearing of dural veins in head injury. There may be no skull fracture. Blood oozes out slowly and causes insidious signs such as headache, lethargy, irritability, vomiting and eventually seizures and cranial nerve abnormalities.

Management is by brain scan and urgent neurosurgery.

Raised intracranial pressure (ICP)

This may present acutely with vomiting, cranial nerve palsies, impaired consciousness and a tense anterior fontanelle in infants. Causes include hydrocephalus and space occupying lesions such as tumour and abscess.

Chronic raised ICP (pseudotumour cerebri) presents non-specifically with headaches, vomiting, diplopia and blurred vision. The most common causes are middle ear or other infections, minor head injuries, withdrawal of steroids, vitamin A toxicity and tetracycline treatment.

INFECTIONS

Bacterial meningitis

Pathology (Box 9.4)

The meninges may be colonised by organisms which have usually spread via the blood stream from a primary focus elsewhere. Rarely meningitis results from direct bacterial invasion from an adjacent structure, e.g. mastoiditis, osteomyelitis, through a fractured skull, via an anat-

---

Box 9.4 Causes of meningitis

Neonates
- Group B streptococci
- *E. coli*
- Rare—*Listeria monocytogenes*, Pseudomonas, Proteus, Klebsiella

Children < 2 years old
- *Neisseria meningitidis*
  —Type B serotypes 70%
  —Type C serotypes 25%
- *Haemophilus influenzae*—Type B (rare since Hib immunisation)
- *Streptococcus pneumoniae*

Children > 2 years old
- *Streptococcus pneumoniae* (carried by 30% of population)
- *Neisseria meningitidis*
- Rare—*Staphylococcus aureus*

---

omical defect (e.g. dermal sinus, spina bifida) or an iatrogenic connection (e.g. lumbar puncture, neurosurgery, ventricular shunt).

Almost any organism can cause meningitis if it gets into the CNS as the internal defence mechanisms are poor and infection can spread quickly. The main protection for the brain is the blood–brain barrier, which usually keeps out organisms as well as many large molecular substances (including drugs).

Clinical features (Box 9.5)

Examination often shows an ill, fractious child. If there is also neck stiffness or a positive Kernig's sign (pain on straightening legs flexed at hips and knees) or Brudzinski's sign (flexion of the hips and knees when the neck is flexed), meningitis must be suspected. The additional presence of a macular or petechial rash is pathognomonic.

Box 9.5 Classical signs of meningitis

- Fever
- Headache
- Irritability
- Impaired consciousness
- Photophobia
- Vomiting
- Neck stiffness
- Rash

Diagnosis in very young children

In infants there may be no classical signs of meningitis. The features are often non-specific with fever, lethargy, failure to feed and a high-pitched cry. The cardinal neurological clinical sign on examination is a tense or bulging fontanelle.

Neonatal meningitis can be even more difficult to diagnose clinically; features include restlessness, apnoeic and bradycardic attacks, hypothermia and jaundice. A lumbar puncture is an essential element of the routine infection screen in neonates.

Management

Suspected bacterial meningitis is one of the relatively few true primary care emergencies. The GP should give an injection (preferably intravenously) of benzyl penicillin and arrange urgent admission to a paediatric unit. In hospital, intravenous penicillin should be administered if it has not already been given. The child needs rapid assessment by an experienced paediatrician who can decide on further management.

Investigations

- Full blood count
- Blood culture
- Clotting studies
- Lumbar puncture unless there is evidence of raised intracranial pressure (papilloedema, bulging fontanelle, coma, focal signs) or the child is so ill that lumbar puncture may precipitate cardiorespiratory arrest.

Turbid CSF confirms the generic diagnosis of bacterial meningitis, and microscopic examination after staining may identify the causative organism (Box 9.6). Antigen detection tests may identify the organism even if the CSF is sterile from antibiotic therapy. Purpuric skin lesions may be aspirated and examined for meningococci.

Treatment

An intravenous line is set up for administration of antibiotics and supportive fluids. The fluid balance should be monitored and intravenous infusion adjusted accordingly.

Antibiotics. Until the organism is identified, the choice of antibiotic to cover the likely culprits depends on the child's age (Box 9.7).

When gentamicin is used drug levels must be monitored to prevent ototoxicity and nephrotoxicity. Haemophilus and meningococcus are increasingly becoming resistant to chloramphenicol and penicillin but at present third generation cephalosporins are effective and recommended by some authorities for first line treatment at all ages. The antibiotic regimen can be modified when the organism has been cultured and sensitivity is known. Intravenous antibiotics should continue for 7 days.

Corticosteroids (dexamethasone) reduce the incidence of complications in Haemophilus and possibly meningococcal meningitis and should therefore be given to all children except neonates.

Fluids. Monitor fluid balance and adjust i.v. infusion.

Complications

Short-term:

- Convulsions. Treat with intravenous phenytoin or phenobarbitone.
- Cerebral oedema. Diagnose by brain scan and monitor by an implanted intracranial pressure transducer. Treat with hyperventilation and/or mannitol.

Box 9.6 CSF microscopy

- Intracellular Gram-negative diplococci—Meningococcus
- Gram-negative coccobacilli—Haemophilus
- Gram-positive spheres—Streptococcus

Box 9.7 Antibiotic therapy in bacterial meningitis

Neonate
- Ampicillin + cefotaxime + gentamicin

> 3 months
- Penicillin + cefotaxime/ceftriaxone/chloramphenicol

- Subdural effusion. Diagnose by brain scan. Consider treatment by subdural taps or neurosurgery.
- Haemorrhage into adrenal glands (Waterhouse–Friderichsen syndrome). Treat for shock with intravenous dexamethasone.

Long-term:

- Deafness—sensorineural type. All survivors must have hearing tests.
- Epilepsy—approximately 5%.
- Cerebral palsy—approximately 2%.
- Learning difficulties—approximately 2%.
- Skin necrosis in areas where there were extensive purpuric lesions—may need grafting. Rarely digits or limbs require amputation.

Prevention

Primary

- Hib immunisation has dramatically reduced Haemophilus meningitis since 1992.
- Group C meningococcal vaccine was introduced in 1999. There is currently no vaccine against Group B which causes 60% of meningococcal infection.
- Pneumococcal vaccine is recommended only for high risk groups (sickle cell disease, splenectomy, nephrotic syndrome).

Secondary. The local consultant in communicable diseases must be informed urgently (do not wait for the Notification procedure). Contacts are treated with rifampicin, which is effective against meningococci and Haemophilus. The index case must also be treated following completion of intravenous antibiotics to prevent long-term carriage.

If there is a vaccine against the specific meningococcus serotype, immunisation should be given to household contacts or other members of a closed community (e.g. nursery, boarding school). The latter is particularly important in an outbreak.

Viral (aseptic) meningitis

The symptoms are similar to bacterial meningitis but less severe. The process is usually a meningo-encephalitis and follows an exanthematous illness.

The diagnosis is made by lumbar puncture which shows clear CSF containing a moderate number of white blood cells, mainly lymphocytes. Bacterial culture is negative but viruses may be seen on electron microscopy or culture. Serology in the acute and convalescent stages of illness shows a rising titre of antibodies against the particular virus.

There is no curative drug treatment. The patient is treated symptomatically with bed rest, analgesia and intravenous fluids if necessary. The prognosis is excellent.

Encephalitis (Figure 9.2)

Encephalitis is uncommon in the UK. A history of foreign travel should therefore be taken in order to exclude infections acquired abroad, e.g. arbovirus, Rickettsia.

Pathology

Invasive encephalitis. This occurs when the organism directly invades the brain substance and is found in biopsy specimens. Cells are destroyed and there is localised inflammation and swelling. The meninges are often also inflamed, causing signs of meningitis (meningo-encephalitis).

Post-infectious encephalitis. This is caused by an immune mediated reaction to an infectious disease (or rarely immunisation) several days earlier. Brain biopsy (or autopsy) shows perivascular inflammation and areas of demyelinisation.

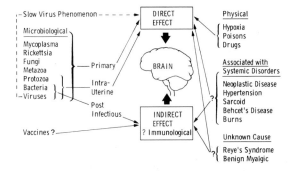

Figure 9.2 Factors associated with encephalitis/encephalopathy.

Clinical features

- Drowsiness, mildly impaired consciousness with confusion and delirium—may progress fairly quickly to coma
- Headache
- Convulsions (focal fits suggest herpes encephalitis)
- Cranial nerve abnormalities
- Motor abnormalities
- Ataxia (especially in chickenpox associated encephalitis).

Management

If herpes virus infection is suspected because of contact or herpes infection elsewhere, antiviral treatment (aciclovir) should be started immediately.

Investigations

- Lumbar puncture (Box 9.8)
- Brain scan—may show cerebral oedema or focal areas of infection in herpes encephalitis
- Full blood count
- Blood culture
- Serology of blood and CSF using polymerase chain reaction (PCR) technology
- EEG.

Treatment

Supportive:

- Set up an intravenous line and maintain fluid/electrolyte balance.

Box 9.8 Lumbar puncture in investigation of encephalitis

- *Avoid* lumbar puncture if there are signs of raised ICP
- Clear CSF with a moderately raised white cell count, mainly lymphocytes, and high protein (oligoclonal banding may show specific antibody fractions)
- Examine CSF for viral particles (electron microscopy and culture)

- Give anti-epileptic drugs if seizures occur.
- Monitor ICP if necessary.
- Give analgesia for headache.

Antiviral therapy. Herpes simplex virus (HSV) is the most important cause of serious viral encephalitis in the UK. It is sensitive to aciclovir, which should be commenced as soon as the diagnosis is suspected and continued for 10 days unless an alternative cause is confirmed.

Prognosis

Most cases of viral encephalitis make a full recovery. Patients with HSV infection may develop persistent neurodisability. Focal deficits are characteristic, e.g. hemiparesis, cranial nerve palsies, epilepsy, deafness and visual impairment. Generalised brain damage with bilateral motor impairment, learning and language difficulties also occurs.

Encephalopathy

- This term is used when a brain illness is not caused by an infectious agent.
- The clinical features are the same as for encephalitis.
- The diagnosis depends on identification of the cause by history or investigation.
- Management consists of treating the underlying cause and supporting the neurological condition symptomatically until resolution occurs.

NEUROMUSCULAR DISEASES

Motor function may be affected by malfunction at any point along the pathway from the brain cortex (e.g. encephalopathy, encephalitis), the upper motor neurone within the brain or spinal cord (e.g. trauma, vascular disease), the anterior horn cells (spinal muscular atrophy), the lower motor neurone (peripheral neuropathy), the neuromuscular junction (myasthenia) to the muscles (muscular dystrophy and myopathy). Impaired sensation can be caused by lesions of the brain, spinal cord or peripheral nerves.

Spinal muscular atrophy (SMA)

(see Table 9.2)

Acute Werdnig–Hoffman disease (SMA Type 1—Box 9.9) is the most severe and frequent form of SMA. All three types of SMA are usually inherited by autosomal recessive transmission and so genetic counselling for families is essential and urgent.

Peripheral neuropathy

Polyneuropathy is a general symmetrical dysfunction of peripheral nerves. Mononeuropathy is when a single nerve is involved.

Clinical features

- Weakness—distal and usually worse in the

legs than in the arms. Foot drop causes a characteristic high stepping gait.
- Sensory impairment of all modalities (pain, temperature, touch and vibration). Worse distally—glove and stocking distribution.
- Absent tendon reflexes.

Investigations

- Electrophysiological testing shows reduced nerve conduction, usually in both motor and sensory nerves.
- Nerve biopsy is often not specific and therefore unhelpful.

Guillain–Barré syndrome

This is the most common type of polyneuropathy, occurring several days after an acute viral infection or rarely after immunisation, because of an immune reaction.

Clinical features:

- History of infection
- Initial sensory loss in hands and feet
- Followed by marked progressive weakness, usually starting in legs and ascending to arms, trunk and cranial nerves (facial palsy in 50% of cases)
- Respiratory muscles affected in 20% of cases
- Autonomic system often affected with CVS changes, flushing, sweating and loss of sphincter control.

Investigations:

- CSF—high protein but no pleocytosis
- Electrophysiology shows slowed nerve conduction.

Box 9.9   Features of acute Werdnig–Hoffman disease

Clinical
- Reduced fetal movements
- Severe floppiness and weakness, often from birth
- Feeding difficulties
- Respiratory difficulty

Examination
- Marked hypotonia
- Symmetrical weakness
- 'Frog leg' posture
- Absent tendon reflexes
- Muscle and joint contractures
- Tongue atrophy and fasciculation

Investigations
- Electromyography
- Muscle biopsy
- CPK—usually normal

Table 9.2   Features of spinal muscular atrophy (SMA)

	Age	Presentation	Prognosis
SMA Type 1 (acute Werdnig–Hoffman disease)	Neonates	'Floppy baby' Respiratory distress	Death from respiratory failure < 3 years
SMA Type 2 (chronic Werdnig–Hoffman disease)	6–12 months	Delayed motor milestones Positive Gower's sign	Most walk with aids until large muscles become too weak Severe scoliosis Death in early adult life
Juvenile SMA (Kugelberg–Welander disease)	5–15 years	Walking difficulties Diagnosed by muscle biopsy	Survive well into adult life

Treatment:

- Supportive—nursing care, physiotherapy, respiratory ventilation if necessary
- Corticosteroids, plasmapheresis and i.v. immunoglobulin are controversial.

Prognosis. Recovery starts after 1–3 weeks and is invariably complete within 2–12 months.

Hereditary motor and sensory neuropathies (HMSN)

These are a group of congenital neuropathies genetically determined by autosomal dominant or recessive inheritance. They are predominantly motor, and there are often postural abnormalities of the feet due to longstanding muscular imbalance (Table 9.3). Genetic counselling must be offered.

Other hereditary neuropathies

- Sensory neuropathy. Mainly distal—causes painless ulcers.
- Familial dysautonomia (Riley–Day syndrome). Recessively inherited, mainly in Jewish families. Involves autonomic system, causing abnormal thermoregulation, hypotension and absence of tears on crying. Presents in infancy with feeding problems. Diagnosed by smooth tongue, lack of pain sensitivity and abnormal

eye findings in context of history. The prognosis is poor.

Toxic neuropathies

Peripheral nerves may be damaged by drugs (e.g. nitrofurantoin, phenytoin, isoniazid, vincristine), insecticides (organophosphates), industrial chemicals (e.g. acrylamide, trichloro-ethylene) and heavy metals (e.g. lead, arsenic, mercury).

Facial (Bell's) palsy

- Lower motor neurone paralysis of facial nerve
- Often associated with an URTI
- Starts with pain in face or ear
- Followed by facial weakness (mouth deviates to opposite side)
- If seen within 72 hours of onset, prescribe oral corticosteroids for 2 weeks
- Patch eye if corneal sensation is impaired.
- Resolves within 3 months
- Check BP as Bell's palsy can be associated with hypertension.

Brachial plexus injuries

The most frequent cause of these injuries is birth trauma, which is now generally rare. The brachial plexus (nerve roots C5, 6, 7, T1) can be damaged by forceful traction when an after-coming head in a breech delivery gets stuck or

Table 9.3 Features of hereditary motor and sensory neuropathies HMSN

	Age	Inheritance	Presentation	Prognosis
HMSN I (peroneal muscular atrophy/ Charcot–Marie–Tooth disease)	First decade	Dominant	Progressive weakness and atrophy of foot and leg muscles —'inverted champagne bottle' legs	Good for ambulation and life expectancy
HMSN II (neuronal type peroneal muscular atrophy)	Second decade	Dominant	Similar to HMSN I	Similar to HMSN I Biopsy shows axon degeneration rather than demyelinisation
HMSN III (Déjérine–Sottas disease)	Infancy	Recessive	Delayed motor milestones Affects proximal as well as distal muscles	Progressive weakness Unable to walk by adolescence
HMSN IV (Refsum's disease)	Primary school age	Recessive	Polyneuropathy, ataxia; retinitis pigmentosa and cardiomyopathy Phytanic acid increased	Diet—reduce dairy products, fish, nuts and chocolate

by pulling hard on the head in a cephalic presentation when the body is stuck (e.g. shoulder dystocia). The nerve roots are damaged by compression from oedema and bruising (in which case recovery may occur) or, rarely, avulsed (when recovery is unlikely). Trauma later in life may also cause brachial plexus injury.

Erb's palsy. The upper roots (C5 and 6) are affected. The arm has a characteristic posture—adducted and internally rotated at the shoulder, elbow extended, forearm pronated and fingers flexed ('waiter's tip' position). The Moro reflex is asymmetrical, but the palmar grasp reflex is normal. Erb's palsy is often associated with bony injuries, e.g. fractured humerus or clavicle, dislocated shoulder. There may be an associated Horner's syndrome (ptosis, miosis and lack of sweating due to sympathetic fibre damage) (see p. 256) or phrenic nerve palsy (diaphragmatic paralysis causing respiratory distress).

Treatment consists of encouraging use, physiotherapy and occupational therapy. The prognosis is good—95% make a full recovery. Microsurgery can be of help in a few cases.

Klumpke's palsy:

- Lower roots (C8, T1) affected
- Rare
- Paralysis of intrinsic muscles of hand
- Absent grasp, but normal Moro reflex
- May be ipsilateral Horner's syndrome.

Myasthenia gravis (MG)

The acetyl choline receptor sites in the motor end plates are blocked by IgG autoantibodies and so cannot receive the impulse from the depolarised motor terminals of the lower motor neurone.

Juvenile myasthenia gravis

Symptoms do not usually appear until about 10 years of age. The female:male ratio is approximately 5:1.

Clinical features:

- Increased fatigability. The onset is usually gradual but may be sudden. The weakness is worse in the afternoon and improves with rest.

- The ocular muscles are often first affected causing ptosis, ophthalmoplegia and diplopia.
- Bulbar weakness causes difficulties of chewing, swallowing and speaking.
- A myasthenic crisis is a sudden severe generalised weakness precipitated by intercurrent infection or other stress.

Diagnosis:

- Tensilon (edrophonium) is a short-acting anticholinesterase that produces a brief improvement in muscle strength in myasthenia gravis (Figure 9.3).
- Acetylcholine receptor antibodies are found in 90% of cases.
- Electromyography (EMG) can be used if the diagnosis is uncertain.

Treatment:

- Anticholinesterase drugs such as pyridostigmine and neostigmine are used. Beware cholinergic crisis in which excessive dosage causes increased weakness with muscarinic symptoms.
- Thymectomy should be considered for antibody positive patients; 80% will improve after thymectomy.
- Corticosteroids—in children only short courses can be used to inhibit the autoimmune process.

Prognosis. The prognosis is good; 25% of cases remit within 2 years.

Transient neonatal myasthenia gravis

This occurs in approximately 15% of infants born to myasthenic mothers because of transplacental transmission of maternal IgG antibodies. The infant presents with floppiness, respiratory distress and feeding difficulties. Usually no treatment is required, but anticholinesterase drugs are prescribed if symptoms are severe. The symptoms gradually disappear over several weeks.

Congenital myasthenia gravis

The condition has its onset at birth or in infancy. It is familial with autosomal recessive inheritance. It is antibody negative as there is no

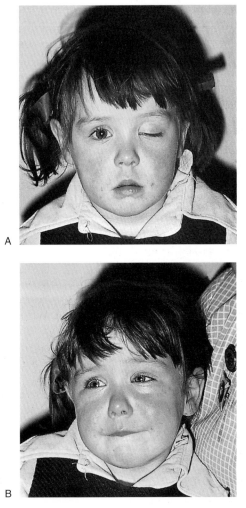

A

B

Figure 9.3 Positive Tensilon (edrophonium) test in myasthenia gravis with unilateral ptosis. A: Before injection. B: After injection.

autoimmune mechanism; treatment is with anti-cholinesterase medication only.

A myasthenic disorder rarely occurs from botulism, drugs (e.g. antibiotics, beta blockers), chemicals (organophosphates) and in malignant disease.

MUSCLE DISEASES

Duchenne muscular dystrophy (DMD)

The incidence is approximately 1 in 3000 male births. DMD is transmitted by X-linked inheri-

tance via a female carrier (who is asymptomatic) to her sons; 50% of her daughters will be carriers. Genetic counselling with carrier detection should be offered, although one third of cases are new mutations.

Clinical features

The condition presents at the age of 3–5 years with motor difficulties, e.g. in going upstairs or getting up off the ground (Figure 9.4) and large calf muscles. There is often a history of late walking. Gower's sign, in which the child pushes with his hands on his knees when arising from lying down (climbs up his legs), is positive (Figure 9.5). There are usually mild learning difficulties (mean IQ 80). Cardiac muscle is also affected.

Investigations

• Creatinine phosphokinase—very high (> 1000).

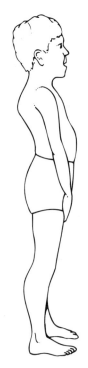

Figure 9.4 Duchenne muscular dystrophy showing pseudohypertrophy of calf muscle and lumbar lordosis.

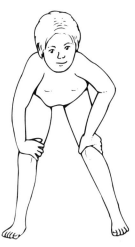

Figure 9.5   Positive Gower's sign.

- EMG—myopathic
- Muscle biopsy.

Prognosis

Inexorable progressive muscle weakness develops and patients are usually wheelchair bound by the age of 12 years. Death occurs from respiratory infection/failure in adolescence.

Becker muscular dystrophy

This has similar features to Duchenne muscular dystrophy but is more benign. It presents between 10 and 12 years of age and progresses slowly; walking is possible into early adult life and patients survive to middle age.

Congenital muscular dystrophy

This has an autosomal recessive inheritance. The muscle cells degenerate at variable rates so fibres are of different sizes within the same muscle.

Clinical features

- Reduced fetal movements
- Weakness and hypotonia from birth (floppy baby)
- Respiratory distress
- Non-progressive
- Joint contractures

- Normal intelligence
- Possibility of neurological involvement with seizures and learning difficulties (Fukuyama type).

Investigations

- CPK—raised (less than DMD)
- EMG—myopathic
- Muscle biopsy.

Prognosis

If the child survives infancy the prognosis is relatively good.

Localised dystrophies

Limb girdle dystrophy. This is usually of autosomal recessive inheritance and affects the pelvic or pectoral muscle girdles.

Facio-scapulo-humeral dystrophy (Landouzy–Déjérine atrophy) is of autosomal dominant inheritance. It presents with weak facial, shoulder and upper arm movements, often asymmetrically. The condition progresses slowly and may arrest.

Myotonic dystrophy (dystrophia myotonica)

This condition is transmitted by autosomal dominant inheritance—invariably through the mother.

Clinical features

The infant presents in the neonatal period with problems such as respiratory distress, hypotonia, facial palsy, CDH and hernias. Mild developmental delay and learning difficulties are present. Myotonia is absent in early childhood.

Prognosis

The prognosis is generally good but dementia may occur in adulthood. Adolescents show the characteristic myotonia (inability to suddenly release voluntary muscle contraction, e.g. grasp). Adults often have cataracts, baldness and endocrine disturbances.

Myotonia congenita (Thomsen)

This is inherited in an autosomal dominant fashion. Myotonia presents in infancy with difficulty in initiating movements. There is only mild weakness and the condition is non-progressive.

Familial periodic paralysis

This condition is of autosomal dominant inheritance. There are three types:

1. Hypokalaemic type. Serum potassium falls when provoked by stress or a high carbohydrate or sodium meal. It presents at 6–10 years of age and improves with advancing age.
2. Hyperkalaemic type. Serum potassium rises. This presents at around 10 years of age.
3. Normokalaemic type. This is provoked by cold and physical exertion.

Treatment of all types is by diagnosis and identification of the triggering factors. Acetazolamide may help.

Metabolic myopathies

Glycogenoses

The glycogenoses are enzymic defects of glycogen metabolism, inherited as autosomal recessives.

Type II (acid maltase deficiency/Pompe's disease) presents as a 'floppy infant' with heart disease and hepatomegaly. The CPK is raised; EMG and ECG are abnormal. There is no treatment and death occurs within one year. A more benign form exists which can be confused with Duchenne muscular dystrophy.

Type III (debrancher deficiency) presents with weakness (poor head control) and hypoglycaemia in infancy.

Type V (McArdle's disease) presents with fatiguability and cramps which usually do not start until late adolescence.

Carnitine deficiency

This presents with progressive weakness and fatiguability. It is diagnosed by measuring carnitine in blood and muscle. Treatment is with oral steroids and/or carnitine supplementation.

Anatomical myopathies

These are a group of congenital myopathies which historically were classified together as 'benign congenital hypotonia'. Recent histochemical techniques have differentiated them; histochemical types include central core disease, multicore disease, nemaline myopathy, myotubular myopathy and congenital fibre type disproportion.

They are usually of autosomal dominant inheritance. The symptoms are mild weakness, hypotonia and sometimes delayed development.

Mitochondrial myopathy

The myopathy is one element of a multisystem disease (mitochondrial cytopathy). The pattern of inheritance is dominant, by cytoplasmic transmission from the mother. Neurological features include weakness, hypotonia, cranial nerve involvement and delayed motor development. Systemic features include short stature and involvement of viscera. The diagnosis is made by the presence of 'ragged red fibres' on muscle biopsy. The prognosis is good.

Acquired myopathy

Inflammatory

Non-infective. Polymyositis is often associated with dermatomyositis. The muscles are tender, swollen and weak. The child is generally unwell and there may be other systemic disturbances. Treatment with high dose corticosteroids, which may need to be continued for several years, produces remission in approximately two thirds of cases.

Infective. Myositis can be caused by a variety of organisms, including parasites (e.g. toxoplasmosis, trichinosis, cysticercosis), viruses (e.g. influenza, adenoviruses) and, less frequently, bacteria (e.g. *Staphylococcus aureus*, Clostridium).

Endocrine

Muscle weakness occurs in association with steroid therapy, Cushing's syndrome, hyperthyroidism and hyperparathyroidism.

Toxic myopathy

This may be caused by drugs, e.g. vincristine and chloroquine, or animal toxins such as snake venom and insect stings.

NEURODEGENERATIVE DISEASES

These are rare but important disorders which cause progressive disabilities including dementia, epilepsy, blindness and motor problems. They are usually inherited as autosomal recessives and so definitive diagnosis and genetic counselling are essential.

Treatment is symptomatic and no cures are available. The natural course is inevitably one of gradual deterioration and is very hard on the whole family involved. Support in the form of respite care, home comforts and attention to siblings is needed.

Neuronal storage diseases

Abnormal lipids accumulate in the grey matter of the brain. The diagnosis is confirmed by biochemical tests on blood.

Gangliosidoses

Infantile GM$_2$ (Tay–Sachs disease). This is most frequent in Ashkenazi Jewish families, in whom the gene frequency is 1 in 30. It presents with delayed motor development and blindness in infancy. Examination shows an exaggerated startle reaction and a cherry red spot in the optic fundi. The prognosis is very poor and most patients die before their fourth birthday. Carriers can be identified and Jewish couples should be screened.

GM$_1$ gangliosidosis. This presents with developmental delay and failure to thrive. A cherry red spot may be seen in the fundi. Diagnosis requires biochemical examination of leukocytes, bone marrow and fibroblasts.

The prognosis is poor with inexorable developmental regression. Death occurs 1–5 years after onset.

Batten's disease (neuronal ceroid lipofuscinosis)

Late infantile form. This, the most frequent form of the disease, presents in the second year of life with loss of developmental skills. Myoclonic epilepsy is common and difficult to treat. Electro-retinogram and visual evoked responses may be diagnostic but rectal biopsy for histology of neural plexuses is usually necessary. Most children deteriorate steadily and die by the age of 6 years.

Juvenile form. This presents with visual failure at the age of 5–6 years because of a pigmentary retinopathy. Seizures, dementia and motor disability occur later and progress tragically slowly to death in adolescence.

Infantile form. This occurs more frequently in Finland than elsewhere. It causes developmental regression and visual loss at approximately one year of age. Ataxia and myoclonic epilepsy may be prominent. The disease often reaches a 'burnt-out' stage by 3 years and children may remain in this severely disabled totally dependent state for a further 5 or 6 years.

Niemann–Pick disease

This disease most commonly occurs in Ashkenazi Jewish children. It often presents as failure to thrive with developmental delay early in infancy. A cherry-red spot my be seen in the fundi, and hepatosplenomegaly and jaundice are frequent findings. X-rays show infiltration of lungs and bones. Bone marrow or rectal biopsy may be required for diagnosis. Affected children usually die by the age of 2–3 years.

Gaucher's disease

Gaucher cells are deposited in the reticulo-endothelial system, including bone marrow, from which a biopsy can be taken. There are several types which present with hepatospleno-megaly, developmental delay and feeding difficulties. Anaemia and bone abnormalities often occur. The disease usually progresses slowly and patients may survive into adult life.

Treatment with bone marrow transplantation or enzyme replacement at an early stage is possible.

Leukodystrophies

Nerve fibres within the brain are demyelinated. These conditions used to be grouped together under the term Schilder's disease but modern investigation has demonstrated that there are several different entities.

MR head scans usually show marked attenuation of the white matter of the brain.

Metachromatic leukodystrophy (MLD)

This affects the spinal cord and peripheral nerves as well as the brain.

The **late infantile type** usually presents at approximately 18 months with delayed walking followed by developmental regression. Death often occurs at 5–6 years of age

The **juvenile type** presents between 5 and 10 years of age and progresses more slowly. Dementia may be more prominent than motor problems. Patients may survive into early adult life.

The diagnosis is made by biochemical examination of urinary epithelial cells and white blood cells.

Globoid cell leukodystrophy (Krabbe's disease)

The infantile type presents with irritability, developmental regression and hypertonia around 6 months of age. Deterioration to a state of cortical rigidity occurs rapidly, followed by death by the age of 18 months.

Children with the late onset type develop well until the age of approximately 2 years then show progressive motor impairment and developmental regression.

Diagnosis depends on enzyme assays of leukocytes or fibroblasts.

Adrenal leukodystrophy (Addison–Schilder disease)

This is a condition of X-linked recessive inheritance. It presents in boys aged approximately 7–8 years. The symptoms include behavioural problems, school difficulties, motor impairment and seizures. There is gradual deterioration in the neurological state with death in adolescence. The condition is diagnosed by finding the characteristic appearance on a brain scan, and

deficient adrenal function in approximately 50% of cases.

Megalencephalic leukodystrophies

Spongiform (Canavan's disease). This is more frequent in Ashkenazi Jewish children. It presents in the first 6 months of life with developmental regression, hypotonia and a large head. It is diagnosed by the combination of clinical features and characteristic brain scan.

Alexander's disease. The onset may be insidious in infancy or early childhood, with developmental delay, epilepsy, motor difficulties and an enlarging head. A brain scan shows attenuated white matter and large ventricles. Brain biopsy is needed for definitive diagnosis. This leukodystrophy is not genetically inherited.

Metabolic encephalopathies

Menke's syndrome (kinky hair disease)

This X-linked recessive disorder presents at around 6 weeks of age with lethargy, feeding difficulties and seizures. The hair is sparse and kinky (like steel wool). Copper and caeruloplasmin serum levels are low and copper is deposited in some viscera.

Wilson's disease (hepatolenticular degeneration)

This autosomal recessive condition presents with rigidity, dystonic movements and liver disease. There may also be behavioural abnormalities and school failure. The diagnosis is made by finding Kayser–Fleischer rings in the cornea, and low serum caeruloplasmin but high copper. Treatment is with D-penicillamine and avoidance of foods with high copper content (e.g. nuts and chocolate).

Lesch–Nyhan syndrome

This X-linked recessive disorder presents by the age of 6 months with developmental delay. Choreo-athetoid dystonic movements and spasms start later and are followed by severe motor difficulties. The distinguishing clinical feature is self-mutilation, which occurs from the age of 4 years and causes severe injuries. The patients die of renal failure in early adulthood. The cardinal pathological finding is a high uric acid due to an enzymic defect. Allopurinol can be used for treatment to reduce the uric acid but does not help the neurological process.

Spinocerebellar degenerations

Friedreich's ataxia

Friedreich's ataxia is inherited as an autosomal recessive trait. The condition has its onset at primary school age with gait difficulties and clumsiness. Scoliosis and heart disease are rare presenting symptoms.

Examination shows ataxia, a wide based gait, absent tendon reflexes and, later, loss of vibration sensitivity, proprioception, and pes cavus. Motor abilities are steadily lost and most patients eventually become unable to walk in early adult life and die before middle age. Investigations include spine X-ray, ECG, and nerve conduction.

Ataxia telangiectasia

This is also inherited as an autosomal recessive trait. It presents with ataxia and susceptibility to respiratory infections in early childhood. The ataxia progresses slowly so that walking ability is lost by about 10 years of age.

Examination reveals ataxia, dyskinetic limb movements, telangiectasia of the eyes, oculo-motor dyspraxia and loss of pharyngeal lymphoid tissue. Investigations include measurement of immunoglobulins and alpha-fetoprotein. Fibroblasts and lymphocytes have increased sensitivity to irradiation because of defective DNA repair systems.

Familial spastic paraplegia

This is usually of autosomal dominant inheritance. It presents as mild 'cerebral palsy' in the second decade of life. Recessive cases present earlier.

Examination reveals classical pyramidal signs in the legs—brisk tendon jerk, extensor plantar reflex, hypertonia and tight Achilles tendons (causing toe walking).

The prognosis is often good with little progression but some cases become non-ambulant.

NEUROCUTANEOUS DISORDERS (PHAKOMATOSES)

These involve pathology of ectodermal tissue (which includes the CNS) and so cause defects of the skin and neurological system. They are inherited by autosomal dominant transmission so accurate diagnosis and genetic counselling is essential.

Neurofibromatosis (NF)

NF-1 (von Recklinghausen disease)

NF-1 accounts for approximately 80% of all cases of neurofibromatosis. 50% of cases arise from new mutations.

Clinical features. Café-au-lait patches are the cardinal feature; they are light to mid brown coloured spots with clearly defined edges. They appear from early childhood and increase in number. Up to 6 small patches can occur in normal individuals but a greater number of patches over 1.5 cm diameter is diagnostic of NF-1. Axillary freckling is often present; this is not seen in normal people.

Neurofibromata form as nodules under the skin or along nerves (plexiform). They may enlarge progressively and cause compression lesions. Bony abnormalities include sphenoidal dysplasia and scoliosis. Optic pathway gliomas may cause visual loss, and children with NF-1 should be screened by brain scanning. Learning difficulties occur in approximately one third of cases.

Prognosis. In many cases the skin café-au-lait patches are the only lesion and the patient remains neurologically well. The neurofibromata may cause problems which are cosmetic if subcutaneous, or neurological if they are in the brain or spinal cord. Surgical removal can be performed if necessary.

NF-2

The gene associated with NF-2 is sited on a different chromosome locus from that of NF-1. There are bilateral acoustic neuromas but usually no skin lesions. The condition presents with deafness, tinnitus and headaches in early adolescence. Diagnosis is by brain scan. Treatment consists of surgical removal of the neurofibromata. Genetic counselling should be offered.

Tuberous sclerosis (TS)

Clinical features

- Epilepsy—tuberous sclerosis commonly presents in infancy with infantile spasms. The EEG shows hypsarrhythmia and the spasms are often resistant to treatment. In later childhood TS presents with major seizures.
- Learning difficulties. These may manifest as developmental delay in early childhood, alone or combined with epilepsy.
- Skin lesions—depigmented patches, adenoma sebaceum (acne-like rash in 'butterfly' distribution on face), shagreen patch on lower back and subungual fibromata.

The condition is diagnosed by finding the characteristic skin abnormalities. Family members should also be carefully examined as these abnormalities may be the only signs of TS.

Investigations

Depigmented patches should be looked for under ultraviolet (Wood's) light with the child fully undressed. A brain scan will identify intracerebral tubers. A body scan may show lesions in other organs.

RETT'S SYNDROME

This is included because it is thought to account for between 1 and 10% of girls with undiagnosed severe learning difficulties. The syndrome is X-linked and may be lethal in males.

Clinical features

Development is normal until onset at around 1 year of age. There is then progressive loss of speech and language skills. Social skills are poor (this feature with the communication deficit causes confusion with infantile autism). There is loss of purposeful hand use with stereotypic hand movements—wringing or tapping. Microcephaly is progressive and seizures may occur.

The prognosis is poor: most children become severely disabled, immobile and totally dependent by late childhood.

BRAIN TUMOURS – see page 288

FURTHER READING

Aicardi J 1998 Diseases of the nervous system in childhood. 2nd edn. Mackeith Press, London
Baxter P S, Rittey C D C 1995 Advances in epilepsy: seizures and syndromes. In: David T J (ed) Recent advances in

paediatrics, 14th edn. Churchill Livingstone, Edinburgh
Dubowitz V 1995 Muscle disorders in childhood, 2nd edn. WB Saunders, London

Internet addresses

http://www.ninds.nih.gov/healinfo/nindspub.htm

Epilepsy
http://bay.ion.bpmf.ac.uk/nsehome/open.html

10

Nephrology and paediatric gynaecology

Martin Moncrieff

RENAL FUNCTION

The function of the kidneys is to maintain the milieu interieur (Claude Bernard). This is achieved by two mechanisms. As the blood passes through the glomerular capillary loops it is filtered into the urinary space leaving only cells and protein. This urine is then modified by selective reabsorption and secretion during its passage along the renal tubules. In the proximal renal tubules, electrolytes, phosphate, bicarbonate, glucose and amino acids are reabsorbed. Water reabsorption takes place mainly in the loop of Henle, and final adjustment of the contents takes place in the distal tubules where H^+ is secreted and potassium and sodium absorbed.

Glomerular filtration is approximately 100 ml per minute for a surface area of 1.73 m^2; as 99% of this is reabsorbed the final urine volume is approximately 1 ml/min. Glomerular filtration depends on renal blood flow, which is 20–25% of cardiac output, and on the blood pressure. Thus a marked fall in cardiac output and blood pressure, as occurs in shock, causes a significant reduction in glomerular filtration. Glomerular filtration and concentrating ability are relatively low in the young infant but mature by one year of age. Sodium reabsorption and urine acidification are well developed at birth. When stressed, the kidney can retain salt and water by increasing tubular reabsorption.

RENAL TESTS

Renal function tests are divided into those that test glomerular function, and those that test tubular function. Tests of glomerular function include the ability to filter, that is the glomerular filtration rate (GFR), and the integrity of the filter. GFR is measured by determining the plasma and urine concentration of a substance which is not absorbed or secreted by the tubules. Creatinine is such a substance, although there is in fact a little tubular excretion of creatinine.

The ratio of urine creatinine (Uc) to plasma creatinine (Pc) multiplied by the urine volume in unit time (V), gives the amount of plasma 'cleared' or filtered of creatinine in a unit time. This is called the creatinine clearance (Cc) and is calculated as $Uc \times V/Pc$. The normal range, corrected for surface area, is 80–120 ml/min/$1.73 \, m^2$. The drawback to this test is that it depends on a timed urine collection. Serial measurements are more useful than one single measurement as any trend will then be revealed. To avoid the problems associated with urine collection, the rate of excretion of chromium-51 labelled EDTA, based on the decline in radioactivity in two blood samples after initial injection, is now often used to measure GFR. The integrity of the glomerular filter to retain blood and protein can conveniently be measured by dip stick. The concept of 'clearance' can be applied to all the substances which are filtered in the glomerulus and appear in the urine (see below).

Proximal renal tubular function can be tested by examining the urine for the presence of glucose and amino acids. Both are normally completely reabsorbed, and so, providing the blood levels are normal, their presence in the urine indicates impaired tubular function. Phosphate is largely reabsorbed in the proximal tubules. The proportion of the filtered load which is reabsorbed is the ratio between the amount in the urine and the amount filtered, which depends on the blood level and the glomerular filtration rate. This is calculated by dividing the phosphate clearance by the creatinine clearance, avoiding the need for a timed urine collection. The proportion reabsorbed is normally greater than 85%;

figures lower than this demonstrate impaired tubular function. Sodium is almost completely reabsorbed in the renal tubules. This function is usually expressed as the fractional excretion of sodium (FE_{Na}). It is calculated in the same way as phosphate excretion and is normally only 1–2%.

The ability of the kidneys to concentrate urine is tested by measuring the urine osmolality after a period of fluid deprivation. After a last drink at 16.00 hours, the osmolality of the second urine passed the next morning should exceed 800 mosmol/kg water.

URINARY TRACT INFECTION

Urinary tract infection (UTI) is a common disorder in childhood. It causes much short-term morbidity and is responsible, in association with vesico-ureteric reflux, for about 20% of the children who develop end-stage renal disease.

UTI is more common in girls, with about 7% of 7-year-old girls having had a UTI compared with only 1.7% of 7-year-old boys. The higher incidence in girls occurs because the short female urethra allows ready access of bowel bacteria to the bladder.

Clinical features

The symptoms vary with age. In the newborn period (when UTI is more common in boys than girls) UTI may be part of a septicaemic illness with fever, anorexia, vomiting, floppiness, cyanosis and sometimes jaundice, or cause a less dramatic illness with fever, anorexia and vomiting. In the first year or two of life the clinical picture remains non-specific as the child is too young to indicate any local symptoms. Over the age of 2, dysuria, frequency, wetting, haematuria and abdominal pain may occur as well as the general signs of infection.

Investigations

The diagnosis should be confirmed by examination of the urine. A midstream specimen can be obtained from older children and a clean catch or bag specimen from younger ones. Providing the genitalia are socially clean no further preparation is necessary. Suprapubic aspiration of urine is often indicated in a child with a septicaemic illness.

Traditionally the urine has been examined for the presence of pus cells, but cell counts are tedious and not always reliable as an indication of infection. Bacteria seen on microscopy are highly suggestive of infection, but microscopic examination of the urine is practised less with the increasing popularity of stick testing. Infected urine contains leukocyte esterase produced by pus cells, and nitrites produced by bacterial breakdown of nitrates in the urine; both can be detected on stick tests. Preliminary results show that if both tests are positive the urine is infected and if both are negative UTI can be excluded. If either of the tests is positive, the urine should be cultured. Infection is present if the number of viable colonies is equal to or greater than 10^5 per ml, and sensitivities can be obtained. A small number of infections (about 5%) have a colony count between 10^4 and 10^5; the results of culture must then be interpreted in the light of the clinical picture. It is important that the urine is cultured within a few hours of collection to avoid growth of contaminants; if this is not possible, urine can be kept for up to 48 hours in a domestic refrigerator before culture without contaminants confusing the result. If the dip stick test is positive, treatment can be started on a best guess basis while awaiting the result of culture. 90% of infections are caused by *E. coli*; 90% of these are sensitive to trimethoprim, which is the initial choice of antibiotic.

Once the diagnosis of UTI has been made it is important to investigate the renal tract, even after only one infection, to look for a cause and for renal scarring. Obstruction, vesico-ureteric reflux, and occasionally a duplex system are the most likely causes. Ultrasound (US) is the best investigation for detecting obstructive lesions such as pelvi-ureteric and vesico-ureteric obstruction, and urethral valves. Ultrasound is harmless, painless and does not involve irradiation; it will show renal scarring in about 90% of cases. A more sensitive test for renal scarring is with ^{99m}Tc-dimercaptosuccinic acid (DMSA) which involves an intravenous injection and mild irradiation. Vesico-ureteric reflux is detected on a cystogram (Figure 10.2). This has numerous disadvantages, including the unpleasantness of urethral catheterisation and moderate irradiation, especially near the gonads.

A reasonable policy for investigating a child after a UTI is an ultrasound examination of the renal tract in all children, and a DMSA in those aged between 6 months and 6 years (an ultrasound scan is more difficult to interpret between these ages). Routine cystography is limited to those under one year of age, when severe reflux is most likely to be associated with renal scarring, and if an abnormality of the renal tract has already been found (Figure 10.1).

Vesico-ureteric reflux, a familial disorder, is caused by a congenital abnormality of the vesico-ureteric junction and is found in approximately half the children investigated after a UTI. It is divided into five grades (see Figure 10.3).

Intrarenal reflux (reflux into the renal substance) is only found in association with grade IV/V reflux in those under 5 years of age, and occurs in areas which can subsequently be shown to develop a scar. Severe reflux, grade IV/V, is found more often in younger children, especially in those under 1 year and improves with age,

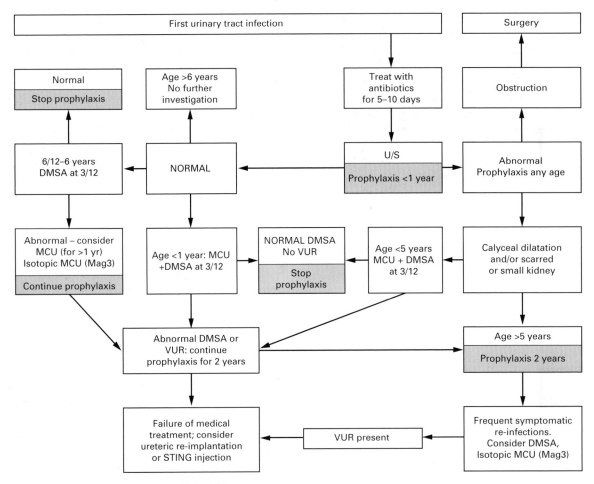

Figure 10.1 Management plan for UTI in children.

usually disappearing in adolescence. There is a close correlation between severe reflux and renal scarring, with four fifths of kidneys showing scars being drained by ureters with grade IV/V reflux. Renal scarring is much less common with lesser grades of reflux. Infection as well as reflux is required for scarring to develop. Vesico-ureteric reflux predisposes to infection, as the refluxing urine is not voided, and it enables infection to reach the kidney, causing renal damage termed reflux nephropathy. Severe renal damage may cause renal failure, and hypertension (see Chapter 5) develops in 10% of cases.

Management

The development of renal scars in a kidney found to be normal on initial investigation is very unusual, especially in those over 5 years of age, and is almost always associated with severe reflux and repeated infections. Therefore, in children over 5 years with a normal renal tract, routine follow-up consultation is unnecessary. If a further infection occurs, which happens in half the children, a further short course of the appropriate antibiotic is indicated. If frequent infections occur with upsetting symptoms, prophylactic antibiotics, usually trimethoprim, for 6 months

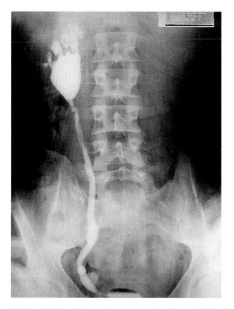

Figure 10.2 Micturating cystogram showing unilateral grade V vesico-ureteric reflux.

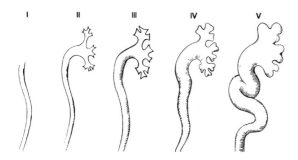

Figure 10.3 International classification of grades of reflux. I—ureter only. II—ureter, pelvis and calyces, no dilation. III—mild or moderate dilation and/or tortuosity of the ureter and mild or moderate dilation of renal pelvis but no, or only slight, blunting of the fornices. IV—moderate dilation and/or tortuosity of the ureter and moderate dilation of renal pelvis and calyces; complete obliteration of sharp angle of fornices but maintenance of capillary impression in majority of calyces. V—gross dilation and tortuosity of ureter, gross dilation of renal pelvis and calyces; capillary impressions are no longer visible in the majority of cases.

may help. In younger children, who are more likely to develop renal damage, it is reasonable to continue regular consultations for a year to institute prophylactic treatment if further infections occur and consider more extensive investigations. The parents of younger children should be told of symptoms which suggest a UTI, given a supply of collecting bags, and asked to supply a urine sample for culture if infection is suspected.

If the child has renal scarring with severe reflux, or severe reflux on its own, prophylactic antibiotics should be given to prevent subsequent infections causing further renal damage. Although a small number of children, usually under 7 years of age, develop fresh renal scars, this only happens in the first two years after diagnosis, so after that prophylactic treatment can be stopped. Long-term antibiotics are as effective as surgery in preserving renal function and preventing infections. Anti-reflux surgery is therefore seldom indicated, being reserved for children who have poor compliance with medical treatment or numerous infections despite prophylactic antibiotics.

Asymptomatic bacteriuria (ASB). In several large surveys involving many thousands of healthy school girls with no urinary symptoms, a small number (between 1 and 2%) are found to have a positive urine culture, called asymptomatic bacteriuria. Investigations usually reveal normal kidneys which are still normal several years later, despite frequent, subsequent positive cultures. As the 'infection' is symptomless and does not cause renal damage, ASB should not be treated. Indeed urine culture is unnecessary in children over the age of 2 years unless they have symptoms suggesting a UTI.

The concept of reflux nephropathy—that is renal scarring in association with severe reflux together with infection, always being the cause of a small irregular kidney—has recently been questioned. With the advent of antenatal scanning, babies with hydronephrosis can be identified before birth (Figure 10.4). Investigations after birth (Figure 10.5) sometimes show severe reflux and a small irregular kidney due to dysplasia. Previously, if a child presented with a UTI and a small kidney was found, this was thought to have been caused by a previous unrecognised infection which might have been prevented by greater parental and medical vigilance. However, dysplasia rather than infection may be the cause in a child with severe reflux and a small irregular kidney. Appropriate management strategies for the dysplastic refluxing

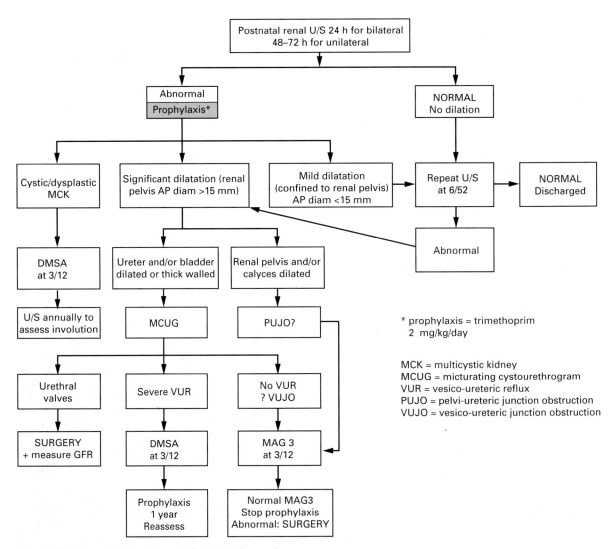

Figure 10.4 Investigation of prenatally detected uropathy.

system have not yet been determined and need to be investigated properly in controlled trials. A suggested protocol for prenatally detected uropathy is shown in Figure 10.4.

ACUTE GLOMERULONEPHRITIC SYNDROME

This consists of macroscopic haematuria, oliguria with a rising blood urea, and hypertension. There are often signs of fluid overload because of normal intake despite reduced urine output.

Classically the syndrome was caused by infection with group A β-haemolytic streptococci, usually in the throat, but in tropical countries often in the skin. Immune complexes are formed and deposited in the glomeruli with complement activation and a marked inflammatory reaction; the disease begins abruptly 7–10 days after the streptococcal infection. Evidence of a preceding streptococcal infection is shown by an elevated ASOT or DNAse, and the C3 component of complement is reduced. These usually return to normal by 6–8 weeks, and renal function almost

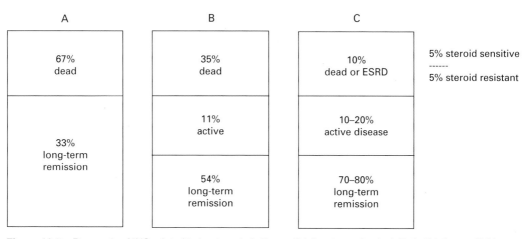

Figure 10.5 Prognosis of INS related to treatment. A. Pre-antibiotics, i.e. untreated. B. Antibiotics available. C. Estimate for present day using steroids and cytotoxics, assuming 10% cases are steroid resistant. ESRD = end stage renal disease. (Reproduced with permission from the Lancet.)

always recovers completely. Management consists of careful fluid balance to avoid fluid overload. Hypotensive drugs for elevated blood pressure are required in 20% of cases. Penicillin is given for 10 days; a low salt, low protein diet is also prescribed.

There is a low incidence of severe complications:

- hypertensive encephalopathy in 3–4% with severe headaches, fits and coma
- marked oliguria or anuria in 3%
- congestive cardiac failure (predominantly fluid overload) in 1%.

Occasionally dialysis is required and referral to a specialist centre is required. Even these patients usually recover normal renal function so the short- and long-term mortality is less than 1%. Haematuria may persist in a few patients for as long as 2–3 years, but chronic renal insufficiency affects only about 1% of cases.

Over the last 20 years, no evidence of preceding streptococcal infection has been found in many cases and the antigen remains unknown. In these circumstances the course of the disease is less predictable and the prognosis more guarded.

HAEMATURIA

In contrast to adults, haematuria in childhood hardly ever heralds serious disease; it has numerous causes. Associated clinical features such as dysuria and fever or oliguria and hypertension suggest the probable diagnosis of UTI or acute nephritis but, in the absence of any obvious cause, an ultrasound examination of the kidneys to exclude a Wilms' tumour and a renal calculus is indicated. Cystoscopy is rarely indicated as it is very unusual to find any abnormality. If no cause is found, a diagnosis of isolated, essential or benign (recurrent) haematuria is made. Some children with isolated haematuria have deposits of IgA in the glomerular mesangium; this is more likely if there is protein as well as blood in the urine. The condition is called IgA nephropathy. An unknown proportion of these children develop renal insufficiency, usually many years later.

Generally, after urine cultures, ultrasound, and measurement of renal function are found to be normal, the parents can be reassured that serious renal disease is very unlikely. A renal biopsy may be indicated to detect IgA nephropathy if haematuria and proteinuria are recurrent; even then renal function may well remain unimpaired.

THE NEPHROTIC SYNDROME

The nephrotic syndrome is defined as heavy proteinuria and a low serum albumin level (less

---

GP Overview 10.2 Haematuria

- Blood in urine needs confirming by microscopy
- Positive dip stick tests may indicate red blood cells, haemoglobin or myoglobin
- Remember factitious causes, e.g. beetroot, food colouring, azo dyes

Causes
- Urinary tract infection
- Trauma to kidneys/genitourinary tract
- Benign recurrent haematuria
- IGA (Berger's) disease
- Glomerulonephritis
  —post-streptoccocal
  —Henoch–Schönlein purpura
  —SLE
  —Alport's syndrome
- Polycystic disease
- Renal stone disease
- Tumours—Wilms' (30% present with haematuria)
- Bleeding disorders/haemolytic uraemic syndrome
- Sickle cell trait
- Munchausen syndrome
- Urethral foreign body
- Renal vein thrombosis
- Tuberculosis, schistosomiasis

Features from history/examination
- Associated fever, dysuria, abdominal pain suggest infection
- Enquire about trauma
- Kidney(s) may be palpable with cystic disease and tumours (Wilms')
- Henoch–Schönlein purpura (HSP)—rash + arthralgia BP must be measured

---

Features requiring immediate referral of a child with haematuria
- Fever, abdominal pain, systemic upset
- Persistent (> 48 h) gross haematuria
- Haematuria following trauma
- Hypertension, oliguria, oedema
- Proteinuria > ++
- Impaired or declining renal function

Investigations
1. Routine dip stick testing of urine with Multistix, hematest, Labstix
2. Follow up of all positive urines and exclusion of false positives (see above)
3. Microscopy to detect significant haematuria (> 10 red blood cells per high power field) and presence or otherwise of casts, suggesting a renal cause of haematuria if positive
4. Urine must be cultured. A bacterial count > 10^5/ml organisms indicates urinary tract infection.
5. Further investigations include:
   - FBC, platelet count, ESR, clotting screen, sickle cell screen
   - Urea, creatinine, electrolytes, serum Ca^{++} PO_4^{--},
   - Throat swab/ASOT
   - Complement levels/ANF/DNA binding
   - Urinary protein/calcium/24 hours
   - Renal ultrasound, plain abdominal X-ray
   - Renal biopsy occasionally indicated

---

than 25 g/l) with or without oedema. Proteinuria can be detected and quantified with dip stick (easy) or on a timed specimen (difficult to collect), when it should not exceed 40 mg/m^2/h, or expressed as the urine protein creatinine ratio, measured on a random sample. The normal level is less than 200 mg of protein/mmol of creatinine. Heavy proteinuria causes a reduction in serum albumin, with a consequent fall in intravascular osmotic pressure. This allows fluid to escape from the circulation causing hypovolaemia and oedema.

In accordance with this definition, the nephrotic syndrome can be associated with a number of recognisable diseases (Box 10.1) but most often is idiopathic. When it is associated with a recognised disease the management and outcome is that of the primary disease. This section is con-

---

Box 10.1 Secondary causes of nephrotic syndrome

- Acute glomerulonephritis
- Rapidly progressive nephritis
- Henoch–Schönlein nephritis
- Systemic lupus erythematosus
- Shunt nephritis
- Quartan malaria
- Amyloid
- Heavy metal poisoning
- Renal venous thrombosis

---

cerned with the idiopathic nephrotic syndrome (INS) of childhood.

Clinical features

The incidence of the INS is 1/100 000 population per year. The peak age of onset is 2–5 years, and the disease is more common in boys than girls. The child presents with generalised oedema, often most obvious periorbitally, and allergy is frequently the initial diagnosis. Oedema progresses with grossly swollen legs, ascites and pleural effusion, although the child often does not feel ill. The finding of heavy proteinuria confirms the diagnosis. Rarely the presentation is with peritonitis, and the diagnosis is revealed on urine testing. A surgical opinion with the possibility of laparotomy to exclude a coincidental perforated appendix may be needed.

Management

Assessment of a new case involves looking for evidence of peripheral circulatory failure due to hypovolaemia, namely pale cold extremities, delayed capillary refill time (normally less than 2 seconds), a rapid thready pulse, low peripheral blood pressure and oliguria (less than 1 ml/kg/h). Abdominal pain and faintness may occur. In a child who is grossly oedematous, with a serum albumin level below 20 g/l, 20% salt poor albumin is given over 2–4 hours in a dose of 0.5–1 g/kg with frusemide 1–2 mg/kg given half way through the infusion.

About 90% of children with the INS respond to steroids; response is more likely in those under 10 years who do not have haematuria, hypertension or an elevated blood urea. Prednisolone in a dose of 60 mg/m², to a maximum of 80 mg, is given daily. A low salt, high protein diet is instituted and prophylactic penicillin given while the child is still oedematous. Accurate fluid balance, best ascertained by daily weighing, is important in order to detect fluid retention which may require further albumin infusions. The mean time to achieve a remission, that is cessation of proteinuria, is 14 days. Once in remission, prednisolone is continued in a dose of 40 mg/m² on alternate days for a further month.

If there is no response in 4 weeks, the disease is termed steroid resistant, and the patient should be referred to a specialist centre where renal biopsy will usually be carried out to categorise the renal pathology. About 10% of children with INS have structural glomerular abnormalities on biopsy and, generally speaking, do not respond to steroids. These are either identified after failing to respond to steroids, or because of suggestive adverse features such as being over 10 years old, female, and having haematuria and hypertension, in which case renal biopsy may be indicated before treatment is started.

Children treated with steroids should have their antibody titres against chickenpox and measles measured, and the parents should be warned of the potentially serious nature of these infections. Those children who are not immune should be given the appropriate gamma globulin if exposed to these infections.

After discharge from hospital the parents should test the urine for protein twice a week and contact the doctor if there are two or more plusses on two successive days. A minority of cases, 10–25%, do not relapse after an initial course of steroids. About half of the remainder relapse occasionally, and should be treated in the same way as for the initial presentation. The others have frequent relapses, usually starting within the first six months. These should be treated in a similar way, but after two relapses a small dose of prednisolone, 0.5 mg/kg on alternate days, can be given to try and prevent further relapses. If there are frequent relapses necessitating frequent courses of high dose steroids, serious side-effects may develop (Box 10.2) and these must be discussed with the parents. If steroid toxicity occurs levamisole (an immunostimulant drug), 2.5 mg/kg on alternate days, can be given for 6–12 months and may reduce the number of relapses.

Cyclophosphamide, 2.5 mg daily for 8 weeks, is used if serious toxic effects of steroids develop. This results in a prolonged remission in about

Box 10.2 Some side-effects of steroids
• Impaired linear growth • Hypertension • Osteoporosis • Obesity • Cataracts • Striae • Susceptibility to infections

half the cases. Cyclophosphamide causes marked immunosuppression with its attendant risk of infection and may cause alopecia and haemorrhagic cystitis. There is an unquantified, but probably small long-term risk of infertility and malignancy. The decision to use cyclophosphamide involves balancing its side-effects against those of steroids; full discussion with the patient and parents is essential and must be fully documented.

The prognosis of the idiopathic nephrotic syndrome has improved enormously over the last 50 years, the impact of antibiotics having had the most dramatic effect, with steroids playing a lesser role and cytotoxics only improving the outlook a little. There still remain patients who are steroid resistant and a small number who frequently relapse, who pose a problem.

When using potentially toxic drugs, it is important to remember to discuss the possible side-effects with the patient and their parents, and to document this fully in the notes. Written instructions to parents about management are also an important part of treatment.

ACUTE RENAL FAILURE

Acute renal failure (ARF) is rare in childhood; it is present when the excretion of urine is less than $300 \, ml/m^2/day$ (0.5 ml/kg/h). ARF may be caused by hypovolaemia with impaired renal perfusion, which responds to fluid replacement, intrinsic renal disease or post-renal obstruction.

Hypovolaemia is caused by loss of blood in severe haemorrhage, loss of plasma in burns or the nephrotic syndrome, and loss of electrolytes and fluid as occurs in severe gastroenteritis. This underlying cause may be obvious from the history and examination. The urine is concentrated, and has a high urea and a low sodium content. Untreated, this condition may progress to intrinsic renal failure in which the urine is not concentrated, the urea content is low and the sodium content high. The distinction is important as the treatment is completely different. Urine and blood examination should clarify the difference (Table 10.1). In pre-renal failure an infusion of 20 ml/kg of blood, plasma, or normal

Table 10.1 Urine and blood abnormalities in acute renal failure

	Pre-renal	Intrinsic renal
Urine/plasma urea	> 5–10	< 5
Urine/plasma osmolality	> 1.1	< 1.1
FE_{Na}	< 1%	> 1%

saline, depending on the fluid lost, should restore renal perfusion and increase urine output. This may be repeated once. If urine output is not increased, intrinsic renal disease, that is acute tubular necrosis, is present.

Intrinsic renal disease causing renal failure occurs after severe renal hypoperfusion as described above or after open heart surgery. Renal failure may also be caused by the haemolytic uraemic syndrome, the acute nephritic syndrome, or nephrotoxic drugs.

The haemolytic uraemic syndrome was first described in Switzerland in the early 1950s. All five of the original patients died. It is now considered to be the most common cause of acute renal failure apart from transient acute tubular necrosis associated with open heart surgery. The disease follows infection with a verotoxin-producing *E. coli*, which initially causes gastroenteritis. The child then develops micro-angiopathic haemolytic anaemia, thrombocytopenia and oliguria. The peripheral blood shows numerous fragmented red blood cells, caused by the cells being damaged by fibrin strands in the glomeruli. With careful management the mortality is now about 15%.

Post-renal causes of renal failure include urethral obstruction by valves, bilateral ureteral obstruction from congenital abnormalities, and calculi. The bladder is enlarged, the urinary stream is poor in boys with urethral valves, and the kidneys may be palpable in bilateral ureteral obstruction. An ultrasound of the renal tract will usually confirm obstruction, and treatment is surgical.

Widespread biochemical abnormalities develop as acute renal failure progresses; acidosis and hyperkalaemia occur. Fluid overload with hypertension (see Chapter 5) and with heart failure may be found. Intrinsic renal failure may be prevented by ensuring adequate hydration and fluid replacement after haemorrhage or burns, and in gastroenteritis, and it is equally important to avoid fluid overload once intrinsic renal failure has occurred. Further management should take place in a centre with adequate experience and facilities, and involves careful management of fluid balance, treatment of hyperkalaemia and, possibly, peritoneal dialysis.

CHRONIC RENAL FAILURE

This is defined as a glomerular filtration rate below 30% of normal; like acute renal failure it is a rare condition in childhood, occurring in approximately 1.5–3.0 children per million total population per year. Congenital causes include obstruction, dysplasia and polycystic disease, and acquired conditions include reflux nephropathy, the nephrotic syndrome with structural glomerular abnormalities and the haemolytic uraemic syndrome. Rare metabolic diseases such as cystinosis and oxalosis also cause chronic renal failure.

Clinical features

The clinical and biochemical abnormalities are complex. The child may already be under medical care, or present de novo with anorexia, growth failure, anaemia, polyuria and polydipsia, rickets and sometimes hypertension. The blood urea and creatinine levels are raised and there is acidosis and phosphate retention. The ability to produce a concentrated urine is often lost, causing polyuria. The kidney also fails to produce 1,25-dihydroxycholecalciferol, causing rickets, and erythropoietin, causing a normocytic normochromic anaemia.

Management is complicated and should be undertaken in a referral centre which undertakes dialysis and transplantation and involves a paediatric nephrologist, transplant surgeon, specially trained nurses, child psychiatrist, dietician, teacher and social workers. The aim is to preserve good health as much as possible with a diet adequate in calories and vitamins but low in protein and salt. Treatment with erythropoietin is usually needed, and sometimes growth hormone and hypotensive drugs are required. When renal function declines to 10% of normal, entry to an end-stage renal disease programme involving dialysis and transplantation occurs. Children from a few weeks of age are now being included. The long-term outlook is encouraging: at least three quarters survive for 5 years, and the majority lead a useful life.

RENAL CALCULI (Figures 10.6, 10.7)

This is a rare problem in childhood. It is more common in boys; three quarters of the cases are under 4 years old. The calculi in 15% of cases are bilateral. The usual aetiological factors are urinary tract abnormality combined with infection, particularly with *Proteus mirabilis* infections. The stones are mixed calcium and phosphate with an organic matrix. Occasionally a metabolic cause such as hypercalciuria, with or without hypercalcaemia, cystinuria, oxaluria and xanthinuria are also found. Structural causes including medullary sponge kidney also occur.

Clinically these children present with a urinary tract infection or haematuria, and sometimes renal colic develops. The diagnosis is confirmed by ultrasonography. Treatment is of the primary condition and surgical removal of the stone or lithotripsy.

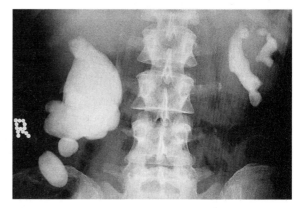

Figure 10.6 Plain X-ray of abdomen showing a staghorn calculus.

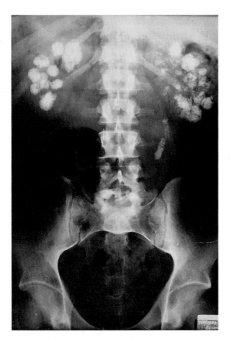

Figure 10.7   Plain X-ray of abdomen showing medullary sponge kidney.

RENAL TUBULAR ABNORMALITIES

The most common of these rare disorders is familial hypophosphataemic hyperphosphaturic rickets, which is inherited as an X-linked dominant. This means that half the children of an affected mother, and all the daughters but none of the sons of an affected father manifest the disease. The primary defect is failure of phosphate reabsorption in the proximal renal tubules, causing heavy phosphaturia and consequent hypophosphataemia. The calcium and phosphate product falls, causing rickets. There are no other proximal renal tubular defects. If the problem is not detected on account of the family history, the child presents with short stature and rickets in the second year of life. The child has bowed legs and metaphyseal swelling at the wrists, ankles and rib ends (the rickety rosary), but does not show the hypotonia and misery of vitamin D deficiency. Phosphate reabsorption is reduced and so the serum phosphate is low, the calcium and vitamin D levels are normal, the alkaline phosphatase is elevated and the urine contains an excess of phosphate as tubular reabsorption of phosphate is less than 85%.

Treatment is with vitamin D in the form of 1,25-dihydroxycholecalciferol, or an analogue such as 1α-hydroxycholecalciferol, and phosphate orally. Although the rickets heal and the deformities resolve, growth is rarely better than the lower centiles. It is important not to over-treat as excessive vitamin D causes hypercalcaemia and nephrocalcinosis with renal failure. Management necessitates frequent measurement of the serum calcium level, aiming to keep it within the normal range. It is often not possible to maintain the serum phosphate at a normal level because this requires more treatment than most children will tolerate. The patients grow up to become healthy adults but they are usually short. The main problem for girls is that, in due course, they will require a Caesarean section at delivery.

POLYURIA AND FREQUENCY

True polyuria, passing large volumes of urine day and night with consequent polydipsia, is rare. Diabetes mellitus must be excluded by testing the urine for glucose if the problem is of recent onset. Serum creatinine and calcium levels are also measured to exclude chronic renal insufficiency and hypercalcaemia respectively. Diabetes insipidus is confirmed by failure to concentrate the urine during a fluid deprivation test. If the diabetes insipidus is central in origin the urine concentration will rise after an injection of synthetic anti-diuretic hormone, but this does not happen in nephrogenic diabetes insipidus. Most children with polyuria concentrate the urine satisfactorily; the polyuria is consequent on polydipsia which has become a mild behavioural problem. The parents are advised to be firm about reducing the child's fluid intake. Some children appear to need to pass urine every few minutes, disrupting their schooling and every social activity within the family. It is usually claimed that the urine volume is excessive, but unlike those with true polyuria these children seldom pass urine at night. A urine concentration test which proves to be normal may be necessary to convince the parents that this is another mild behavioural problem.

GP Overview 10.3 Polyuria

Causes
- Diabetes mellitus
- Compulsive drinking
- Diabetes insipidus
  —hypothalamic
  —nephrogenic

History
Diabetes mellitus—thirst/weight loss/abdominal pain and vomiting
Compulsive drinking—excess drinking and other behavioural aspects including attention seeking

Diabetes insipidus
- Hypothalamic
  —history of pituitary tumour
  —leukaemia
  —meningitis/encephalitis
- Nephrogenic
- —obstructive uropathy
- —chronic renal failure
- —tubular disorders, e.g. Fanconi syndrome
- —nephrotoxins

Investigations
GP
- Urine dip stick to exclude glycosuria or check blood sugar
- MSU, urea, creatinine
- Urine for amino acid screen

Hospital
- Water deprivation test using DDAVP to distinguish the types of diabetes insipidus if appropriate

Treatment
- Diabetes mellitus—joint care between paediatric diabetic team and primary care team
- Diabetes insipidus—use of DDAVP/fluid balance control
- Compulsive water drinking—behavioural management, GP/child mental health services

---

Enuresis. See Chapter 8, page 189.

INCONTINENCE

True incontinence, which usually takes the form of constant dribbling, is extremely uncommon relative to enuresis and is caused by a neurological lesion or anatomical defect in the urinary tract. Evidence of a spinal cord lesion with impaired sacral sensation and weakness, together with abnormal reflexes in the legs, should be sought. Anatomical lesions include an ectopic ureter and urethral obstruction with an enlarged bladder and poor urinary stream. Ultrasound examination of the kidneys and bladder should be performed and imaging of the spinal cord may be indicated.

PAEDIATRIC GYNAECOLOGY

As a result of transplacental transfer of maternal oestrogens there are several signs which may be present in normal newborns; these will resolve over a short time. They include:

- breast swelling in male/female infants
- vulval congestion
- prominent hymen and white vaginal discharge
- vaginal bleeding.

Other newborn problems include:

- Labial adhesions. These are common and can be separated with the use of oestrogen cream for 1–2 weeks. If this is unsuccessful then probing may be advised following referral to a gynaecologist.
- Hydrocolpos (with an imperforate hymen). This may later lead to delayed menarche. It may also cause abdominal pain and urinary retention. Treatment consists of incision of the membrane and release of the fluid.

VULVOVAGINITIS

After the first few weeks of life the protective effect of maternal oestrogen is lost and the vulva and vagina become prone to infections. The absence of lactobacilli (as in adults) leads to the vaginal pH being less acidic; bacteria and fungi can grow and cause vulvitis or vaginitis. Other factors contributing to infection are:

- short distance between anus and vagina
- incorrect wiping after defecation
- threadworms
- poor hygiene.

The most common organisms include haemolytic streptococci, Gardnerella, *Trichomonas vaginalis*, *Candida albicans* and threadworms (*Oxyuris vermicularis*). The discharge is often copious, smelly and sometimes bloodstained. (Blood should raise the possibility of a foreign body.) Management includes:

- gentle examination
- swab for bacteriology
- appropriate antibiotic/antifungal/anti-helminthic
- advice to parents on avoidance of bubble baths
- avoidance of perfumed soap
- avoidance of tight fitting clothes (use cotton).

Sometimes the use of a topical oestrogen cream is sufficient when cultures are negative. Continuing problems require further investigation to exclude a foreign body and child sexual abuse in particular.

SKIN DISORDERS IN INFANTS AND YOUNG CHILDREN

These may include the following conditions:

- Lichen sclerosus. This is a vulval dystrophy causing white plaques and leading to pruritus/scratching. Treatment includes good hygiene and treatment for secondary infection.
- Eczema—emollients and mild steroid creams.

- Psoriasis and seborrhoeic dermatitis may also be present in the vulval area.

VAGINAL BLEEDING IN PREPUBERTAL GIRLS

This always needs to be investigated to establish the cause:

- trauma, both accidental and non-accidental in sexual abuse
- foreign body (may require a general anaesthetic for removal)
- vaginal or cervical tumour (e.g. botryoid sarcoma)
- precocious puberty (see Chapter 11)
- urethral prolapse.

PROBLEMS IN PUBERTAL GIRLS

These include heavy and painful periods. It is not unusual for the first six or so periods to be heavy and/or painful. The first cycles are often anovulatory. Analgesics such as paracetamol and mefenamic acid (a prostaglandin inhibitor) and, in some cases, oestrogen in the form of an oral contraceptive may be needed.

FURTHER READING

Fitzpatrick M M, Dillon M J 1991 Current views on aetiology and management of haemolytic uraemic syndrome. Postgraduate Medical Journal 67: 707–709

Lieberman E, Donnell G N 1965 Recovery of children with acute glomerulonephritis. American Journal of Diseases of Childhood 109: 398–407

Working Group of the Research Unit, Royal College of Physicians 1991 Guidelines for the management of acute urinary tract infections in childhood. Journal of the Royal College of Physicians of London 25: 36–42

Workshop by the British Association for Paediatric Nephrology and Research Unit, Royal College of Physicians 1994 Consensus statement on management and audit potential for steroid responsive nephrotic syndrome. Archives of Disease in Childhood 70: 151–157

Internet address
http://www/mc.vanderbilt.edu/peds/pidl/nephro/index.htm

11

Endocrinology and metabolic disorders

Derek Johnston

GROWTH

Growth is at the core of paediatrics, and its measurement is an essential step in assessing whether or not an individual child is achieving his or her potential within the spectrum of family and society. Subnormal growth may be the first manifestation of an environmental or health disorder, and normalisation of growth is a primary target in the management of social adversity or disease.

Physiology of growth

It has been calculated that the fertilised human ovum undergoes some 42 cycles of cell division before birth and only a further 5 cycles from birth to adult size. The dynamic phase of fetal growth and tissue organisation is especially susceptible to transplacental influences, notably nutrition, and there has recently been renewed interest in the nature of fetal programming and its impact on adult health.

It is convenient to divide postnatal growth into three main components—infancy, childhood and puberty—the 'ICP' model of growth.

- *Infancy growth* is a continuation of fetal growth in which nutrition is the dominant control although the growth hormone–insulin-like growth factor (GH–IGF) axis is also operative.
- *Childhood growth.* Dominant control shifts to endocrine pathways during childhood, and the height growth rate gradually declines until it reaches a nadir in the prepubertal period.

• *Pubertal growth* represents temporary acceleration superimposed on the linear decline of childhood growth, and is determined by sex steroid release which in turn amplifies growth hormone (GH) secretion and the tissue responsiveness to the GH–IGF axis. Pubertal growth occurs relatively earlier in girls, with peak height velocity matching the emergence of breast buds (breast stage 2), while in boys the slowing childhood phase continues until the second half of puberty, and acceleration is signalled by testicular volumes of 8 ml or greater. The adult height advantage of boys reflects longer childhood growth and a pubertal surge which has a greater component of trunk growth.

Growth hormone release is regulated by complex neuroendocrine pathways which act through the hypothalamus to release growth hormone releasing hormone (GHRH) and somatostatin. It is the balance between stimulatory GHRH and inhibitory somatostatin which determines the frequency and amplitude of GH pulses. The normal secretory pattern is for higher amplitude GH pulses to occur in deep sleep. Pulse amplitude is maximal in parallel with the pubertal growth spurt. GH acts primarily on hepatocytes to generate the production of IGF-1, which in turn promotes chondrocyte hyperplasia in the growth plates. The resultant GH–IGF-1 axis is further modified by an interplay of binding proteins, cell receptors, nutrition and other endocrine pathways.

GH production varies considerably within and between individuals. Childhood growth is not linear, as suggested by population growth charts, but is based on short- and medium-term periods of slowing and acceleration, so-called stasis and saltation. Season, general health (both physical and emotional), and nutrition influence GH release. Tall children produce greater total GH than short children. Assessment of GH adequacy or insufficiency is further complicated by the relatively poor precision of GH provocation tests, and the limitations of laboratory-based evaluation of the GH–IGF axis reinforce the place of detailed clinical interpretation of abnormal growth.

Measurement techniques

In normal paediatric practice the core measurements are:

• weight
• height or length (stature)
• head circumference.

An accurate weight is provided by reliable electronic scales; infants should be naked and children only minimally dressed. A range of reliable, low cost, portable or static equipment is available for length and height measurement. The equipment must be regularly calibrated against a standard rule. Supine length, measured by two people with head and foot boards, is used until a child can be consistently placed in the required standing position, usually after the age of 2 years. The technique to provide accurate, reproducible lengths or heights needs training and review to ensure that the level of variation of repeat measurements falls within ± 3 mm. Measurement of height requires that the child stands with naked feet together and flat on the floor, and with heels, buttocks and shoulder blades touching a vertical measure. The measurer uses both hands to position the child's head with the auditory meatus in the same horizontal plane as the lower border of the eye socket (the Frankfurt plane), and exerts gentle upward pressure on the mastoids to achieve maximum extension. The measuring plate is brought down to make firm contact with the scalp. Measurements should be recorded to the nearest completed millimetre.

In older children, growth measurement should include pubertal assessment using the Tanner grades 1–5 for female breast, pubic hair and male genital changes. Testicular growth may be calibrated against a Prader orchidometer, which comprises beads of volumes 1–25 ml; the onset of puberty matches a volume of 4 ml and greater.

Growth charts

UK cross-sectional reference data charts were revised in 1994. The new standards reflect a modest secular trend towards greater stature, and the revised format is based on 9 centiles to facilitate more discriminating referral criteria. Each intercentile band of the height chart is equivalent to 0.67 standard deviations (SD) so that the 2nd centile and the 0.4th centile are equivalent to -2.0 and -2.67 SD respectively. The 0.4th centile (4 per 1000) is a considerably more specific threshold for detecting children with organic disorders.

Simple inspection of height and weight charts will show that the height centile bands are symmetrically distributed around the 50th centile, a normal distribution. By contrast, weight centile bands show increasing width with increasing weight reflecting a population bias towards obesity, a feature which increases with age.

Measurements should be plotted as discrete points, ensuring that age is calculated correctly and appropriately for either decimal or duodecimal scales. A series of accurate points, without the unnecessary embellishment of circles, makes it easier to visualise whether growth parallels normal centiles. Infancy plots need to take account of prematurity, and it avoids confusion if the date of the measurement is noted on the chart.

UK growth charts provide instructions for plotting corrected parental heights, deriving midparental height and calculating the target centile range (Box 11.1). Specialist growth centres make use of the statistical expression, standard deviation score or SDS, to describe a child's growth parameter in comparison to the population mean; for example

$$\text{height SDS} = \frac{(\text{individual height} - \text{mean population height corrected for sex and age})}{\text{SD}}$$

Box 11.1 Midparental height corrected
Boys Target height (cm) = $\dfrac{\text{FH (cm)} + \text{MH (cm)} + 7}{2}$
Girls Target height (cm) = $\dfrac{\text{MH (cm)} + \text{FH (cm)} - 7}{2}$
FH = Father's height; MH = Mother's height

Detection of abnormal growth

For the general childhood population, growth assessment is part of health surveillance. Growth also needs to be checked when children present with persisting health problems, or when families or professionals express concern. *Health For All Children* makes the following recommendations.

Infancy

- As a minimum, neonatal length should be measured in infants of low birth weight or with abnormality.
- At age 6–8 weeks length should be measured in infants of low birth weight and infants with abnormality, or if there is concern over growth or feeding pattern.
- Head circumference should be measured shortly after birth, at 6–8 weeks, and subsequently if there is concern about head or general growth.

Early childhood

- Height and weight should be measured at the ages of 18–24 months, 36–42 months, and at school entry (around 5 years).
- An additional measurement at the age of 7–8 years is preferable and should be insisted upon if previous height data are incomplete or there is concern about the child's general health or growth rate.

The case for pre-school measurement is accepted, but firm national guidelines on later childhood growth monitoring await evidence of effectiveness.

Action thresholds in early childhood:

- A single height measurement below the 0.4th or above the 99.6th centile requires referral to a specialist clinic.
- A height in the 0.4–2.0 or the 98–99.6 centile band requires repeat measurements at 6 and 12 months.
- If serial height plots show abnormal deviation, action depends on the age and the time scale of observations. The following recommendations reflect current consensus:
  —For children aged less than 5 years, referral

is needed if, between two height measurements usually separated by 18–24 months, the plot crosses two major centile bands (1.34 SD). If height crosses one band (0.67 SD) then measurement should be repeated after 18–24 months and referral made if a further band is crossed.

—For children aged between 5 and 9 years the referral criterion is the crossing of one centile band over 12 months. Deviation across the equivalent of half a band merits community assessment and measurement after a further 12 months. This strategy, based on accurate plotting, avoids emphasis on calculated height velocities and the use of growth velocity charts which have potential pitfalls.

- Any child whose height falls outside the parental target height merits referral.
- Height/weight discrepancy has attracted less attention; referral criteria remain provisional, for example a discrepancy between stature and weight of more than 3 centile bands. Body mass index (weight, kg/height, m^2) reference curves have been derived from recent population data.

Late childhood and adolescence

The interpretation of growth in older children is complicated by the variable timing of the transition from the declining height velocity of late childhood to the acceleration which coincides with early puberty (breast stage 2) in girls and late puberty in boys.

Primary assessment of a child with growth failure

The history must include a review of pregnancy, birth and early infancy in order to identify causes of intrauterine or infancy growth failure (Box 11.2). 80–90% of small-for-gestation age (SGA) infants achieve normal range stature by the age of 4 years; those who fail to catch up by this age are destined to remain small. The endocrine basis of children programmed to be small may represent a spectrum of relative GH insufficiency

---

Box 11.2 Causes of growth failure

Fetal
- Chromosomal and genetic
  - autosomal chromosome disorders, e.g. trisomies, deletions
  - sex chromosome disorders, e.g. 45XO and variants
- Syndromic intrauterine growth retardation, e.g. Russell–Silver, Prader–Willi
- Congenital infections
- Skeletal disorders
- Utero-placental disorders
- Maternal disorders

Infancy
- Continuation of fetal growth failure
- Organ and systemic disorders
- Malnutrition

Childhood
- Familial short stature
- Social and environmental problems
- Organ and systemic disorders
  - conspicuous, e.g. severe asthma
  - inconspicuous, e.g. coeliac or Crohn's disease

Endocrine disorders
- Growth hormone (GH) deficiency
  - congenital: familial, e.g. gene deletion, idiopathic, multiple pituitary hormone deficiency
  - acquired: tumours, e.g. craniopharyngioma, dysgerminoma, optic nerve glioma; irradiation, trauma, inflammation
- GH receptor defects, e.g. Laron syndrome
- Insulin-like growth factor (IGF) receptor defects
- Hypothyroidism
- Adrenal failure

Adolescence
- Constitutional delay of growth and puberty
- Hypogonadism

---

and GH–IGF end-organ resistance. A minority of SGA infants have syndromic features, for example pedal oedema and facies indicating Turner's syndrome, or the clinodactyly and body asymmetry of Russell–Silver syndrome.

Family stature, health, and age of onset of puberty need to be recorded (Box 11.3). An abnormally short parent may share the same but previously unrecognised disorder, for example a mild skeletal dysplasia such as hypochondroplasia, or a metabolic bone disease such as X-linked hypophosphataemic rickets. Alternatively parents may also have been victims of a recurrent cycle of deprivation.

Primary care health workers are well placed to

> **Box 11.3** Preliminary assessment of growth failure confirmed by two or more accurate height measurements
>
> **Child's history** (refer to parent-held record)
> * Pregnancy and birth size
> * Infancy health and growth
> * Development and schooling
> * Diet and eating behaviour
> * General health
>
> **Family**
> * Structure and stability
> * Height
> * Age of puberty
> * General health
>
> **Examination**
> * Height, weight, head circumference
> * Body proportion, sitting height
> * Pubertal stage
> * Dysmorphic features
> * General review
> * Visual acuity, fields and fundoscopy
>
> **Optional investigations,** guided by history and examination
> *Imaging*
> * Left hand bone age
> * Ovarian ultrasound
> * Cranial MRI
>
> *Blood*
> * FBC, ESR
> * Electrolytes, urea, creatinine, Ca, P, LFT
> * Gliadin and endomysial antibodies
> * Ferritin
> * Thyroxine, TSH
> * Karyotype
>
> *Urine*
> * Microscopy, culture

identify environmental and emotional problems, but it is easy to overlook psychosocial short stature or to confuse it with chronic malnutrition. Characteristic features of stress related growth failure include hyperphagia with gorging and vomiting linked to polydipsia.

The majority of non-endocrine organic health disorders likely to result in growth failure will be apparent from a comprehensive history and examination, but targeted investigation may be required to exclude coeliac disease, chronic inflammatory bowel disease, or chronic renal failure. Karyotyping is warranted in all girls whose stature falls below that anticipated from parental heights. General review must incorporate

fundoscopy, visual acuity and field assessment to rule out a mass lesion in the hypothalamic–pituitary area, but the probability is that lesions such as craniopharyngioma will present with symptoms of raised intracranial pressure.

Causes of short stature amenable to diagnosis and management in primary care

Familial or idiopathic short stature

This can usually be managed by explanation and counselling, but parents who have experienced the stigma of short stature and who have been exposed to media revelations about the claimed benefits of GH may request specialist assessment and intervention. They should do so in the knowledge that, although GH in supra-physiological dosage does increase short-term growth, it is unresolved whether the final height advantage is sufficient to justify years of costly, invasive therapy and the uncertainty about long-term side-effects.

Constitutional delay of growth and puberty (CDGP)

Children are genetically equipped to reach their adult height at different rates. Those with CDGP remain in the declining phase of late childhood growth for longer, so that by comparison with cross-sectional height standards they appear to deviate below normal centiles. Their pubertal growth takes place later and is less pronounced although the majority have acceptable catch-up growth. The general rule for CDGP is that height matches that expected for pubertal stage and bone age. The diagnosis is more convincing when there is a family history; any concern about the child's general health merits further investigation to exclude covert organic disease or gradual onset hypothyroidism or GH deficiency.

Boys are more likely to present with concerns about short stature or delayed sexual maturation. Alternatively they may divert their lack of self-confidence into aggressive behaviour and other school conduct disorders. In girls, anorexia nervosa and exercise-induced amenorrhoea enter the differential diagnosis.

Explanation and a realistic forecast of future growth is adequate for most boys but a minority may benefit from specialist advice on the use of short-term growth promoting androgen therapy, either oral oxandrolone 2.5 mg daily or intramuscular testosterone depot 50–100 mg monthly, both for 3–6 months.

Causes of short stature requiring specialist referral for diagnosis and management

Suspected GH insufficiency

GH deficiency is relatively easy to confirm when it is severe and results in early childhood growth failure, truncal obesity, an immature facies, micropenis and pronounced bone age delay. Early diagnosis is also more likely in multiple pituitary hormone deficiency, when it will be accompanied by one or more of the following: persistent neonatal hypoglycaemia, prolonged neonatal unconjugated or conjugated jaundice, failure to thrive with polyuria and hypernatraemia (diabetes insipidus), or collapse associated with hyponatraemia (ACTH, cortisol deficiency). A midline facial malformation, for example a central cleft palate, or congenital visual impairment due to optic nerve hypoplasia suggests a structural lesion of the hypothalamus with secondary panhypopituitarism. High resolution imaging with MRI defines the anatomical status of the hypothalamic–pituitary axis and can for example identify congenital failures of migration of the pituitary stalk.

Certain well-defined acquired disorders such as postoperative craniopharyngioma have a high likelihood of rendering the child panhypopituitary and hence in need of full pituitary hormone replacement, including GH. A growing number of children are survivors of intensive treatment programmes which have salvaged them from acute leukaemia or intracranial malignancy. The combination of cranial irradiation and intracranial pathology places them at risk of neurosecretory dysfunction with relative GH deficiency.

The majority of short children who may potentially benefit from biosynthetic GH therapy have isolated partial deficiency without an obvious anatomical basis, and they are not readily differentiated from children with familial or idiopathic short stature. In practice, GH insufficiency is confirmed by the exclusion of other growth restraints, by demonstrating a subnormal height velocity over at least 6–12 months, and by one or more tests which meet accepted criteria of defective GH secretion. Widely used tests include glucagon, clonidine and arginine stimulation tests but their limitations include variability of response, potential hazards such as delayed hypoglycaemia after glucagon, and the necessity for multiple blood samples. It is especially difficult to interpret low responses during the phase of relative GH deficiency which parallels the transition from late childhood to early adolescence. Less invasive tests include single blood sample measurement of IGF-1 and IGFBP3 which reflect downstream action of GH, and urinary GH measurement, but it has to be emphasised that no single measurement can fully define GH status.

The growth specialist uses national guidelines to establish whether the child warrants GH therapy; in some borderline situations the therapy will be offered as a therapeutic trial with continuation dependent on the growth response. The specialist will then enter into a shared care agreement with the family practitioner to enable the supply of GH. Biosynthetic GH has an excellent safety profile and is available in formulations for pen injector device administration. It is administered as a once-daily subcutaneous injection in a dose of 0.5–0.7 units/kg body weight/week (14–20 units/m^2 surface area/week). The high cost of GH therapy demands that its use is properly targeted and effectively audited, and that families are fully supported to ensure compliance.

Turner's syndrome

Turner's syndrome is relatively common, occurring in 1 in 2500 female live births. There is a misconception that most affected girls have conspicuous dysmorphic features which lead

Table 11.1   Turner's syndrome: main clinical features and approximate frequency

Problem	%
Short stature	> 90
Ovarian failure	> 90
Webbed neck	70
Inverted widely spaced nipples	70
Narrow, hyperconvex nails	75
Multiple pigmented naevi	75
Cardiac:	
—coarctation	10–20
—bicuspid aortic valves	40–50
Renal malformations	40–50
Scoliosis	10
Eustachian tube dysfunction	common
Progressive sensorineural deafness	common
Ptosis, strabismus, refractive errors	common
Autoimmune thyroiditis	50 (by adult life)
Relative insulin resistance and hyperlipidaemia	
Normal IQ but increased visuospatial problems and attention deficit disorder	

to early recognition (Table 11.1). The reality is that diagnosis is often delayed despite the girls having greater than average family doctor and specialist clinic attendance because of feeding problems, middle ear disease, strabismus and amblyopia. Karyotyping should be performed in all girls who are inappropriately short compared to midparental height, bearing in mind that approximately 25% have heights within the normal population range during the pre-school years. The pubertal growth acceleration fails to emerge although around 30% of girls have a spontaneous partial puberty with early breast development. The net result is a mean final height of 143 cm compared to the normal population mean of 163 cm; the distribution of heights is similar in that 95% fall within 12 cm of the mean, emphasising the genetic importance of parental heights despite the X chromosome abnormalities. The growth failure represents intrinsic programming and a mild skeletal dysplasia rather than identifiable endocrine deficiency. Body mass index increases disproportionately from late childhood.

Management needs to encompass initial explanation and counselling, general health review, educational and behavioural issues, growth promotion and hormonal replacement.

Several multicentre studies have established that high dose GH therapy accelerates height growth in Turner's syndrome, and uncontrolled results show final height gains of 5–8 cm. The best height gain results from GH treatment in the age range 4–12 years. The GH dose range is 0.6–1.0 unit/kg/week (18–28 units/m^2/week) given as a daily subcutaneous injection. Adverse events are modest with initial fluid accumulation which may precipitate headaches and aggravate pedal oedema. Cutaneous pigmented naevi are reported to increase in size. There are potential long-term issues of carbohydrate intolerance and altered lipid profiles.

Oestrogen replacement is designed to give the girls pubertal changes to match those of their peer group, to promote uterine growth which may facilitate later ovum transfer programmes, and to preserve skeletal integrity. From the age of 14 years, ethinyloestradiol is introduced at an initial dose of 2 µg daily. Depending on responsiveness the dose is increased at 6–12-monthly intervals to an adult dose of 20 µg/day. A progesterone is introduced to the cycle after 12–18 months, guided by uterine ultrasound appearance.

Around 5% of girls have mosaicism incorporating Y chromosome fragments and resultant testicular tissue. This predisposes to virilisation and gonadoblastoma, and prophylactic gonadectomy is indicated.

The long-term implications of Turner's syndrome, notably hormone replacement, access to IVF, an increased incidence of autoimmune hypothyroidism, osteoporosis, and a possible requirement for cardiovascular monitoring justify a multidisciplinary team extending care through adult life.

Tall stature

The majority of tall children match their tall parents; the main problem relates to a small minority of girls who are considered by their families to be at risk from unacceptable adult stature. A family history consistent with constitutional advance of growth and puberty, and a moderately advanced bone age suggest that final height is likely to be within acceptable limits. A tall girl with long limbs, no bone age advance and a mother who had late menses is at greater risk, but it is still a highly individual decision as to what is a challenging height. Although there are established methods for height prediction, these are based on models of normal growth and become less reliable in atypical growth patterns. Treatment to reduce residual growth needs to be introduced near the onset of puberty so that it may subtract from the end of childhood growth before the inevitable height gain which accompanies puberty.

In girls, relatively high dose oestrogen, for example ethinyloestradiol 50 μg daily combined with a progesterone agent, is claimed to provide useful height reduction with an acceptable safety profile.

Pathological causes of excessive stature are uncommon but there is an overlap between children with long limbs and those with the criteria which match Marfan's syndrome. The diagnosis of Marfan's syndrome is supported by family history and major features in the skeletal, ocular and cardiovascular systems. Key clinical features include joint laxity, chest deformity and scoliosis. Around one third have echocardiographic evidence of aortic root enlargement or mitral valve prolapse. The basis is an autosomal dominant fibrillin gene mutation on chromosome 15, but 25% of cases represent new mutations.

Homocystinuria is a rare (1 in 50 000) recessive disorder of methionine metabolism in which children have a Marfanoid appearance. Diagnostic features include high myopia accompanied by lens dislocation, learning delay and early onset thromboembolic events.

Klinefelter's syndrome, karyotype 47XXY, occurs in around 1 in 600–1000 live-born males. The mean height lies near the normal 75 centile and presentation is more likely to be with cryptorchidism, delayed puberty and learning delay.

Beckwith–Wiedemann syndrome is characterised by intrauterine overgrowth, macroglossia, exomphalos, visceromegaly, hemihypertrophy and an increased incidence of embryonal tumours. Adult height is not excessive. There is an association with over-expression of paternally imprinted insulin-like growth factor 2 on chromosome 11.

PUBERTY

Physiology of puberty

Sexual maturation is part of a continuum of events initiated during fetal life but suppressed by ill understood mechanisms during childhood. The hypothalamic pulse generator of gonadotrophin releasing hormone, GnRH, is reactivated after the age of 6–8 years, resulting in increasing frequency and amplitude of nocturnal gonadotrophin (LH, FSH) pulses. This reactivation is programmed by neural networks which are under the control of both genetic and environmental influences. Pelvic ultrasound imaging demonstrates ovarian and uterine changes prior to the onset of detectable breast maturation, and this is a valuable tool in the assessment of female puberty.

Adrenal cortical maturation usually parallels gonadal changes, and the resultant increase in androgens, dehydroepiandrosterone and androstenedione produces pubic hair and skin changes.

Ages of normal puberty

Normal UK girls reach breast stage 2 at mean age 11.5 years, and menarche at age 13.5 years with peak height velocity (PHV) near pubertal onset at 12 years. Boys start puberty with genital stage 2 at a similar age, 11.6 years, and reach full maturity at 15.2 years but the male PHV is later at 14.1 years.

Precocious puberty

Precocious puberty is generally accepted as sexual development appearing in a girl before age 8 years, and in a boy before 9 years, but it is more important to consider the nature of the puberty (Box 11.4) and its impact on the child and family.

Early puberty which matches the normal pattern in combining sexual maturation, pubic hair growth and growth acceleration in the usual order is likely to have a central origin with premature activation of the hypothalamic GnRH pulse generator. Pelvic ultrasound scanning will confirm bilateral ovarian maturation with multicystic changes and matching uterine growth. The equivalent in boys is symmetrical testicular growth, 4 ml or greater. In girls, central precocious puberty is commonly familial or constitutional, and it is not necessary to perform cranial imaging unless there are additional features

---

Box 11.4   Differential diagnosis of early puberty

Complete precocious puberty
- Constitutional
- Organic brain disease: tumours, trauma, inflammatory, irradiation

Incomplete precocious puberty
- Ovarian cysts and tumours
- Leydig cell tumours
- Adrenal tumours
- Congenital adrenal hyperplasia
- hCG secreting tumours
- McCune–Albright syndrome
- Familial testotoxicosis
- Hypothyroidism
- Exogenous sex steroid exposure

Partial forms of precocious puberty
- Premature thelarche
- Premature adrenarche

---

such as recent onset headache, behaviour change or eye signs. Skin pigmentation suggestive of neurofibromatosis increases the likelihood of a hypothalamic or optic nerve glioma. Central precocious puberty is 20 times less common but is considerably more ominous in boys. A pathological basis such as a pineal area tumour must be excluded by detailed pituitary area imaging, preferably MRI.

The spectrum of early puberty in girls is such that explanation and sympathetic support is appropriate management for many. Intervention may be justified if sexual maturation and menses are unacceptable within the child's overall capacity to cope, and if parallel bone age advance threatens adult height. In appropriate children, LH and FSH production may be suppressed using long-acting injectable gonadorelin analogues (LHRH superagonists). Some girls with predominantly breast and uterine maturation have ultrasound evidence of ovarian cysts which prove to be independent of LH, FSH control. These autonomous cysts may be linked to the McCune–Albright syndrome combining irregular skin pigmentation and fibrous dysplasia of bones.

Early puberty which follows an abnormal pattern with, for example inappropriate virilisation in a girl, or penile and pubic hair growth without matching testicular volume increase in a boy is termed 'incomplete'. The causes are late-presenting congenital adrenal hyperplasia and adrenal or gonadal tumours. Key investigations include bone age assessment, gonadal and adrenal imaging, adrenal androgen, sex steroid and gonadotrophin measurement.

Partial precocious puberty

Breast development (premature thelarche)

Isolated, usually self-limiting and often asymmetrical breast development is relatively common in young girls, especially under 2 years. Investigation is unnecessary if height growth is appropriate and there is no other sexual development. Transient elevations of FSH paralleled by ovarian follicular activity are responsible.

Pubic and axillary hair growth (premature adrenarche)

This is relatively common, especially in girls over the age of 6 years. It is accompanied by apocrine activity and modest height and bone age acceleration; it reflects accentuation of the normal increase of adrenal androgen production.

Delayed puberty (Box 11.5)

Pubertal delay warrants review when the first signs are delayed beyond 13.5 years in girls and 14.0 years in boys. An incomplete or unusually prolonged puberty lasting over 5 years may also be abnormal.

Boys present at least 20 times more commonly than girls, and the vast majority who are otherwise healthy have constitutional delay of growth and puberty (CDGP). The family history and a delayed bone age are important guides, and it is usually evident from growth records that the child has had a slow tempo of maturation. Without a positive family history it is important to rule out eating disorders, insidious systemic illness such as coeliac or Crohn's disease, or endocrine deficiency, notably hypothyroidism.

Box 11.5   Differential diagnosis of delayed puberty

Constitutional delay of growth and puberty (CDGP)
- Familial, non-familial

Hypogonadotrophic hypogonadism
- Isolated gonadotrophin deficiency (with hyposmia in Kallman's syndrome)
- Multiple pituitary hormone deficiency
- CNS disorders, e.g. congenital, tumours, irradiation
- Syndromic, e.g. Noonan, Prader–Willi
- Chronic systemic disease or malnutrition
- Anorexia nervosa, exercise amenorrhoea

Hypergonadotrophic hypogonadism
- Females
  — ovarian dysgenesis, including Turner's syndrome
  — ovarian damage, e.g. irradiation, chemotherapy
  — autoimmune oophoritis

- Males
  — seminiferous tubular dysgenesis including Klinefelter's syndrome
  — testicular damage, e.g. surgery, irradiation, chemotherapy
  — anorchia, e.g. fetal vascular accident

Turner's syndrome needs to be excluded by karyotype and pelvic ultrasound.

A positive family history of infertility and a background of cryptorchidism or micropenis may be clues to gonadotrophin deficiency. This may be accompanied by relative impairment of olfactory sensation—Kallman's syndrome. In practice it is difficult to differentiate this from CDGP; a pragmatic approach is to treat substantial delay with escalating sex steroid replacement until individuals match their peer group. Persistent LH, FSH deficiency merits more detailed investigation of the hypothalamic–pituitary–gonadal axis.

In boys with probable CDGP and emotional problems sufficient to merit intervention, a reasonable strategy is to give intramuscular depot testosterone 50 mg per month for 3–6 months. This should initiate secondary sexual development and a sustained growth spurt so long as the testes have reached a volume of 8 ml or more. Persisting small testes call for specialist guidance and more prolonged replacement regimens. A girl requiring short-term intervention can be given very low dose ethinyloestradiol, 1–2 μg daily, for 3–6 months.

THYROID DISORDERS
Congenital hypothyroidism

The addition of TSH measurement to neonatal capillary blood screening has revolutionised the detection and prognosis of infants with congenital hypothyroidism. The incidence is in the range 1 in 3500–4500, and 90% of cases are sporadic failures of differentiation (agenesis, hypoplasia) or migration (ectopic). In most populations, errors of thyroid hormone synthesis account for less than 5–10%.

It is essential that health professionals have an agreed protocol for initial explanation about the significance of an elevated TSH and for arranging prompt confirmation at specialist centres, and that they understand the long-term strategy of thyroxine replacement. The majority of affected infants have an unequivocally raised TSH both at screening and on repeat sample. The plasma thyroxine may be normal or subnormal; those with initial levels below 60% of the lower limit of normal are at greater risk of long-term learning problems. Some centres arrange for isotopic thyroid scans at diagnosis, but others reserve this for the minority who present management problems, or where the family background increases the probability of a biosynthetic defect. TSH screening is sensitive but cases may still be missed and there remains a need for thyroid function tests in prolonged jaundice or otherwise unexplained growth failure. TSH measurement will not detect hypopituitary-based hypothyroidism, a rarer problem which usually manifests in other ways, for example hypoglycaemia or micropenis and cryptorchidism.

Thyroxine replacement should be commenced by the age of 14–21 days, the usual starting dose for term infants being L-thyroxine 25 µg/day. Infants readily tolerate crushed tablets and it is possible to titrate the dose using 12.5 µg increments so that TSH levels are suppressed to the normal range. In the longer term, children usually require replacement in the dose range 100–110 µg/m^2/day, the treatment aims being to achieve normal activity, development and growth while avoiding overtreatment-induced irritability and sleep disturbance. This strategy results in fewer than 10% of children requiring specialist education compared to reports of 40% prior to screening. It needs to be emphasised that treatment is lifelong; after children mature beyond paediatric specialist supervision there should be secure arrangements for review by family practitioners. Some regions have thyroid registers to facilitate shared care.

Childhood-onset hypothyroidism

The majority of later onset hypothyroidism is caused by autoimmune thyroiditis. This usually has an insidious onset and is more common in adolescent girls. A palpable goitre is common and may be the presenting feature before hypothyroidism emerges. A positive family history is common and there may be other autoimmune manifestations such as vitiligo or diabetes. The duration of hypothyroidism determines whether there is growth failure and a delayed bone age. Girls may present with premature breast development despite growth delay because of overlap between elevated TSH and FSH.

Laboratory confirmation includes elevated TSH, a low or borderline thyroxine level, and a high titre of anti-microsomal thyroid antibodies. Management is based on thyroxine replacement, young persons normally tolerating a rapid dose escalation to 100 µg/m^2/day. The resulting physical and behavioural changes may be substantial, and the introduction of a normal, active adolescent into a household may need preparation.

The natural history of autoimmune thyroid disease is variable; initially obvious cases are likely to persist, but patients with borderline findings such as a minimal goitre and marginal TSH elevation need reassessment before commitment to lifelong therapy.

Juvenile hyperthyroidism

Hyperthyroidism is rare in childhood and the incidence rises during adolescence, especially in girls. The presentation is usually typical with a symmetrical smooth goitre (Figure 11.1), proptosis, tremor and tachycardia. There may be a long unrecognised phase of concentration problems, sleep disturbance and growth acceleration.

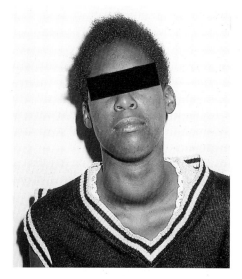

Figure 11.1 Pubertal goitre.

Juvenile hyperthyroidism is part of the spectrum of autoimmune thyroid disease related to TSH receptor-stimulating immunoglobulins. Elevated free thyroxine and a suppressed TSH confirm the diagnosis. Medical management with carbimazole, initial dose 0.4–0.6 mg/kg/day up to a maximum of 30 mg/day and maintenance 0.1–0.3 mg/kg/day, is the favoured option in young patients. Prominent autonomic symptoms merit additional β-adrenergic blocking agents, propranolol 0.75–2 mg/kg/day. Approximately 60% enter permanent remission but if active disease persists for more than 4–5 years or antithyroid drugs cause problems then there is a place for either partial thyroidectomy or radioactive iodine.

ADRENAL DISORDERS

Adrenal disorders are relatively rare in paediatric practice and can be categorised under three main headings:

- congenital adrenal hyperplasia
- adrenal overactivity
- adrenal underactivity.

Congenital adrenal hyperplasia (CAH)

Disorders of adrenal steroid biosynthesis present with the following features:

- ambiguous genitalia, notably a masculinised female because of 21-hydroxylase deficiency
- adrenal salt-losing crisis (hyponatraemia and hyperkalaemia), more threatening in the otherwise unrecognised male infant
- incomplete precocious puberty in boys; penile and pubic hair growth without testicular enlargement
- virilisation, hirsutism and acne in girls
- the features of polycystic ovarian syndrome in young women.

Over 90% of children with CAH have 21-hydroxylase deficiency; this is associated with salt loss in around 75%. The incidence in most populations is in the region of 1 in 5000–15 000 live births.

CAH presenting as masculinisation of a newborn female is the most common cause of ambiguous genitalia in which the gonads are impalpable. Current imaging, biochemical and genetic resources allow prompt diagnosis so that the girl's parents can be counselled that masculinisation is limited to the external genitalia, and that the upper vagina, uterus, fallopian ducts and ovaries are intact. Surgical and endocrine management can provide an unequivocally female lifestyle with the potential for fertility. A corrective genitoplasty is performed in the first months of life although later procedures may be required to ensure vaginal patency.

Typical maintenance treatment consists of hydrocortisone 20 mg/m^2/day in three divided doses, and for salt losers fludrocortisone 50–200 μg/day as a single dose. Infants with more severe salt loss require added sodium chloride 5–15 mmol/kg/day until weaned. Families must have guidance on increasing the hydrocortisone dose at the onset of coincidental illness, and should be provided with injection hydrocortisone for emergencies. Young children with congenital adrenal hyperplasia are also vulnerable to hypoglycaemia. Longer-term monitoring of both sexes consists of careful growth measurement; an active child with a normal height velocity is likely to be appropriately treated.

The 1 in 4 risk of recurrence necessitates genetic counselling. There is a place for maternal dexamethasone treatment from 3–4 weeks' gestation to reduce masculinisation of affected females. 21-hydroxylase is controlled by a large gene area on chromosome 6 and a range of mutations are responsible for the deficiency; it is therefore necessary to perform family studies before attempting fetal diagnosis.

Adrenal underactivity

Primary adrenal failure or Addison's disease is rare in childhood, and the early features of lethargy, weight loss and delayed recovery from coincidental illness may be overlooked until an emergency arises because of circulatory collapse. Clinical clues include abnormal skin and mucosal pigmentation, vitiligo and a family history of autoimmune disease. A low plasma sodium calls for cortisol measurement and, if possible, a sample promptly separated and frozen for ACTH assay. Hyperkalaemia is less evident but if present it points to primary adrenal pathology rather than to secondary or hypopituitary failure. Positive adrenal cytoplasmic antibodies confirm an auto-immune cause. A synacthen test may clarify equivocally low cortisol levels.

Emergency treatment includes correction of circulatory failure and hypoglycaemia, and intravenous hydrocortisone 50 mg followed by 5 mg/ kg/day before reduction to a maintenance dose of 15 mg/m^2/day. Fludrocortisone 100–200 µg/ day is the usual aldosterone substitution. Monitoring therapy places more emphasis on energy and quality of life than on blood cortisol and ACTH levels. Families must have written guidelines on the need to increase the dosage at the onset of coincidental illness and for surgery.

Adrenoleukodystrophies are rare inherited peroxisomal disorders in which intellectual or behavioural deterioration and other neurological deficits may present before adrenal failure.

Adrenal overactivity

Although adrenal overactivity is sometimes suggested in children and adolescents with escalating obesity, it is readily excluded when height growth is intact, pubertal development is appropriate, and the obesity is generalised rather than centripetal or truncal. Innocent although cosmetically troublesome striae may accompany weight gain in pubertal girls.

Pathological adrenal overactivity is rare and is usually linked to the less common varieties of congenital adrenal hyperplasia or to adrenal adenoma/carcinoma. A mixed pattern of virilisation, hirsutism and acne, combined with features of cortisol excess, is suggestive of a tumour and requires specialist biochemical and imaging definition. A key issue in boys is whether the apparent pubertal progress is accompanied by appropriate testicular enlargement; prepubertal testes point to adrenal pathology. Long established height acceleration and an advanced bone age favour a late presenting form of congenital adrenal hyperplasia; the presence of hypertension would further consolidate a clinical diagnosis of 11-hydroxylase deficiency.

Cushing's disease or ACTH-dependent adrenal hyperactivity is very rare in childhood.

DISORDERS OF SEXUAL DIFFERENTIATION (Box 11.6)

Uncertainty about the gender of a newborn is an extreme test for parents and health professionals. In a majority of cases an experienced multidisciplinary team can provide a prompt diagnosis and an authoritative recommendation on gender assignment, but a challenging minority require detailed and time-consuming evaluation before a decision can be reached.

The functional gender of a child is determined at several levels:

- Genetic—usually signified by the karyotype but there are exceptions, e.g. XX males.
- Gonadal—testes, ovaries, mixed or incompletely differentiated gonads.
- Internal and external genitalia—complete male differentiation is dependent on intact testosterone and Müllerian inhibitory factor (MIF) pathways while female differentiation is to

---

Box 11.6 Classification of more common causes of ambiguous genitalia

Virilised female (no palpable gonads), XX karyotype
- Congenital adrenal hyperplasia
- Transplacental androgen exposure

Undervirilised male (gonads may or may not be palpable), XY karyotype
- Disorders of testicular differentiation
  — Leydig cell hypoplasia (gonadotrophin unresponsiveness)
  — pure or mixed gonadal dysgenesis
- Disorders of testicular function
  — enzyme defects in testosterone and/or corticosteroid synthesis
- Disorders of androgen dependent target tissues
  — 5α-reductase deficiency
  — complete and partial androgen insensitivity

Varied karyotypes with malformed, streak or mixed gonads
Malformation syndromes associated with gonadal and genital anomalies

a large extent independent of functioning ovaries (the default mechanism).

• Psychological—the end result of both genetic and environmental influences.

The medical priorities are to make an aetiological diagnosis which will guide management of the individual child and provide the basis for genetic counselling, to anticipate and prevent further problems such as a salt-losing crisis, and to develop a care plan which will support child into adult life. Final decisions on gender assignment must also take account of the parents' religious and cultural background.

Congenital adrenal hyperplasia (21-hydroxylase deficiency), the most common cause of the masculinised female newborn, is discussed above.

The investigation of an undervirilised male is more complex, one of the key issues being to establish whether the fault lies with gonadal hormone production which is potentially amenable to correction with testosterone replacement, or with target organ insensitivity which is likely to be refractory to hormone replacement.

Androgen insensitivity

Androgen insensitivity encompasses a wide spectrum from relatively mild undervirilisation through to a fully female phenotype albeit with a blind-ending vagina and no uterus, the so-called testicular feminisation syndrome. A child with a poorly developed phallus and androgen insensitivity is unlikely to have a satisfactory life in a male role, and will be more appropriately raised as a girl. Once a female gender is assigned to a XY child, rearing must be unequivocal with genitoplasty, gonad removal and hormone replacement designed to allow as normal a life as possible.

XY girls with complete androgen insensitivity may present with hernias which contain testes, or later in life because of primary amenorrhoea despite full breast development, the latter being a consequence of aromatisation of endogenous testosterone to oestrogen.

Patient support groups have highlighted the deficiencies of the counselling provided by doctors, and there is a tendency to conspire with parents to delay full explanation beyond an age when girls wish to know the truth about their own bodies. If the disorder is recognised in childhood there will also have to be a decision as to gonad removal. Early removal is indicated if there is partial androgen insensitivity so that the girl does not run the risk of unwanted virilisation at puberty. Early removal also removes the low risk of germ cell cancer in intra-abdominal testes. The early gonadectomy policy has to be matched by a strategy of escalating oestrogen replacement to provide an artificial puberty. Other authorities favour gonadectomy after puberty so that the girl has the benefit of a more natural puberty and is better informed to provide consent for such a fundamental procedure. The genetic counselling of families also requires expert knowledge and sensitivity. As this is an X-linked disorder, apparent sisters of the proband may also be affected XY individuals, and XX females have a 50% risk of being carriers. There are parallel implications for the mother's sisters.

Micropenis and cryptorchidism

An anatomically intact but small penis (Figure 11.2) suggests that testicular function was quali-

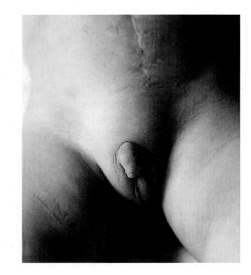

Figure 11.2 Micropenis.

tatively normal during genital differentiation but that there is a relative deficiency of gonado-trophin, LH and possibly growth hormone. More severe LH deficiency results in cryptorchidism. There may also be a family history of similar problems, including infertility. An interesting subgroup of LH deficiency is combined with defective olfactory sensation, Kallman's syndrome, an X-linked disorder.

Confirmation of LH deficiency is difficult in childhood; a pragmatic option for boys with micropenis is to prescribe one or more short courses of low dosage testosterone supplementation. A definitive diagnosis and hormone replacement programme can be devised at or after puberty.

Impalpable or inguinal testes should be assessed for orchidopexy by a paediatric surgeon. Preliminary investigation including karyotyping, LH and testosterone measurement (with hCG stimulation) and imaging may be required to assess the functional viability of intra-abdominal testes. Testes capable of releasing testosterone in early fetal life may subsequently atrophy, and these agonadal boys require hormone replacement from around age 12 years, prosthetic testes insertion and counselling.

Klinefelter's syndrome (47XXY)

This is a relatively common disorder, 1 in 600–1000 male births, and encompasses a wide spectrum. Many individuals do not appreciate that there is a problem until sterility is confirmed. Some present in childhood with undescended testes or delayed puberty, but the majority have pubertal progression within an acceptable time scale although the testes remain small and atrophy in adult life. The low testosterone levels may contribute to a more retiring personality with reduced academic and social drive. Defective verbal and co-ordination skills are characteristic, but overall performance scores are close to controls. There is a place for offering gradually escalating testosterone replacement to selected patients, as well as counselling and contact with support groups. As XXY boys are increasingly recognised in fetal life it is essential that parents are offered informed counselling based on objective studies of large cohorts.

CHILDHOOD DIABETES

Insulin-dependent diabetes is the most common paediatric endocrine disorder, having a prevalence of 1 in 400–500 of the population under 15 years of age. Family practitioners will infrequently encounter a newly diagnosed case but they need to be alert to the diagnosis so that confirmation and treatment may be initiated before the problems of ketoacidosis arise. They also need to be familiar with the district strategy for ensuring that children and their families are supported by a diabetes team capable of meeting nationally agreed criteria which emphasise a family centred approach and the promotion of independent self-care.

Although the peak incidence occurs in early adolescence, there has been a trend towards presentation at an earlier age with 20–25% arising before the age of 5 years. The rising incidence in industrial societies emphasises that environmental factors are becoming more prominent in causation. The genetic basis for susceptibility to presumed dietary or viral triggers has been linked to the DQ region on chromosome 6, but it is likely that there are at least two further control loci. Insulin-dependent diabetes is preceded by several years during which markers of islet cell autoimmune injury are present; symptoms arise when the beta cell reserve falls to 10% or less of normal. Current research is attempting to consolidate the suggestion that breast feeding is protective, and other studies are focusing on modification of the immune system of at-risk individuals.

The onset of diabetes is usually typical with thirst, polyuria and weight loss but, especially in the young child, initial symptoms may be masked and the presentation confused by prominent abdominal pain, hyperventilation or collapse. Parents and health professionals are increasingly making the diagnosis early, so the introduction to diabetes and its management can be conducted as a primarily home-based exercise. For the minority with symptomatic ketoacidosis treatment must take place in a centre with well rehearsed diabetic ketoacidosis protocols.

Modern management incorporates an at least twice-daily insulin regimen, often based on pre-mixed insulin formulations injected with a pen device. The prepubertal child seldom requires a total daily insulin dose above 0.8 units/kg body weight. Puberty generates an increased requirement, sometimes exceeding 1.5 units/kg, and lifestyle pressures may justify conversion to a four injection regimen based on short-duration insulin before meals and medium-duration at bedtime. Dietary advice tends to be qualitative rather than quantitative with the emphasis on a regular mealtime pattern based on a healthy eating plan. The aims are an active lifestyle with normal growth and development without the disruption of hyper- or hypoglycaemia. Home monitoring targets can be set at pre-meal blood sugars in the range 4–10 mmol/l but the reality is that profiles are often variable and not readily amenable to correlation with insulin dose. Clinic targets are guided by HbA1c levels; the DCCT (Diabetes Control and Complications Trial) study suggested that sustained control matched by values less than 8.0% (for a normal upper limit of 6%) is protective against retinopathy and nephropathy. The challenge is to translate this objective for a childhood population supported by average resources and with the potential penalties of an increased incidence of severe hypoglycaemia. Apart from the disruption of recurrent hypoglycaemia, episodes can lead to long-term erratic control, loss of awareness of low blood sugar and potential neurological problems. Faced with this dilemma, control is a compromise dictated by the circumstances of the individual child. Other key lifestyle issues are the avoidance of smoking and preparation for the adult pressures of work, alcohol and sexual activity.

Structured review (Box 11.7) is essential to long-term care, and each district should have a diabetes register supported by an information system which promotes shared care between family practitioners and paediatric and adult diabetes teams.

Box 11.7 Review of the diabetic child or adolescent

Symptoms
- Hyperglycaemia
- Hypoglycaemia
- Other problems

Lifestyle
- Home
- School
- Sport and leisure

Education and self-directed management
- Insulin injection and capillary sampling techniques
- Sick day rules
- Hypoglycaemia and exceptional activity

School liaison
Insulin regimen
- Formulation(s)
- Injection frequency and timing
- Insulin dose, units/kg/day
- Injection device

Diet
- Meal pattern
- Snack plan
- Dietician review

Monitoring
- Home blood sugar diary (validity?)

Growth
- Height, weight, puberty

Examination
- Injection sites, distribution and hypertrophy
- Finger sampling sites
- Finger flexion deformity, skin elasticity
- Skin, e.g. necrobiosis
- Feet
- Blood pressure (plotted against standards)
- Fundoscopy (dilated after age 12 years)
- Coincidental disease, e.g. goitre, vitiligo

Laboratory screening
- HbA1c
- Microproteinuria
- Urine microscopy and culture
- Thyroxine, TSH (autoimmune thyroiditis)
- Gliadin and endomyseal antibodies (coeliac disease)
- Creatinine
- Lipid studies

Excessive drinking and diabetes insipidus

Genuine polydipsia is a potentially important symptom, but in the assessment of young children it is important to recognise that behavioural drinking is the main cause in otherwise healthy toddlers who assert themselves by constantly demanding the comfort provided by bottle or beaker. The majority can tolerate nights without fluid intake or can be diverted by play strategies. A minority are more worrying, especially if their diet is also deficient and growth is borderline. These children may justify a more extensive assessment including early morning plasma electrolyte, urea and osmolality measurement combined with urinary osmolality. It is seldom necessary to have to go to the lengths of formal fluid deprivation studies in an attempt to confirm cranial or nephrogenic diabetes insipidus.

METABOLIC DISORDERS
(Table 11.2 and Box 11.8)

The range and complexity of metabolic disorders is daunting but their combined prevalence and potential impact on children and families make them an important area of paediatrics. The primary care based paediatrician needs to be familiar with local neonatal screening programmes and the availability of regional specialist metabolic and genetic services.

Metabolic disease seldom enters the top rank of differential diagnosis when a previously healthy child becomes acutely ill but there may be important clues such as a family history of previous unexplained infant death, recent change in diet, hepatomegaly, hypoglycaemia or metabolic acidosis. Surveys have established that even potentially fatal disorders such as medium chain fatty acyl-CoA dehydrogenase deficiency

---

Box 11.8 Clinical and laboratory features suggestive of a metabolic disorder

Family history
- Consanguinity
- Unexplained infant death
- Unexplained neurodevelopmental disorder

Feeding
- Problems after onset of feeding
- Problems after change of diet, e.g. introduction of sucrose
- Apparent recovery with interruption of feeds

Presenting problem
- Apparent life-threatening event
- Multiple fits
- Encephalopathy
- Developmental deterioration
- Prolonged jaundice
- Haemorrhagic disease (underlying liver disease)

Examination findings
- Dysmorphic, abnormal facies
- Abnormal hypo- or hypertonia
- Cataracts or abnormal fundoscopy
- Hepatosplenomegaly
- Unusual smell

Laboratory findings
- Hypoglycaemia
- Metabolic acidosis
- Abnormal LFTs, elevated NH_3
- Positive metabolic screen (blood, urine)

(MCAD) may remain asymptomatic until coincidental illness provokes metabolic decompensation. All too often the sudden presentation and potential death mimics sudden infant death syndrome or leaves a damaged child labelled as having unexplained cerebral palsy. The prompt collection of blood and urine samples during the acute phase may be the key to the diagnosis,

---

Table 11.2 Laboratory screening in infancy

Test	Disease	Incidence
Phenylalanine	Phenylketonuria	1 in 10 000
Bacterial inhibition assay (Guthrie test)		
Amino acid fluorometry or chromatography	Potential for detecting other aminoacidopathies	
TSH	Congenital hypothyroidism	1 in 3000
Immunoreactive trypsin (IRT) linked to DNA technology ΔF508	Cystic fibrosis	1 in 2500
Haemoglobin analysis	HbS, C and others	Common in selected groups
Electrophoresis, isoelectric focusing, chromatography, monoclonal antibody	Thalassaemias	

which may in turn lead to specific therapy as well as genetic counselling.

In more chronic progression, the features may be those of a multisystem disease with the emphasis on neurological symptoms and deterioration, for example fits, axial hypotonia and limb hypertonia. Hepatosplenomegaly is seldom the sole presenting feature of a metabolic storage disease, although it may be the case in non-neuronopathic Gaucher and Niemann–Pick disease. Glycogen storage disease produces massive soft hepatomegaly without splenomegaly; there are usually additional major features such as fasting hypoglycaemia or profound hypotonia and developmental delay. It is all too easy on casual abdominal examination to miss the ill-defined liver edge in the lower quadrant!

CALCIUM DISORDERS

Apart from the receding problem of nutritional rickets, it is rare for calcium related problems to present in primary care paediatrics. It needs to be emphasised that vitamin D deficiency does not usually present with hypocalcaemia; more discriminatory biochemical markers are an inappropriately elevated alkaline phosphatase level and a low plasma phosphate.

Hypocalcaemia

After the neonatal period, and in children who do not have renal or liver disease, the combination of hypocalcaemia and hyperphosphataemia suggests hypoparathyroidism which may be isolated or part of a syndrome complex. The abnormal biochemistry may be discovered as part of the investigation of atypical seizures or tetanic spasms including intermittent stridor. DiGeorge syndrome needs to be considered in dysmorphic infants who present with hypocalcaemia, cardiac anomalies and thymic hypoplasia causing T cell immune deficiency.

Another group of usually older children present with short stature, round facies, brachydactyly and learning difficulties, features of parathyroid hormone (PTH) resistance or pseudohypoparathyroidism. Hypocalcaemia requires specialist assessment including PTH measurement. Management is based on the vitamin D analogue alphacalcidol, in the dose range 40–50 ng/kg/day, aiming to provide relief from neuromuscular symptoms and a plasma calcium in the low normal range.

Hypercalcaemia

This is an even rarer problem in children. A positive family history of hyperparathyroidism and multiple endocrine neoplasia provides a major clue. The symptoms are non-specific: poor feeding, failure to thrive, thirst and polyuria and exceptionally abdominal pain due to renal calculi.

Syndromic hypercalcaemia (Williams' syndrome)

Hypercalcaemia is one component of this variable autosomal dominant contiguous gene syndrome caused by mutations involving the elastin gene on chromosome 7. Other features include supravalvular or valvular aortic stenosis, an elfin facies, lacy or stellate iris and learning problems.

Hypoglycaemia

Hypoglycaemia, defined as a plasma glucose of less than 2.6 mmol/l, is an uncommon problem after the neonatal period other than in diabetic children. The detection of a low blood glucose using a blood stick may be an important clue to the diagnosis of a child presenting with fits or impaired consciousness. Hypoglycaemia, preferably confirmed by laboratory measurement and accompanied by matching plasma and urine samples, may point to the following:

• An unrecognised metabolic disorder. An important example is medium-chain acyl-CoA dehydrogenase deficiency (MCAD), a mitochondrial defect which interferes with hepatic metabolism of acetyl-CoA and $NADH_2$ which are essential to gluconeogenesis and ATP synthesis. There is also a block in ketone production which aggravates energy starvation to key tissues such as brain and cardiac muscle. Affected children may be entirely asymptomatic until stressed by illness which within hours precipitates collapse or encephalopathy associated with hypoglycaemia and deranged liver function. It is suspected that undiagnosed MCAD is relatively common, 5–10 per 100 000 and that it contributes to unexplained infant mortality and devastating brain insults. The diagnosis has been simplified by the application of gene probe methodology and can be applied to dried blood on filter cards, opening up the option for population screening. Recognition and measures to ensure adequate feeding during illness can protect these children.

- An evolving endocrine deficiency. Examples such as panhypopituitarism and adrenal failure are described above.

- Inappropriate drug administration. Family practitioner prescribing records may assist in recognising accidental or deliberate oral hypoglycaemic drug ingestion. Insulin administration has also to be considered and can be confirmed in the specialist laboratory.

- Ketotic hypoglycaemia. Lean young children with borderline energy reserves may develop mild hypoglycaemia and pronounced ketosis when fasted or ill. They seldom provide a diagnostic problem because of the absence of other features of disease and their prompt recovery on being fed. This is, however, a diagnosis based on careful review and exclusion of the problems listed.

Hyperlipidaemia

Family practitioners have a key role in the selection of children who warrant serum cholesterol measurement. The United Kingdom emphasis is on selective rather than population screening for the detection of major inherited disorders of lipoprotein metabolism. The British Hyperlipidaemia Association recommends that total cholesterol is measured in children when the family history demonstrates a first or second degree relative with hyperlipidaemia, notably familial hypercholesterolaemia (FH), or there is premature onset ischaemic heart disease. The age cutoff for the latter may be arbitrarily defined as 50 years in men and 55 years in women. Cholesterol measurement is not usually justified before the age of 2 years, after which there is scope for dietary modification, and it is preferably performed before the age of 10 years on the basis that earlier recognition promotes better compliance. The age of blood testing and lifestyle intervention will obviously be influenced by the family's attitude and the extent to which they are already adhering to a healthy diet.

Age and sex related population data for lipid and lipoprotein levels in childhood are available from the US. These show a progressive rise in serum cholesterol levels through childhood, reaching a peak at around age 10 years, after which there is a temporary decrease in early adolescence before a progressive and substantial rise in adult life. Although the mean cholesterol levels alter during childhood, the 95th centile remains stable and it has been possible to define useful action thresholds. If an initial random total cholesterol on either capillary or venous blood exceeds 5.5 mmol/l then a further fasting venous sample should be assayed for total and HDL cholesterol and triglyceride. A total serum cholesterol of above 6.7 mmol/l correctly identifies 95% of FH heterozygotes and misclassifies only 2.5% of unaffected children. The further definition of a FH heterozygote includes an LDL cholesterol of above 4.0 mmol/l.

Children with elevated lipid levels require specialist referral for confirmation of the diagnosis and guidance on intervention. Drugs have a limited role in childhood and are rarely introduced before the age of 10 years. The emphasis is on dietary control, recognising that the intake of dietary energy should be adequate to allow normal growth and development but that our young population is at risk of moderate obesity which amplifies morbidity from hyperlipidaemia. The main recommendations are that total fat intake should be in the range 30–35% energy with minimal saturated and trans-fatty acid intake.

Steps to detect and manage childhood hyperlipidaemia are important but have to be set against the greater challenge of the *Health of the Nation* targets to reduce the death rates for coronary heart disease and stroke. The targets on obesity and teenage smoking are especially challenging.

FURTHER READING

Barker D J P 1994 Mothers, babies and disease in later life. BMJ Publishing Group, London

Brook C G D 1995 Clinical paediatric endocrinology, 3rd edn. Blackwell Science, Oxford

Buckler J M H 1994 Growth disorders in children. BMJ Publishing Group, London

Kelnar C J H 1995 Childhood and adolescent diabetes. Chapman and Hall Medical, London

Neil A, Rees A, Taylor C 1996 Hyperlipidaemia in childhood. RCP Publications, London

Additional information
1990 UK Charts, published by the Child Growth Foundation. Available from Harlow Printing, Maxwell Street, South Shields, Tyne and Wear NE33 4PU, UK

Internet addresses

Growth
http://www.cgf.org.uk

Diabetes
http://www.idi.org.au/frameset6.htm

12

Eyes, ENT and common emergencies

Andrew W. Boon

EYES

Congenital abnormalities

Coloboma of the iris

This is a sector-shaped deficiency, usually involving the lower part of the iris. It may extend backwards to involve the ciliary body and choroid, and may be associated with other ocular abnormalities or occur as part of a syndrome (see Box 12.1).

Heterochromia

In heterochromia one iris is of a different colour from the other. Sector heterochromia involving part of the iris of one eye is of no significance. Heterochromia may be associated with Horner's syndrome and with Waardenburg's syndrome (heterochromia, white forelock, patches of skin hypopigmentation and deafness).

Box 12.1   Syndromes including coloboma

- CHARGE association—Coloboma, Heart disease, choanal Atresia, Retarded growth and development, Genital abnormalities, Ear anomalies/deafness
- Aniridia–Wilms' tumour association
- Cat-eye syndrome—coloboma of iris and anal atresia
- Goltz syndrome—poikiloderma with focal dermal hypoplasia, syndactyly and dental anomalies

Blocked lacrimal duct

This occurs in 2% of babies. It is usually caused by delay in canalisation of the duct and presents with recurrent sticky eyes. It usually resolves spontaneously. Treatment consists of bathing the eyes with cooled boiled water. Repeated application of local antibiotics should be avoided because of the risk of sensitisation. Some cases may require probing of the duct under general anaesthesia towards the end of the first year of life.

Ptosis

This may be an isolated finding or part of a syndrome. It is generally bilateral and is often hereditary. There is concern if the pupil is occluded because of the risk of amblyopia developing. Surgery is indicated mainly because of the risk of visual impairment or the presence of compensatory posturing. Surgery may later be indicated for cosmetic reasons. Syndromes including ptosis are listed in Box 12.2. Ptosis may be a presenting feature of neuromuscular disease, e.g. myasthenia or myopathy.

Horner's syndrome

In this condition the sympathetic nerve supply to the eye is disturbed. Clinical features include miosis (a small pupil that is reactive to light) because the parasympathetic supply to the pupillary constrictor muscle remains intact, a drooping eyelid, absence of sweating over the ipsilateral side of the face and apparent enoph-

thalmos. Congenital Horner's syndrome may also be associated with heterochromia of the iris.

Acquired Horner's syndrome should prompt a search for a tumour or other compressive lesion. It may also occur in cluster headaches.

No treatment is required for congenital Horner's syndrome.

Nystagmus

Nystagmus is a rhythmic oscillation of the eyes which is described by the direction of the fast phase, rate and amplitude.

Physiological nystagmus

Physiological nystagmus may be optokinetic or induced by rotation or caloric stimuli.

Congenital nystagmus

This is usually horizontal. It may be associated with compensatory posturing of the head. There are a number of patterns of inheritance, including dominant, recessive or X-linked. The cause is generally unknown.

Nystagmus secondary to reduced vision

This typically occurs in albinism and in aniridia, corneal opacity, optic nerve hypoplasia and high refractive errors. Generally, the worse the vision the slower the speed of the nystagmus. Syndromes including nystagmus are listed in Box 12.3.

Box 12.2 Syndromes including ptosis

- Turner's syndrome
- Noonan's syndrome
- Moebius syndrome—VIth and VIIth cranial nerve palsies
- Smith–Lemli–Opitz syndrome—anteverted nostrils, ptosis, syndactyly of second and third toes, hypospadias and cryptorchidism; failure to thrive
- Aniridia–Wilms' tumour association
- Aarskog's syndrome—hypertelorism, brachydactyly, shawl scrotum, short stature

---

Box 12.3 Syndromes including nystagmus

- Aniridia–Wilms' tumour association
- Septo-optic dysplasia—absent septum pellucidum, hypoplasia of the optic nerves, hypopituitarism
- Chediak–Higashi syndrome—partial albinism, cytoplasmic inclusions in leukocytes
- Cerebro-oculo-facio-skeletal (COFS) syndrome—reduced white matter in the brain leading to hypotonia and areflexia; deep-set small eyes with cataracts and nystagmus; prominent root of the nose; upper lip overlapping the lower lip; mild arthrogryposis; rocker bottom feet.

Nystagmus secondary to neurological lesions

Acquired nystagmus requires prompt and thorough investigation. It may be associated with lesions of the brainstem, cerebellum and vestibular apparatus.

Cataracts

A cataract is an opacity of the lens which results in an absent or partial red reflex on ophthalmoscopy. This is an essential element of the routine neonatal examination and at 6 weeks.

Hereditary (primary) cataracts

Cataract is present at birth and is usually bilateral. The cataracts are frequently incomplete and may not interfere with vision. The usual pattern of inheritance is autosomal dominant. Early surgery is required (within 3 months of birth) when vision is seriously reduced, to prevent permanent visual loss. Any child with suspected cataracts should therefore be referred immediately to an ophthalmologist. Following surgery the child will require spectacles or contact lenses.

Secondary cataracts

Rubella during the first 3 months of pregnancy may cause cataracts; the virus can be cultured from the lens following surgery. There may be other features of congenital rubella. Galactosaemia is a rare cause of cataract but all children with congenital cataracts should be screened for this disorder.

In later childhood, Down's syndrome is associated with a greatly increased incidence of lens opacities, although they are generally small and do not interfere with vision.

Trauma to the eyes and prolonged treatment with systemic corticosteroids (for more than 1 year) may also cause cataracts.

Squint

Squint, or strabismus, results from misalignment of the visual axes. Squint is important for three reasons:

1. It may show that the acuity of the eye is impaired because of ocular disease.
2. The squint itself may result in amblyopia.
3. The squint may be a sign of a life-threatening condition.

Pseudo-squint

The presence of prominent epicanthic folds may give the impression of a squint. The child should be carefully assessed using a cover test (see p. 37). Referral to an orthoptist or ophthalmologist is indicated in cases where doubt remains.

Concomitant (non-paralytic) squint

Non-paralytic squints are commonly associated with hypermetropia (long-sightedness). The child develops a convergent squint in order to accommodate. Refractive errors may be familial. The squint may be manifest (present all the time) or latent (apparent when the child is tired or ill, or on testing).

Incomitant (paralytic) squint

This is much less common and is usually secondary to a cranial nerve palsy. Acquired squint is an ominous sign and may be caused by an intracranial tumour or hypertension.

Testing for squint

History:

- A positive family history is a strong risk factor for the development of squint.
- Squints are more common in children with neurological disorders such as cerebral palsy.
- Perinatal problems and developmental delay increase the likelihood of a squint.
- Parental concern about a squint should always be taken seriously and the child should be carefully assessed for the presence of a squint.

The child should be referred to an orthoptist

or ophthalmologist if there is any continuing doubt about the possibility of a squint.

Before testing for squint, the visual acuity should be assessed using letter matching if the child is old enough (over the age of 3 years). The position of the child's eyes should be observed. Large squints should be immediately obvious. Wide epicanthic folds may give the impression of a squint; it is important to remember, however, that these children may also have true squints.

Two tests are used:

1. *The corneal light reflex.* The positions of the corneal reflexes (reflections of light) are noted when a small light is directed towards the child's face. The reflections should be symmetrical.

2. *The cover test.* This consists of covering and uncovering one eye and repeating the process with the other eye. Ideally the child should fix on a distant object and then a near object. With a latent squint the covered eye takes up the squinting position behind the cover and moves back to the central position when the cover is removed. With a manifest squint the uncovered squinting eye moves to the fixing position when the other eye is covered.

Squint amblyopia

The presence of a squint in childhood is rapidly followed by suppression of vision in the squinting eye which soon leads to permanent loss of central vision (amblyopia). Mild squinting may occur soon after birth, but a severe squint within the first month of life requires an ophthalmological opinion. Any child over the age of 3 months should be carefully assessed and referred if there is any doubt. It is always important to act on a parent's concerns about a possible squint, particularly if there is a family history of squint.

ACUITY PROBLEMS

Severe visual handicap is relatively uncommon (only 1 in 4000 children is registered blind). Refractive errors are much more common, affecting 50 per 1000 children.

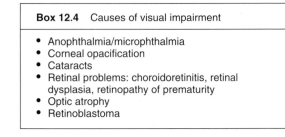

Box 12.4 Causes of visual impairment

- Anophthalmia/microphthalmia
- Corneal opacification
- Cataracts
- Retinal problems: choroidoretinitis, retinal dysplasia, retinopathy of prematurity
- Optic atrophy
- Retinoblastoma

The blind child

Severe visual handicap may be caused by a lesion anywhere in the visual pathway. Most of these will be within the eye itself (Box 12.4). Cortical blindness may result from intrauterine infections, perinatal insults (hypoxia, intracerebral haemorrhage), cardiac arrest, trauma and meningitis later in life.

It is important to remember that severe visual impairment is often associated with other problems such as learning difficulties, epilepsy, behavioural problems, deafness and cerebral palsy.

Refractive errors

Hypermetropia (long sight) is the most common refractive error; it occurs because the eye is relatively short. Mild hypermetropia is the rule before the age of 3 years. Severe hypermetropia may present with a squint; this can be corrected by the use of appropriate spectacles which relax the ciliary muscles and remove the drive to over-converge.

Children rarely complain of poor vision, and so regular screening of visual acuity is very important. Refractive errors can usually be readily corrected with spectacles.

Needs of visually impaired children

Vision is one of the main ways in which the young child learns about the world. Gross motor development is often delayed because of an impaired awareness of space. The blind baby is often relatively hypotonic. Fine motor development, object permanence and social development may also be affected and there may be feeding problems.

Registration of blindness (normally undertaken by an ophthalmologist) is optional but may help in obtaining benefits.

Management of visually impaired children and services

Peripatetic teachers are particularly helpful in advising parents of pre-school visually impaired children how to facilitate their child's development. Children with mild to moderate visual impairment should cope with mainstream schooling, often with the help of some extra support at school and low vision aids. Placement in a special school may be necessary if the child has severe visual impairment or other disability. The severely visually impaired child will need to be taught Braille.

ACUTE EYE PROBLEMS

Glaucoma

Intraocular pressure is raised and the main clinical features are photophobia, blepharospasm, corneal haziness from oedema, and progressive enlargement of the eye (buphthalmos).

Congenital glaucoma

This is caused by an abnormality in the angle of the anterior chamber which results in impaired drainage of aqueous humour. It may be an inherited autosomal recessive condition.

Secondary glaucoma

Any condition resulting in impaired drainage of the aqueous humour may cause glaucoma, e.g. uveitis, ocular tumours, trauma and the Sturge–Weber syndrome.

Glaucoma is a serious condition; any child with apparently enlarged eyes should be examined carefully by an ophthalmologist. Treatment is surgical. Untreated, the condition results in blindness.

Conjunctivitis

Conjunctivitis is common throughout childhood.

It is generally infectious but may also be caused by allergies and chemical irritants as well as trauma.

Neonatal conjunctivitis (ophthalmia neonatorum)

The most common bacterial causes are *Staphylococcus aureus*, *Chlamydia trachomatis*, *Neisseria gonorrhoeae* and other Gram-positive and Gram-negative organisms. Ophthalmia neonatorum is a notifiable condition.

Gonococcal conjunctivitis

This usually presents early in the newborn period with a profuse greenish discharge and marked inflammation of the lid and conjunctiva. It can lead to corneal damage and blindness. The diagnosis may be made by Gram staining of the pus and culture on chocolate agar. Treatment consists of penicillin eye drops, initially every 25 minutes, and systemic penicillin.

Chlamydial conjunctivitis

This usually presents later in the newborn period, after the first week. The conjunctivitis and discharge may be relatively mild. The clue to its cause is often that the conjunctivitis does not resolve with chloramphenicol drops. The diagnosis is made by obtaining a swab from the upper and lower palpebral conjunctiva which is then placed in 2SP or another chlamydial transport medium. Chlamydial conjunctivitis may also result in corneal scarring. Treatment is with tetracycline eye drops and systemic erythromycin.

Other bacterial conjunctivitis

In general, a purulent discharge implies bacterial origin. Treatment is with a topical antibiotic such as chloramphenicol or fusidic acid.

Conjunctivitis in older children

Conjunctivitis is one of the most common causes of an uncomfortable red eye. It has many causes including bacteria, viruses, Chlamydia and allergies. It may be associated with a purulent or clear discharge which is most noticeable on waking when the lids are often stuck together.

Allergic conjunctivitis

This produces injection of the conjunctivae, often with profuse watering of the eyes (epiphora). It occurs particularly in atopic children during the pollen season. A characteristic feature is itching of the eyes. Topical cromoglycate and systemic antihistamines may be helpful. Topical steroids should only be used under the supervision of an ophthalmologist because of the danger of enhancement of herpes simplex corneal infection and a risk of producing glaucoma. Topical antibiotics may cause an allergic conjunctivitis.

Viral conjunctivitis

Viral conjunctivitis is commonly associated with upper respiratory tract infections, usually caused by an adenovirus. It may produce outbreaks of pink eye in schools. There is usually a watery discharge from the eyes and the child often complains that the eye feels gritty and uncomfortable. In older children there may be follicle formation and there is often corneal involvement. Viral conjunctivitis is generally self-limiting, and bathing of the eyes is often all that is required. Chloramphenicol eye drops and ointment provide symptomatic relief, however, and may help to prevent secondary bacterial infection. Viral conjunctivitis is highly contagious; strict hand washing by the doctor, parents and child is very important to prevent spread of the infection.

Blepharitis

Inflammation of the lid margins is either staphylococcal or crusted seborrhoeic; bathing of the lid margins is part of the treatment of both forms. A topical anti-staphylococcal antibiotic should be used for staphylococcal blepharitis. In seborrhoeic blepharitis the associated seborrhoea of the scalp must also be treated.

Orbital cellulitis

Orbital cellulitis usually results from spread of infection from a paranasal sinus—in infants most often the ethmoid sinus but in older children from the ethmoid, frontal or maxillary sinuses.

The clinical features include proptosis, limitation of ocular movement, conjunctival oedema (chemosis) and inflammation and swelling of the eyelids. The child is often toxic with a high fever. Untreated the infection may lead to loss of vision, meningitis and cavernous sinus thrombosis. Urgent hospital admission is therefore essential to initiate treatment with intravenous antibiotics. Drainage of an infected sinus may also be required.

Eye injuries

Eye injuries account for about a third of all cases of blindness in children. Even apparently trivial injuries require prompt treatment. The history of how the injury was sustained is crucial as it gives clues to the type of injury and focuses the examination. A high velocity injury suggests that there may be a penetrating injury. Signs of a 'blow out' fracture should be sought if there has been a forceful blunt injury. There may be important medico-legal implications so the findings must be carefully documented. For all but the most trivial of eye injuries the child should be seen in the eye casualty department for a thorough examination of the eye.

Corneal abrasions

These cause acute pain and watering of the eye. It is mandatory to use fluorescein strips, otherwise abrasions will be missed. Padding the eye speeds healing and protects the eye. Chloramphenicol ointment prevents secondary infection, and pain can be relieved using cycloplegic drops (e.g. homatropine 2%) with oral analgesia if necessary. Minor abrasions heal promptly without complications.

Lacerations of the eyelid

These usually require specialist treatment, particularly if the lid margins have been torn or the lacrimal ducts have been damaged. There may be muscle involvement and an associated foreign body or penetrating injury to the eye.

Lacerations of the cornea and sclera

Large wounds may result in escape of vitreous and haemorrhage. Emergency treatment consists of padding the eye; this is followed by repair under general anaesthesia.

Penetrating injuries of the eye

These may be caused by high velocity injuries such as from using a hammer and chisel and also from objects such as darts, pencils and thorns. If there is any suspicion of a penetrating injury the child requires urgent referral to an eye casualty department where the eye should be examined very gently with no pressure to the globe. The signs of a penetrating injury can easily be missed because the injuries may seal themselves, producing very subtle signs. Signs of a penetrating injury include a distorted pupil, cataract and vitreous haemorrhage. Unless there is an associated head injury the pupil should be dilated and a thorough search made for an intra-ocular foreign body. An X-ray of the orbit may also help in identifying a foreign body. The main complication of penetrating wounds of the globe is sympathetic ophthalmia.

Foreign body

Small, loose conjunctival foreign bodies can be removed using the edge of a tissue or cotton wool bud, or they may be washed out with water.

Corneal foreign bodies are often more difficult to remove but metallic objects in particular must be removed as they will prevent healing and produce permanent staining of the cornea. Care must be taken not to damage the cornea when removing a foreign body: if there is any doubt the child should be referred to an eye casualty department. The symptoms are sudden pain associated with lacrimation and conjunctival congestion. Most foreign bodies can be located using a good light, but sometimes X-rays may be helpful in identifying radio-opaque foreign bodies.

RETINOBLASTOMA

About 30% of cases are bilateral and dominantly inherited; about 15% of unilateral tumours are inherited. Retinoblastoma usually presents with a white pupil (leukocoria) or the 'cat's eye reflex'. There is often a squint involving the affected eye. The tumour is not usually painful. Prompt ophthalmological referral is required followed by examination under anaesthesia and imaging. Depending on the staging of the disease, treatment includes photocoagulation, radiotherapy and chemotherapy. The families of children with retinoblastoma also require genetic counselling.

EARS

Congenital abnormalities

Low set ears

The ears are low set if the upper border of the ear is below a line drawn from the outer canthus of the eye to the external occipital protuberance. Low set ears are found in Down's and other syndromes.

Accessory auricles

These usually require excision by a plastic surgeon.

'Bat' ear

Abnormally protruding ears may cause a child to be the object of teasing by his peers and result in emotional problems. The deformity therefore should be corrected before the child starts school, i.e. about the age of 5 years. Pinnaplasty is simple and effective.

Microtia

Apart from the cosmetic problems, microtia may be associated with deafness. Microtia may also be part of a syndrome, e.g. Goldenhaar and Treacher–Collins.

Auricular pits and tags may indicate the presence of sensorineural or conductive deafness but are of no other significance.

OTITIS MEDIA

Acute otitis media

This is one of the most common diseases of childhood with peaks between 6 and 24 months and again on school entry. Most cases are primarily viral infections with secondary bacterial invasion.

Clinical features

The symptoms are often non-specific, particularly in younger children, with crying, fever, poor feeding and irritability. Older children complain of earache. It is important to examine the ears of any child with a febrile illness. The drum is dull, red, bulging, thickened and immobile. There may be a perforation of the drum.

Management

Analgesics and antipyretics should be given. Most doctors will administer antibiotics such as amoxycillin or trimethoprim directed towards the most common bacterial pathogens (*Strep. pneumoniae*, *Haemophilus influenzae* and group A streptococci) but a number of studies have failed to show a clear benefit for their use.

The ears should be re-examined two to three weeks after treatment and the hearing checked.

Glue ear (otitis media with effusion, serous otitis media, secretory otitis media)

The pathogenesis of glue ear is poorly understood but the basic pathology is accumulation of fluid secreted into the middle ear because of obstructed drainage and ventilation through the Eustachian tube.

Causative factors include recurrent upper respiratory tract infections (with or without treatment with antibiotics), atopy, air pollution (especially cigarette smoke) and institutional care (e.g. day nursery). Glue ear is very common in Down's syndrome and universal in cleft palate. It is asymptomatic apart from hearing impairment which often goes undetected. The tympanic membrane is dull, retracted and immobile with a bluish discolouration.

Impedance tympanometry is helpful in confirming the diagnosis, and audiometry can be used to demonstrate the hearing loss. Glue ear is very common and occurs in up to 30% of children in the pre-school period.

Treatment

This remains controversial as the natural history is one of eventual complete resolution in the vast majority of cases. A 3–6-week course of pro-

---

GP Overview 12.1 Earache (otalgia)

Causes—50% viral, 50% bacterial (*Streptococcus pneumoniae, Haemophilus influenzae*, group A β-haemolytic streptococcus, *Moraxella catarrhalis*)
- Otitis externa
- Otitis media
- Glue ear (secretory otitis media)

Complications
- Glue ear (secretory otitis media)
- Chronic suppurative otitis media
- Mastoiditis
- Intracranial abscess
- Meningitis
- Lateral venous sinus thrombosis

History
- Preceding URTI/nasal catarrh
- History of eczema for otitis externa

Examination
- Otitis media—red, bulging, non-reflective tympanic membrane
- Glue ear—dull, indrawn, non-reflective tympanic membrane

Investigations
- Otitis media—none
- Otitis externa—swab for bacteriology may be helpful (remember Candida)
- Glue ear—audiometry/tympanometry

Management
- Otitis externa—antibiotics (topical/oral) + anti-fungals
- Severe/resistant otitis externa—consider aural toilet
- Underlying eczema may respond to steroid drops
- Otitis media—oral antibiotics, e.g. amoxycillin, co-amoxiclav
- Glue ear—consider decongestants/antibiotics/grommets

N.B. Analgesia for pain relief is important

phylactic antibiotics (e.g. amoxicillin or trimetho-prim) may be helpful in preventing further infection and to allow the effusion to resolve. Decongestants (nasal or oral) are frequently used but are of unproven value. It is important to look for an underlying aggravating cause such as allergy, sinus disease or adenoidal hypertrophy. Glue ear commonly causes a mild to moderate hearing loss (40–50 dB). In most children this is intermittent and does not interfere with language and educational development. However, if hearing remains persistently impaired (longer than 2 months), there is a significant risk of language difficulties and myringotomy may be required. The tympanic membrane is incised and the gelatinous fluid is aspirated from the middle ear. This is usually accompanied by the insertion of grommets to allow re-aeration of the middle ear. Some ENT surgeons advise that a child with grommets may go swimming in shallow water but must not dive; others disagree or advise wearing commercial ear plugs or home-made ones made from cotton wool and Vaseline. Adenoid-ectomy may be performed at the same time as myringotomy to aid Eustachian tube function.

DEAFNESS

Mild deafness (hearing threshold 35–50 dB) is relatively common, affecting 13 out of every 1000 children. Moderate deafness (threshold 50–70 dB) and severe deafness (threshold greater than 70 dB) are much rarer, affecting 2 children and 1 child in 1000 respectively.

Parental concern about a child's hearing should always be taken seriously and a hearing test arranged.

Box 12.5 Causes of conductive deafness

- Acute otitis media
- Glue ear
- Middle ear malformation, e.g. Treacher–Collins syndrome
- Ossicular damage after head injury
- Otosclerosis—rare in children
- Wax—rare in children

Conductive deafness (Box 12.5)

The most common cause in children is glue ear. The diagnosis is made by finding a mild to moderate deafness on air conductors but a nor-mal threshold with bone conduction (Fig. 12.1A). Tympanometry shows a flat impedance curve which is diagnostic.

Sensorineural deafness (Box 12.6)

Diagnosis

Infants are routinely screened for hearing im-pairment (see p. 37).

Deafness is often first identified by parents (or grandparents) because of deficient hearing responses. These include lack of startle to sounds, sleeping through loud noise and failure to re-spond to everyday sounds such as telephones and doorbells. Parents' complaints must always

---

Box 12.6 Causes of sensorineural hearing loss

Genetically determined
Isolated
- Autosomal dominant or recessive
- X-linked

Part of a syndrome, e.g.
- Usher's (deafness with retinitis pigmentosa)
- Waardenburg's (deafness with white forelock)
- Pendred's (deafness with goitre)
- Alport's (deafness with progressive renal failure)
- Jervell–Lange–Neilsen (deafness with prolonged Q-T interval)

Inner ear malformations
- Abnormal cochlea
- Widened vestibular aqueduct

Craniofacial malformations
- Cleft palate
- Treacher–Collins syndrome
- Goldenhaar syndrome

Infections
- Intrauterine infections
- Meningitis
- Mumps
- Measles

Perinatal problems
- Perinatal asphyxia
- Hyperbilirubinaemia

Drugs
- Aminoglycosides

be taken very seriously. It is essential to remember that vocalisation and babbling in the first year of life do not exclude deafness. Any child with delayed language should have audiometry as part of the assessment.

Hearing tests

Hearing can be tested by various methods throughout life (Table 12.1).

Oto-acoustic emissions (OAEs) detect the 'cochlear echo', which is only present if the cochlea is functioning normally. The test requires co-operation and can be done on sleeping babies or older children who can keep quiet and still. OAEs cannot be done if there is middle ear dysfunction. The OAE equipment consists of an ear probe attached to a portable computer and can be easily operated. It has been used extensively in the neonatal period on high risk babies (Box 12.7). In the US, OAEs are used for universal screening, and this approach is being introduced in the UK.

Brainstem evoked responses (BSER)/auditory brainstem response (ABR) examine the electrical transmission of nerve impulses through the brainstem region between the cochlea and the cerebral cortex. The impulses are detected by simple electrodes that are stuck onto the surface of the head. There are five waves, which have characteristic amplitudes and latencies. Specific abnormalities indicate lesions at different levels of the auditory pathway. A BSER test can be done on a sleeping baby or co-operative older child but requires general anaesthesia in unco-operative children. It requires a high level of technical expertise and is used for diagnostic purposes in difficult cases or if a screening test such as the neonatal OAE was failed.

Table 12.1 Hearing tests

Method	Age
Oto-acoustic emissions	from 48 hours
Brainstem evoked response	from birth
Parent questionnaire	from birth
Distraction test	7–12 months
Co-operation (conditioning) test	2–4 years
Speech discrimination test	2½–4 years
Pure tone audiometry	from 3 years

Box 12.7 High risk factors for deafness
• Family history of childhood sensorineural deafness
• Intrauterine infection
• Birth weight < 1500 g
• Severe birth asphyxia
• Mechanical ventilation for > 10 days
• Craniofacial abnormalities, including external ear
• Severe hyperbilirubinaemia
• Ototoxic drugs (aminoglycoside antibiotics)
• Bacterial meningitis

Parent questionnaires (e.g. the McCormick checklist) can be given out by health visitors in order to structure parental observations. In some areas of the UK they are used to supplement or replace the distraction test.

The distraction test is only reliable if performed under good conditions by well trained personnel. If these ideals cannot be attained then an alternative technique should be considered. A better strategy is to use universal OAE testing in the neonatal period, and parental questionnaire and language surveillance in the second year of life with specific hearing tests in audiology centres for high risk children (Box 12.7).

Visual reinforcement audiometry (VRA) is a distraction test with additional visual rewards for a correct response. It is a useful clinical technique for children with learning difficulties or others (at any age) who cannot co-operate with usual tests.

Pure tone audiometry (PTA) is delivered by a machine (audiometer) which produces single tones of selected frequency and intensity. It can be performed in the Free Field to test hearing in both ears together but is better when delivered through headphones so that hearing in each ear can be evaluated separately. This test is possible from the age of 3 years and is performed by trained audiologists. PTA can distinguish between conductive and sensorineural deafness by administering sounds firstly through an ordinary headphone (air conduction) and then through a bone conductor (to bypass the middle ear). In conductive deafness bone conduction is normal but air conduction is impaired (air–bone gap) whereas in sensorineural deafness both audiograms are equally impaired (Figure 12.1).

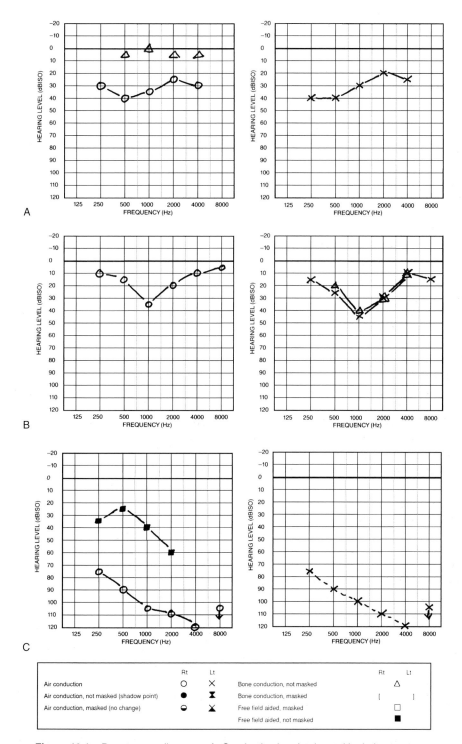

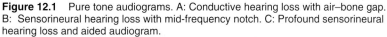

Figure 12.1 Pure tone audiograms. A: Conductive hearing loss with air–bone gap. B: Sensorineural hearing loss with mid-frequency notch. C: Profound sensorineural hearing loss and aided audiogram.

Management of sensorineural deafness

Accurate diagnosis is very important as management must be carefully individualised. Many paediatric audiology units have a standard protocol for the investigation of sensorineural deafness. This often includes full history, paediatric and ophthalmological examination, biochemistry and chromosome analysis. It is important to look for associated disorders such as renal disease. Imaging is becoming increasingly helpful and minute abnormalities of the inner ear (e.g. cochlear atresia, widened vestibular aqueduct) can be identified. Genetic abnormalities are responsible for around 50% of all cases of sensorineural deafness, and genetic counselling should be offered if no alternative diagnosis is made. In the absence of a specific diagnosis or family history, inheritance is usually autosomal recessive and, allowing for natural variance, a recurrence risk of 1 in 6 is quoted.

Hearing aids

Residual hearing is amplified using hearing aids. A wide range of powerful hearing aids is available and must be individually customised according to each patient's exact requirements by a specialist paediatric audiology unit. The aids can be frequency specific and modify sound input so that the user obtains maximal benefit. Two 'behind the ear' aids are usually best for children but other models include 'in the ear', body worn and bone conductors. They now come in various colours as not all children prefer skin coloured hearing aids.

Hearing aids cannot restore hearing input to normal. Despite their ability to select frequencies, background noise is also amplified and hearing aids are of limited benefit in noisy surroundings. This is often the situation in a classroom and teachers need careful guidance about how to manage deaf children. A radio aid worn by the child and a microphone worn by the teacher overcome the distance effect suffered by ordinary aids and enable the child and teacher to move about freely. Hearing aids should be fitted as soon as possible after identification of the hearing impairment.

Cochlear implants are increasingly being used in children with sensorineural deafness, particularly in circumstances where the hearing has been lost because of meningitis. These are inserted surgically into the cochlea and a surface electrode connects the microphone to a subcutaneous receiver. The results can be very good.

A teacher of the deaf is involved at an early stage to encourage the use of residual hearing, aid communication, maintain the hearing aids and advise the school teachers about appropriate strategies.

Deaf children should also start speech and language therapy as soon as possible in order to promote language development. There is much debate about the merits of signing versus the oral approach. The most important aspect however is the efficiency of total communication: a combination of methods is usually best.

Most children with useful residual hearing are integrated into mainstream schooling, often in special units for the hearing impaired in normal schools, but a minority need to attend a special school. Some children will require signing as their form of communication.

OTITIS EXTERNA

Pain in the ear is the main symptom, and is often preceded by itching. There may be a conductive hearing loss caused by soft tissue swelling and purulent secretions. On examination the canal is oedematous and inflamed with a greenish discharge. Treatment with topical antibacterial agents and topical corticosteroids produces rapid resolution.

NOSE

EPISTAXIS

Nose bleeds are common in childhood but rare in infancy and less common after puberty. They are usually caused by trauma such as picking the nose and foreign bodies. Hyperaemia of the nasal mucosa from an upper respiratory tract infection may predispose to nose bleeds. They

---

GP Overview 12.2 Epistaxis

Causes
- Idiopathic
- Infection in Little's area with associated nasopharyngitis
- Trauma
- Foreign body
- Bleeding disorder
- Allergy

GP tests
- Inspection of nares
- Nasal swab
- FBC, platelets, clotting screen (if coagulopathy suspected)

Hospital tests
- Endoscopic rhinoscopy

Management
- Firm pressure
- Nasal packing
- Cautery to Little's area
- Topical treatment of *Staph. aureus* infection
- Intranasal steroids/antihistamines for allergic rhinitis
- Sometimes needs blood transfusion

---

are also associated with enlarged adenoids, rhinitis and polyps. Profuse epistaxes may occur with bleeding disorders and thrombocytopenia.

Treatment

Minor epistaxes usually require no treatment, but if bleeding continues the nostrils should be compressed with the child in an upright position with the head tilted forwards. Topical adrenaline and thrombin followed by packing may be required if the bleeding persists.

RHINITIS
Viral rhinitis

The most common cause of rhinorrhoea is the common cold. In older children a persistent nasal discharge associated with fever, pain and frontal headache suggests acute sinusitis. Although antibiotic treatment is traditional, there is little objective evidence that this produces a more rapid resolution of the symptoms than symptomatic treatment with analgesics.

Allergic rhinitis

Allergic rhinitis is very common: its incidence increases from around 10% in children to about 20% in young adults. 75% of children with asthma also suffer from rhinitis. Seasonal allergic rhinitis is less common under the age of 5 years. Glue ear often results from blockage of the Eustachian tube.

The timing of the symptoms gives a useful clue to the likely offending allergen. Symptoms in the early spring suggest tree pollen allergy, grass pollen allergy occurs between May and July, and allergy to moulds and spores produces symptoms in the autumn. Exposure to animal danders, feathers and dust may sometimes produce acute symptoms. There is little evidence that any foods are a common cause of rhinitis.

Exposure to the allergen produces sneezing, profuse watery rhinorrhoea, itching of the nose and palate and watering of the eyes.

Sensitivity to an allergen may be confirmed by skin testing specific IgE antibodies or nasal provocation testing. Treatment consists of allergen avoidance, if possible; non-sedating antihistamines are also helpful, together with topical (nasal) steroids. Hyposensitisation is no longer recommended because of the risk of provoking an anaphylactic reaction.

Chronic rhinitis

In perennial allergic rhinitis the patient is symptomatic throughout the year. It is usually caused by allergens to which the patient is continually exposed, such as house dust and the house dust mite. Feathers and animal danders may also produce chronic rhinitis, and mould spores may be the cause in some children. The clinical features, investigations and treatment are essentially as for acute allergic rhinitis but allergen avoidance often proves to be impractical; reasonable attempts should be made, however, to reduce concentrations of house dust mite in the home (see p. 129).

Hay fever (grass pollen allergy)

Treatment with antihistamines should be started before the anticipated rise in the grass pollen count, i.e. at the beginning of May, and can usually be stopped at the beginning of August. The symptoms can also be controlled by the use of topical corticosteroids, drops or sprays or sodium cromoglycate. Occasionally, for severe symptoms interfering with examination performance, etc., a short course of prednisolone may be indicated.

UPPER RESPIRATORY TRACT INFECTION (URTI)

Children under 5 in the United Kingdom contract around 3–6 upper respiratory infections per year. These are usually viral infections: rhinoviruses, adenoviruses and parainfluenza viruses are among the most common agents. URTIs tend to occur most commonly in winter and their frequency is influenced by the number of contacts within and outside the family that a child may have. Thus a firstborn child may be relatively spared these infections until entering school whereas the youngest infant in a large family tends to contract them early in life. Both situations may give rise to concern to a parent anxious that the child is getting an excessive number of infections. The infections are characterised by moderate fever, rhinitis, pharyngitis, cough and, in the younger child, diarrhoea. The illness is self-limiting, lasting 3–4 days. In a small infant that is predominantly milk fed, feeding may be made difficult by a blocked nose. This may be treated with saline or short-term 0.5% ephedrine nose drops.

NASAL POLYPS

Nasal polyps are uncommon in children, but up to 10% of children with cystic fibrosis develop polyps. They present with obstruction of the nasal airway, often with a profuse nasal discharge. They need to be distinguished from the turbinates; these appear pink or red whereas polyps are grey, grape-like structures between the turbinates and the septum.

Cystic fibrosis needs to be excluded. Treatment of polyps is by surgical excision.

INDICATIONS FOR ADENOIDECTOMY

Infection of the adenoids resulting in enlargement occurs mainly in pre-school children. Mouth breathing and persistent rhinitis are the main symptoms. The hypertrophied adenoids may also interfere with drainage of the Eustachian tube, leading to glue ear.

The symptoms produced by enlarged adenoids are very similar to those of rhinitis. A trial of treatment with nasal steroids may therefore avoid the need for surgery. There is some evidence that adenoidectomy may improve Eustachian tube function and relieve catarrhal symptoms but surgery requires general anaesthesia and hospitalisation and the benefits are disputed.

Adenoidectomy may be undertaken for persistent nasal obstruction and is often combined with insertion of grommets. It is important that a child with a cleft palate or submucous cleft (often associated with a bifid uvula) should not have adenoidectomy because of the risk of aggravating nasal speech caused by pharyngo-palatal incompetence when the splinting effect of the adenoids is lost.

SLEEP APNOEA

Enlargement of the tonsils and adenoids may result in severe upper airway obstruction which is particularly marked during REM sleep. Symptoms of obstructive sleep apnoea (Box 12.8) are generally worse during upper respiratory tract infections. Sleep apnoea from adeno-tonsillar hypertrophy usually occurs in children between 1 and 3 years old.

The diagnosis can be confirmed by pulse oximetry during sleep, when the episodes of apnoea are associated with desaturation. Adeno-

---

Box 12.8 Symptoms of sleep apnoea

- Snoring
- Episodes of stopping breathing
- Restlessness
- Disturbed sleep with frequent waking
- Mouth breathing
- Tiredness during the day

tonsillectomy in this group of children results in immediate resolution of the upper airway obstruction, together with an improvement in the child's general health, energy levels, appetite and growth.

THROAT

PHARYNGITIS

Pharyngitis is often associated with other features of URTI such as a fever and nasal discharge. The child may sometimes complain of dysphagia and there may be a painful barking cough. Clinically it is impossible to distinguish a viral pharyngitis from a streptococcal sore throat. Symptomatic treatment with anti-pyretics is usually all that is required.

TONSILLITIS

Infection of the tonsils, like the adenoids, occurs particularly in younger children in the 3–8-year age group. It presents with fever, sore throat, minor constitutional upset and occasionally vomiting. The tonsils appear enlarged and inflamed, sometimes with exudate and haemorrhages. There is often associated enlargement of the cervical lymph nodes. Approximately 90% of cases are viral in origin. The most common bacterial cause is the β-haemolytic streptococcus. Glandular fever may present with tonsillitis; diphtheria remains endemic in parts of the former USSR.

Treatment remains controversial: adequate fluid intake and an anti-pyretic analgesic is probably sufficient. If a streptococcal infection is suspected the child should be treated with oral penicillin, or with erythromycin if there is a history of penicillin allergy. Complications of bacterial tonsillitis are rare; immediate complications include peritonsillar abscess and acute cervical adenitis. Late complications of streptococcal infection include rheumatic fever and acute glomerulonephritis.

Quinsy

Peritonsillar abscess is uncommon in childhood; nearly all cases are caused by the group A β-haemolytic streptococcus. Following an attack of tonsillitis the child develops a severe sore throat associated with difficulty in opening the mouth, often resulting in a refusal to swallow or speak. The child is often toxic and unwell with a high fever. The affected tonsillar area is very swollen and inflamed with displacement of the uvula to the opposite side. Treatment with penicillin at an early stage may halt the progression of the abscess but incision is indicated once it has become fluctuant. Further attacks should be prevented by tonsillectomy three or four weeks after the abscess has resolved.

Indications for tonsillectomy

Tonsillitis reaches a peak when children start at playgroup or nursery, falling to adult levels by the age of 7–8 years. The tonsils form an important part of the first line of defence against URTIs and it is therefore somewhat illogical to

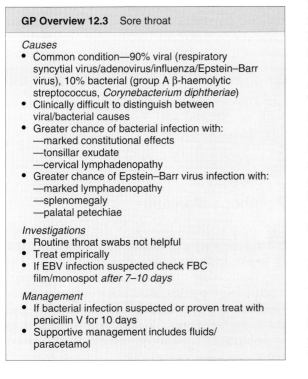

GP Overview 12.3   Sore throat

Causes
- Common condition—90% viral (respiratory syncytial virus/adenovirus/influenza/Epstein–Barr virus), 10% bacterial (group A β-haemolytic streptococcus, *Corynebacterium diphtheriae*)
- Clinically difficult to distinguish between viral/bacterial causes
- Greater chance of bacterial infection with:
  —marked constitutional effects
  —tonsillar exudate
  —cervical lymphadenopathy
- Greater chance of Epstein–Barr virus infection with:
  —marked lymphadenopathy
  —splenomegaly
  —palatal petechiae

Investigations
- Routine throat swabs not helpful
- Treat empirically
- If EBV infection suspected check FBC film/monospot *after 7–10 days*

Management
- If bacterial infection suspected or proven treat with penicillin V for 10 days
- Supportive management includes fluids/paracetamol

remove them merely because they have become inflamed. Occasionally recurrent tonsillitis may interfere with growth and weight gain, in which case tonsillectomy is indicated. Other indications include sleep apnoea (combined with adenoid-ectomy), peritonsillar abscess (see above), recurrent cervical adenitis and suspected tonsillar tumour. The presence of large, asymptomatic tonsils is not an indication for tonsillectomy and neither is parental pressure on the doctor.

MOUTH

CONGENITAL ABNORMALITIES
Cleft lip/palate

Cleft lip and palate occur in about 1 in 600 births. About a third of cases involve the palate only.

Aetiology/genetics

The clefts result from failure of fusion of the facial processes; this usually occurs between the 5th and 12th weeks of pregnancy. Clefts vary in severity from a notch in the upper lip or bifid uvula to bilateral clefts of the lip and palate. A bifid uvula is often associated with a submucous cleft. The cleft palate associated with the Pierre Robin syndrome is a direct consequence of under-development of the mandible, with the tongue being pushed up and preventing fusion of the palate.

There is a family history of a cleft in about a third of patients. If one sibling is affected the risk in a subsequent sibling is approximately 1 in 25, rising to 1 in 8 if a parent also had a cleft. Midline clefts are uncommon but are important as they may be associated with other midline defects, including absence of the posterior pituitary gland and corpus callosum. Repair of the lip is usually delayed until around 3 months of age, and is followed by closure of the palatal defect at around a year. Parents of children with cleft lip and palate require sympathetic counselling. Photographs of children with cleft lip before and after surgery are very helpful.

Associated problems

Feeding. An isolated cleft lip with an intact palate should not cause any feeding problems. Sucking is not possible with palatal defects except with modified teats. A few babies, particularly pre-term babies, with a cleft may require tube feeding.

Speech. Speech usually develops without any major problems after satisfactory closure of a cleft palate, and any minor speech defects can be improved by speech therapy. Cleft palate is frequently associated with Eustachian tube dysfunction, with resultant middle ear infections and hearing impairment which may lead to further speech problems. It is therefore essential that a child with a cleft palate receives regular audiological and ENT supervision. Involvement of the orthodontist is also important to correct any incisor malocclusion.

Tongue tie

A short lingual frenum causes anxiety in parents and grandparents, particularly in the belief that it may interfere with language development. In practice, tongue tie rarely gives rise to any speech or feeding difficulties but, in cases where there is doubt, assessment by a speech therapist may be helpful in assessing tongue function towards the end of the second year of life. If tongue movement is so restricted as to cause problems with speech and oral hygiene, division of the frenum is a simple surgical procedure.

STOMATITIS
Aphthous stomatitis

Recurrent painful ulcers of the oral mucous membranes are common. There may be single or multiple lesions involving the mucosa. The lesions usually resolve within 10–14 days. Aphthous stomatitis often has a cyclical presentation. It is not caused by herpes simplex and may have an immunological basis. Treatment is symptomatic. Topical corticosteroids may speed the resolution of the lesions.

Herpetic stomatitis

Acute herpetic gingivostomatitis

This affects children between 1 and 3 years of age. It presents with a high fever and irritability followed by reluctance to eat or drink. The mouth becomes swollen and red with white plaques or shallow ulcers involving the buccal mucosa, lips, tongue, palate and fauces. There may also be satellite lesions around the mouth and on the anterior chest wall caused by drooling saliva. There is often associated cervical lymphadenopathy. The acute phase of the illness lasts 4–9 days. Treatment with aciclovir has been shown to shorten the course of the illness and should be started at presentation. There may be super-added bacterial infection with *Staphylococcus aureus* or streptococcus requiring additional antibiotic therapy. During the acute phase of the illness children may require intravenous fluids and analgesics.

Recurrent stomatitis

70–90% of adults have antibodies to the herpes simplex virus. The virus frequently remains latent and produces recurrent clinical symptoms, particularly in association with a febrile illness. Cold sores usually involve the lips, together with the adjacent mucosa. Treatment with topical aciclovir speeds the resolution of the lesions.

EMERGENCIES

MAJOR INJURY

The most common causes of multiple trauma are road traffic accidents and falls. The 'ABC' of resuscitation should be followed.

At the scene

1. Airway

- Check that the mouth, nose and pharynx are clear.
- If necessary, open the mouth carefully (try not to move the neck in case of cervical spine damage) and remove any obstruction manually, with forceps or by suction.
- If equipment is available, insert an oropharyngeal airway or intubate.
- If an oral airway is impossible, perform tracheostomy.

2. Breathing

- Give 100% O_2 if available.
- Assess the adequacy of respiration by observing chest movement and listening for air entry with a stethoscope.
- Pneumothorax is diagnosed clinically by unilateral reduction of air entry, hyper-resonance on percussion and asymmetrical trachea. This emergency should be treated by urgent insertion of a chest drain through the second intercostal space in the mid-clavicular line on the affected side.
- Flail chest from multiple rib fractures prevents active chest wall movement. Positive pressure ventilation is required.

3. Circulation

- Control haemorrhage by pressure.
- Monitor heart rate, blood pressure, skin colour and capillary filling after blanching.
- Establish venous access, preferably with two lines.
- Take blood for group and cross matching and baseline haematology and biochemistry.

- If venous access is impossible, interosseous infusion by syringe into a tibia is a good alternative.
- Infuse crystalloid (e.g. normal saline) or artificial colloid fluid at an initial rate of 20 ml/kg.

In hospital

The child must be transferred as quickly as possible after stabilisation by a paramedical transport team. In hospital the 'ABC' procedure will be repeated and, if necessary, more sophisticated support treatment administered.

- Respiration—mechanical ventilation.
- Shock—low blood pressure arising from severe hypovolaemia from haemorrhage is treated with blood transfusion. Inotropic drugs, e.g. dopamine, dobutamine, improve blood flow and cardiac output.
- Metabolic acidosis can be corrected with sodium bicarbonate.
- Examination for injuries, e.g. head, chest, abdomen, bones.

A surgical opinion must be obtained if there are penetrating injuries, abdominal signs or evidence of internal haemorrhage.

DROWNING

High risk places

- Poorly supervised swimming pools, ponds, rivers, etc.
- Infants can drown in a bath.

Pathological effects

1. Hypothermia
2. Hypoxia.

The 'diving reflex' is weakly present in infants and young children and gives some protection by selective vasoconstriction diverting blood to the brain and heart.

Management

1. Immediate

- Asystole occurs in severe hypothermia. Ventricular fibrillation is more likely to occur during the warming up phase.

- Respiratory arrest—artificial ventilation with 100% O_2 if available (beware cervical spine injury after a diving accident).
- Transfer urgently to hospital.

2. In hospital

- Monitor core body temperature with a low reading thermometer.
- If body temperature is > 30°C, passive or gentle external warming is sufficient.
- If temperature is < 30°C the patient can be warmed by gastric, rectal or peritoneal lavage or intravenous infusion with carefully warmed fluids.
- Give O_2.
- Monitor ECG and perform chest X-ray.

BURNS

Most burns and scalds occur at home. Health education about the dangers of fire, heaters, kettles, cookers, hot drinks, etc. should be given to parents at every appropriate opportunity. The severity of a burn depends upon the degree of heat and the duration of exposure.

First aid

- Pour cold water onto the burned area immediately for several minutes. This rapidly reduces the temperature.
- Do *not* apply any cream or ointment.
- Cover with clean non-adherent material.
- Transfer to hospital unless the burn is trivial.

In hospital

Examination

- Area—assess using standard charts.
- Thickness:
  — superficial: unbroken red skin
  — partial thickness: epidermis burned off but dermis intact; blisters usually appear.
  — full thickness: dermis burned through;

nerve endings destroyed so burned area is anaesthetic.

Management

- Pain relief—most burns are very painful and require morphine, preferably intravenously.
- Paracetamol may be sufficient for minor burns.
- Fluid replacement should be given intravenously for burns covering more than 10% of the body area. In the first 4 hours, plasma or artificial colloid should be given according to the formula:

$$\text{Volume (ml)} = \frac{\% \text{ burn} \times \text{weight (kg)}}{2}$$

Follow this with maintenance fluids at 25 ml/ kg using normal or dextrose saline and monitor electrolytes, urine output and cardiovascular status.
- Prevent infection—the burn will have sterilised the skin and this sterile state should be maintained.
- Secondary infection must be treated vigorously with topical and systemic antibiotics.
- Transfer to a specialised burns unit in the following circumstances:
  — burns covering more than 10% body area
  — full thickness burns as these will probably require skin grafting
  — burns to the face, hands, feet or perineum
  — electrical burns.

POISONING

Accidental poisoning occurs most commonly in young children aged 1–4 years. Intentional self-poisoning occurs with increasing frequency in older children, particularly girls. The diagnosis is usually obvious, although children may present with impaired consciousness or abnormal behaviour without a clear history of ingestion.

Management

The principles of the ABC of resuscitation should be followed if the child has an impaired level of consciousness. If there is respiratory insufficiency the child may require endotracheal intubation and mechanical ventilation. The child's general condition should be assessed and the level of consciousness monitored using the AVPU scale (Alert, responds to Voice, responds to Pain, Unresponsive) together with pupillary responses.

Attempts should be made to identify what poison has been ingested, when the poison was ingested and how much has been ingested. The MIMS colour identification chart is helpful in identifying drugs. The parents may know how many tablets were in the bottle as a guide to how much has been ingested.

Poisons information services located around the country provide advice on all aspects of poisoning, day or night. The telephone numbers are listed in the British National Formulary.

Activated charcoal

Activated charcoal reduces the absorption of poisons through binding and enhances elimination if given within 1–2 hours of the ingestion. It is widely used in cases of poisoning but will not absorb some substances, including iron and alcohol. Repeated doses of activated charcoal are required to interrupt entero-hepatic cycling of poisons such as aspirin, theophylline and barbiturates. The dose of activated charcoal is 1 g/kg. Aspirated charcoal produces a severe pneumonitis which can be avoided by protection of the airway in the child with a depressed level of consciousness.

Emesis

Although traditionally vomiting has been induced using ipecacuanha syrup 15 ml with water, there is evidence that little of the poison will be eliminated unless emesis occurs within 1 hour of ingestion of the poison. A few drugs, such as salicylates, slow gastric emptying and therefore emesis or gastric lavage may be effective for up to 4–6 hours after ingestion. No attempt should be made to induce vomiting for corrosive or volatile substances such as petrol or paraffin and in general there is little, if anything,

to be gained by inducing emesis for poisons which are bound by charcoal. Haemodialysis and haemoperfusion are very rarely needed.

Even when there are no apparent ill effects from the ingestion, the child should be observed in hospital for 6 hours. The child should always be admitted if symptomatic or after ingestion of iron, tricyclic antidepressants, aspirin or paracetamol. Blood, urine and gastric contents should be obtained for drug identification and medicolegal purposes in any child with suspected poisoning.

Specific poisons

Paracetamol

Young children rarely swallow enough paracetamol elixir for it to be dangerous but older children frequently self-poison with paracetamol. The main danger is hepatic necrosis. There are usually no clinical features apart from vomiting on the day of ingestion. Subsequently there may be abdominal pain and features of hepatic failure on days 2–7.

Oral charcoal should be given; a paracetamol level should be measured at 4 hours after ingestion and up to 15 hours to identify patients at risk of liver damage.

Liver function tests and prothrombin time should be measured in all patients requiring treatment. If the level is below the toxic line no treatment is required but if it is above the line the child is at risk of hepatic toxicity and should be treated with intravenous acetylcysteine, which is effective up to 48 hours after ingestion. Oral methionine can also be used but is less effective than acetylcysteine. Advice should be obtained from the National Poisons Information Service if there is any doubt about whether the child should be treated.

Aspirin

Aspirin poisoning has become much less common in children as salicylates are no longer recommended for children under the age of 12 years because of the risk of Reye's syndrome. Clinical features include nausea, vomiting, epigastric pain, fever, sweating, sighing respirations and dehydration.

Aspirin causes delayed gastric emptying; ipecac or gastric lavage can therefore be used up to 4 hours after ingestion. Repeated doses of activated charcoal should be given to patients who have ingested a sustained release preparation. The plasma salicylate level should be measured, initially at 2 hours after ingestion, together with the urea and electrolytes and blood sugar, but repeated 2-hourly measurements should be obtained until they start to decline. The peak salicylate level usually occurs at around 6 hours.

The arterial blood gases should also be measured if the child is acutely ill or has impaired consciousness. Children who are symptomatic or whose salicylate levels are greater than 250 mg/l should be admitted for observation. Treatment is required if the salicylate level exceeds 300 mg/l, particularly in children under the age of 2 years. An intravenous infusion of dextrose saline with added potassium chloride should be started. Alkalisation of the plasma and urine with bicarbonate (sodium bicarbonate 1 mmol/kg infused over 4 hours) improves excretion of salicylate. Haemodialysis may be required if the serum levels exceed 700 mg/l or if there is renal failure or pulmonary oedema.

Tricyclic antidepressants

Clinical features of poisoning occur soon after ingestion because of rapid absorption. Central nervous system clinical features include restlessness, hallucination and seizures followed by depressed consciousness and coma. Respiratory depression is common. Cardiovascular effects include hypotension and arrhythmias, which may be fatal. Activated charcoal should be administered. The child should always be admitted for close monitoring, including ECG monitoring. Alkalisation using a sodium bicarbonate infusion (1 mmol/kg) reduces the available free drug and reduces the toxic effects on the heart. Phenytoin is the drug of choice for treating arrhythmias (15 mg/kg over 15–30 minutes).

Emesis is worth attempting up to 8 hours after ingestion, provided that the child is fully conscious, followed by activated charcoal. The child should always be admitted for close monitoring, including ECG monitoring. Hypoxia, acidosis and hypovolaemia may all potentiate arrhythmias. A pressor agent such as dopamine may be required, together with specific treatment of cardiac arrhythmias.

Corrosive agents

Many poisonous agents, such as caustic alkalis, paint remover, drain cleaner and bleach, are common in the home. Effects of ingestion include damage to the lips, mouth and oesophagus. Emesis and gastric lavage are contraindicated. The child should be encouraged to drink milk.

Alcohol

Alcohol is often accessible in the home; additionally there is an increasing problem of underage drinking affecting children as young as 11 years. Features include ataxia, dysarthria, nystagmus and drowsiness which may progress to coma with hypotension and acidosis. Hypoglycaemia is a particular hazard in children and may be severe and life-threatening. For this reason, children with alcohol poisoning should be referred for possible hospital admission.

Emesis should be induced if the child is fully conscious. The blood alcohol level should be measured, together with regular monitoring of the blood glucose until the child has regained consciousness. If consciousness is impaired the child should be given an intravenous infusion of 10% dextrose.

Prevention

There is still a need to educate parents about the risks and dangers of accidental poisoning in young children. There is a clear link between accidental poisoning and family psychosocial stress but unfortunately families under stress are unlikely to remember safety propaganda.

Child resistant containers have been associated

with a fall in the incidence of accidental drug ingestion. A number of potentially toxic household products such as white spirit and bleach are also now sold in child resistant containers. Unfortunately no child resistant container is completely childproof and it is therefore important that parents store any potentially toxic substance out of the reach of young children.

FURTHER READING

Colton R T, Myer C M III eds 1999 Practical pediatric otolaryngology. Lippincott-Raven, Philadelphia
Froom J, Culpepper L, Jacobs M et al 1997 Antimicrobials for acute otitis media? British Medical Journal 315: 98–101
Khaw PT, Elkington AR 1994 ABC of eyes, 2nd edn. BMJ Publishing Group, London
Northern J L, Downs M P 1991 Hearing in children, 4th edn. Williams and Wilkins, Baltimore
O'Donoghue GM, Bates GJ, Narula AA 1992 Clinical ENT and illustrated textbook. Oxford University Press, Oxford
The British National Formulary. British Medical Association and Royal Pharmaceutical Society of Great Britain, London

Internet addresses

ENT disorders
http://icarus.med.utoronto.ca/carr/manual/outline.html

Poisoning
http://www.peds.umn.edu/divisions/pccm/teaching/acp/poison.html

CHAPTER CONTENTS

13

Haematology, oncology and immunology

Anthony Robinson

HAEMATOLOGY

INTRODUCTION

Haemoglobin is an iron-containing protein, essential for transferring oxygen to tissues. It is manufactured in the bone marrow in adults and children but there may be extra-medullary sites in liver and spleen if the rate of loss exceeds production. Its concentration is high at birth and falls at about 4 months as placentally transferred iron is used up. At this age iron-containing foods are essential to maintain normal values. Although iron is well absorbed from breast milk this eventually diminishes. Absorption from cow's milk is only one fifth that of human milk. Formula milk is supplemented with iron and therefore, from this perspective, provides satisfactory nutrition.

Normal haemoglobin values, dependent on the number of red cells, vary in the first year, but thereafter 11 g/dl is accepted as normal.

The **haematocrit** (HCT) also depends on the number of red cells and is calculated from the mean corpuscular volume (MCV) and red blood cell (RBC) count. The MCV, dependent on the size of the red cells and the red cell dispersion width (RDW), provides information about cell size variability which may be undetected by simply visualising the blood film.

The mean corpuscular haemoglobin (MCH) and its concentration (MCHC) provide information about the quantity of iron in the red cells.

Ferritin is an iron storage protein and may be

low if the child's iron is largely deposited in haemoglobin. It is usually at the lower range of adult normal and may be difficult to increase.

Reticulocytes are detected by staining their high RNA content. They live for only one day and reflect red cell production.

Dietary iron deficiency is the most common abnormality found by measuring the above indices but iron deficiency anaemia may be the initial finding in coeliac and chronic inflammatory bowel disease.

THE ANAEMIAS

Iron deficiency

Skin pallor is an unreliable sign of iron deficiency anaemia unless the haemoglobin is under 6–9 g/dl. Koilonychia in children is usually familial. However, diminished learning skills and some behavioural problems, e.g. tiredness, poor appetite, pica and breath holding, have been shown to relate to low haemoglobin values.

The prevalence of iron deficiency anaemia in the UK ranges from 12–40% of 1–2-year-olds if deprived populations are included.

Screening is not universally acceptable but it was found that, after counselling, parents strongly approved of it at the time of MMR immunisation if haemoglobinopathy tests were also included. The accuracy of 'field equipment' is questioned, however, and use of the haemoglobin value alone will underestimate the true incidence of iron deficiency. Additional tests such as ferritin, red cell protoporphyrins and transferrin are expensive and compound the difficulties by not being instantly available.

Iron deficiency is frequently discovered only by direct measurement, though clues to its existence may be present when the history is that s/he 'won't eat', or s/he will 'only drink milk or juice, or eat biscuits'. If iron deficiency is found, blood loss should be considered (Table 13.1); Helicobacter peptic ulceration as well as traditional causes, e.g. nose bleeds, Meckel's diverticulum and polyps, should be excluded. Splenomegaly may be clinically detectable in about 10% of cases, and systolic flow murmurs are frequent.

Treatment consists of correction of the blood

Table 13.1 Typical indices

Iron deficiency anaemia	Anaemia of inflammation and chronic disease
Hb < 10.5 g/dl	Hb 6–9 g/dl
MCV microcytic	normocytic
MCH hypochromic	normochromic
Ferritin low	may be raised

loss, if present, and replenishment of the body's iron stores. This may take several months with iron medication or much longer by improved diet. Recommended iron-containing foods are red meat, poultry, sardines, eggs, pulses (peas, beans, lentils), iron-fortified cereals and breads, and sesame seed paste (tahini). These should be taken with vitamin C, e.g. orange juice, to convert ferrous to ferric iron and thereby improve absorption, which is impaired by tannin in tea.

Iron therapy with 5 mg/kg of elemental iron will be required until the diet improves. A 6-week course at a minimum is needed to replete the iron stores. Several liquid preparations of iron are available such as Plesmet (1 ml/kg/day) or Sytron (1 ml/kg/day).

The anaemia of inflammation and chronic disease

This anaemia is widely prevalent; whilst juvenile chronic arthritis provides a typical model, it is more frequently seen in association with acute infectious states such as upper respiratory tract infections, diarrhoea, orbital cellulitis, septic arthritis, meningitis (especially *Haemophilus influenzae* type B) and Mycoplasma infection. It is also seen in other chronic conditions, e.g. cystic fibrosis, inflammatory bowel disease and malignancy.

This anaemia is the consequence of decreased red cell survival, impaired release of stored iron and decreased erythropoietin production, resulting in depressed bone marrow response.

Treatment is to address the infective cause; blood transfusion may be considered.

The thalassaemias

In these anaemias the globin moeity of haemoglobin is defective; haemolysis may occur, depending on the degree and type of abnormality. These anaemias are most frequently found in those of Asian, Mediterranean and African descent.

Of the varieties likely to be encountered, α thalassaemias are more common than β thalassaemias, while haemoglobin E variants have a world-wide distribution and are even more common and second only to haemoglobin S variants. There may be co-existent iron deficiency.

Haemoglobin A (adult type) contains two α and two β chains ($\alpha_2\beta_2$). Defects of these chains cause reduced numbers of microcytic cells to be produced, and the defective red cells are then haemolysed. α chain synthesis requires 4 genes on chromosome 16 ($\alpha\alpha/\alpha\alpha$).

- The carrier state lacks one gene ($-\alpha/\alpha\alpha$) and is asymptomatic.
- α thalassaemia trait lacks 2 genes ($--/\alpha\alpha$) and produces mild anaemia with microcytes.
- HbH disease lacks 3 genes ($--/-\alpha$) with microcytes, hypochromia and raised Hb Barts.
- Homozygous α thalassaemia ($--/--$) is incompatible with life.

β chain synthesis requires two genes, one on each chromosome 11. β thalassaemia **trait** is caused by inheriting one defective gene and **homozygous** β thalassaemia is caused by inheriting two defective genes.

Clinical features

Frank haemolytic anaemia occurs from about 6 months of age when adult haemoglobin (HbA) begins to be formed. It presents with tiredness, diminished exercise tolerance, growth delay and lethargy. Microcytosis and hypochromia are severe, reticulocytes are reduced, nucleated RBCs are present, there is hyper-unconjugated bilirubinaemia and the HbA2 and HbF are raised. Extramedullary haematopoiesis causes enlargement of liver and spleen, and an increase of bone marrow space is seen clinically in the face.

Management

Blood transfusions are required approximately every month to maintain the haemoglobin level at around 10 g/dl. The donated iron will accumulate in the heart, adrenals and pancreas if it is not removed by chelation. Desferrioxamine is infused subcutaneously overnight, vitamin C promotes iron excretion, and folic acid is also given. Bone marrow transplantation may be very successful.

The serum ferritin is measured frequently and the patient regularly screened for hepatitis B. Pneumococcal vaccine is given if hypersplenism requires splenectomy.

The haemoglobin E variant which occurs in South East Asia may be protective against malaria and is asymptomatic in its pure heterozygous and homozygous state, however it may be doubly heterozygous with β thalassaemia and clinically result in a syndrome resembling homozygous β thalassaemia.

Sickle cell disorders

A simple modification of the β chain of haemoglobin (replacement of valine for glutamic acid) results in deformity of the red cell so that it assumes the shape of a sickle under conditions of deoxygenation. Dehydration and cold are also triggers.

The defective gene can co-exist with other genes, e.g. β thalassaemia or HbC, and produce clinically important disorders.

Clinical features

In the heterozygous state (HbAS) the sickle gene is benign and confers protection against malaria. Low oxygen levels in high flying unpressurised aircraft may produce symptoms seen in the homozygous state.

True sickle cell disease, homozygosity for the HbS gene (HbSS), shortens the life span of red cells with persistent haemolytic anaemia, mild jaundice, gallstones, aplastic bone marrow crises and sequestration crises. Short stature and delayed puberty are also common.

Vaso-occlusive crises cause considerable pain of muscles and abdominal organs but occur more commonly in the fingers, which also swell. The most serious painful crises are those of cerebro-vascular occlusion when resulting stroke can be devastating. Priapism, chest and kidney ischaemia and bone necrosis may also occur.

Clinically the spleen is at first enlarged and then shrinks because of infarction. When this happens immunisation against *H. influenzae*, Pneumococcus and Meningococcus should be given. Lifelong oral penicillin is required and folate supplements are also given.

Management

Treatment consists of the provision of adequate hydration, analgesia and appropriate antibiotics for febrile episodes. Opinion is divided on the value of exchange transfusion but it is recommended for priapism; blood transfusion should be given for aplastic and acute neurological crises. Following stroke syndrome, repeat transfusions are given to suppress bone marrow production of HbS to 30% and thereby reduce the risk of recurrence to 10%.

Hypoxia can cause sickling, even in patients with the trait. Homozygous patients are therefore simply transfused before a short operation, but for operations longer than 15 minutes blood viscosity is reduced by exchange transfusion in order to produce approximately half HbA and half HbS. Oxygen is administered preoperatively and antibiotic cover is also given.

Bone marrow transplantation is curative if successful but is usually reserved for children with severe symptoms because of the uncertain and sometimes benign course of the natural disease.

Megaloblastic anaemias

Folic acid deficiency occurs when absorption from the small intestine is impaired as in coeliac disease or chronic inflammatory bowel disease. It also occurs in states of chronic haemolysis (e.g. sickle cell disease) but replacement is unnecessary if the dietary intake is adequate. Other causes include prematurity and drug therapy, e.g. phenytoin.

Dietary vitamin B$_{12}$ deficiency is uncommon in children but may be seen if no dairy or animal products are eaten. Treatment is with oral B$_{12}$.

A macrocytic anaemia can occur in the juvenile form of pernicious anaemia when gastric intrinsic factor is not produced in the presence of normal gastric acid. The symptoms are the same as in adults (irritability, listlessness, anorexia) but only occur when transplacental stores are exhausted at about 4 years. Treatment is with parenteral B$_{12}$.

HAEMOLYTIC STATES OTHER THAN DEFECTS OF HAEMOGLOBIN
(see also p. 58)

Red cell enzyme deficiencies

Glucose-6-phosphate dehydrogenase deficiency

G6PD deficiency impairs chemical reduction of glutathione which would otherwise protect red cells from oxidant induced haemolysis. There are two types:

- acute, induced by infection and, less frequently, by drugs
- chronic non-spherocytic haemolytic anaemia (rare).

There are about 100 enzyme variants, and a large number of abnormal alleles are found on the X chromosome. Homozygous females can be as seriously affected as males, and when the X chromosome is randomly inactivated (Lyon hypothesis) the heterozygotes have intermediate enzyme activity.

G6PD is the most common enzyme deficiency and variably affects Mediterranean, Middle East, African and Oriental populations. The first symptom is neonatal jaundice; world-wide, G6PD deficiency is the most common reason for exchange transfusion and kernicterus if treatment is delayed.

Haemolysis does not occur until 2–4 days after exposure to a precipitant, and the haemoglobin may fall to 2 g/dl. The diagnosis depends on demonstrating reduced G6PD activity, but results may be misleadingly normal or high during an acute crisis. The blood film may show many round inclusions of denatured precipitated haemoglobin (Heinz bodies) which disappear after a few days to be replaced by reticulocytes when recovery takes place. Recovery is usual.

Treatment is directed at the cause, i.e. infection, hyperbilirubinaemia in the neonate, the very low haemoglobin and the consequences of haemolysis, e.g. renal failure, in older children. Avoidance of antimalarials such as primaquine, chloroquine and dapsone should be discussed but these drugs may be safe in therapeutic doses. Sulphonamides, e.g. in co-trimoxazole, and also aspirin are to be avoided but are no longer widely used. Ciprofloxacin and some penicillins may initiate attacks. Naphthalene in mothballs, formerly used to protect towelling nappies, and the dietary staple fava bean may be very potent triggers.

Pyruvate kinase deficiency

This is much less common and occurs in children homozygous for the abnormal autosomal recessive gene. Pyruvate kinase levels are low. Red cells leak potassium and are depleted of ATP; their survival is reduced, resulting in increased haemolysis.

The clinical expression is variable with jaundice in the neonate but seldom with kernicterus. In later childhood there is pallor and enlargement of the spleen, which may require removal.

Spherocytes are not seen. The diagnosis rests on demonstrating reduced activity of red cell pyruvate kinase.

Red cell membrane disorders

Spherocytosis

This is an autosomal dominantly inherited defect of red cell sodium transport whereby the unusually small cells absorb water, become spherical and, because they are osmotically fragile when they pass through the spleen, are destroyed. The increased loss of cells results in anaemia, jaundice and reticulocytosis.

There is usually a family history. Symptoms can begin in infancy or even in the neonatal period. Gallstones may be troublesome later in life, and aplastic crises precipitated by the human

parvovirus B19 may be fatal. The diagnosis is confirmed by demonstrating increased osmotic fragility.

Splenectomy is curative but is delayed for as long as possible because of the risk of infection. Folic acid supplements are given daily. Immunisation against H. influenzae, Pneumococcus and Meningococcus type C, together with regular penicillin administration is advocated.

Elliptocytosis

This is also an autosomal dominantly inherited condition but is much more benign than spherocytosis and may only cause mild jaundice, however gallstones can occur as can aplastic crises.

NEUTROPHIL DISORDERS

Neutropenia

A transient reduction of neutrophils below $2.0 \times 10^9/l$ occurs in many acute illnesses and as a toxic effect of several drugs (see Box 13.1). When this has lasted more than 6 months the condition is said to be chronic.

The causes may be reduced bone marrow production, failure of release into the circulation

---

Box 13.1 Causes of neutropenia

Infection
- Viral
  —hepatitis
  —influenza
  —exanthemata
- Bacterial
  —septicaemia

Drugs
- Antibiotics, e.g. chloramphenicol
- Anticonvulsants, e.g. carbamazepine
- Antineoplastics

Chemicals
- Benzene
- Insecticides

Irradiation
Bone marrow infiltration
- Leukaemia
- Secondary malignancy
- Storage disease

and an autoimmune process of destruction. The risk of bacterial infection occurs if the absolute count is less than $1 \times 10^9/l$, when Staphylococcus, Klebsiella, *E. coli* and Pseudomonas may become invasive.

Chronic benign neutropenia is the most common form of neutropenia. It is non-cyclic and has no identifiable underlying disease association. Cellulitis and upper and lower respiratory tract infections with otitis media are seen but susceptibility to infection is less than in malignancy because the bone marrow can produce an acute response.

Cyclic neutropenia occurs at approximately 20-day intervals and is suggested by the periodic occurrence of mouth ulcers and febrile illnesses with a very low neutrophil count.

Intermittent neutropenia can be a feature of Schwachmann-Diamond syndrome and is fairly frequently seen. There is associated pancreatic insufficiency, an increased incidence of infection, especially of the lungs, failure to thrive, metaphyseal dysplasia and the possibility later in life of the development of aplastic anaemia or leukaemia. It has an autosomal recessive inheritance.

Neutrophil dysfunction (see Immunology, p. 291)

PLATELET DISORDERS

Transient thrombocytopenia

This is frequently asssociated with viral illness, especially with the increasingly common human parvovirus B19. The reported prevalence of IgG antibodies to this virus in children aged 5–19 years ranges from 15–60%. The accompanying symptoms are febrile illness, arthropathy, red face and a fluctuating widespread rash which may persist for 2–3 weeks.

Idiopathic thrombocytopenia (ITP)

Acute type

This is usually caused by antibodies induced by viruses binding to glycoprotein IIb-IIIa on the platelet membrane, which is then destroyed by macrophages in the spleen. Megakaryocyte production in the bone marrow is increased but there is insufficient production to balance the loss.

Clinical features. Blood indices and clotting studies are normal but the bleeding time is prolonged and the platelet count is less than $150 \times 10^9/l$. The clinical presentation may be preceded by a viral illness one or two weeks earlier and usually consists of spontaneous bruises, epistaxis or petechiae which, if they occur around the head and neck, may be the result of vomiting. The liver and spleen are not enlarged. The children are not usually ill and there is no lymphadenopathy, all of which might otherwise suggest leukaemia.

Intracranial haemorrhage is rare but is the usual cause of death. It is fear of this which is the most frequent reason for treatment. Adolescents are more at risk than young children; head injury may be a precipitating factor but the occurrence of haemorrhage is often spontaneous when the platelet count is less than $20 \times 10^9/l$.

Management. Bone marrow aspiration is unnecessary if leukaemia is not suspected but is advocated if steroids are to be given. The prognosis is usually excellent, with or without treatment.

Steroids block destruction of the antibody coated platelets and may also stabilise fragile capillaries. They need only be given when there is frank haemorrhage and should be discontinued when the underlying process has resolved after around 2–3 weeks. The action of steroids is relatively slow and if there is no response at this time it is unlikely to occur subsequently.

Intravenous immunoglobulin produces a very prompt rise in platelet count within 2–3 days but it is uncertain whether it affects bleeding, which is much less than in children with malignancy. Immunoglobulin is also expensive and invasive and has attendant risks of transmitting infection.

Chronic type

This is arbitrarily defined as thrombocytopenia lasting more than 6 months after the acute presentation. The platelet count is frequently greater than $30 \times 10^9/l$.

Recovery without splenectomy can take years, and long-term treatment with cytotoxic and immunosuppressive drugs should be avoided. Early onset autoimmune disease should be considered.

Congenital thrombocytopenia

This may be associated with other anomalies (e.g. absent radius syndrome—TAR) or can be an isolated phenomenon. Transmission may be autosomal dominant or recessive.

Qualitative dysfunction

Sometimes, when the platelet count is normal, excessive bleeding and the occurrence of petechiae may be associated with platelets which are large and also functionally abnormal. Inheritance may be autosomal recessive (e.g. Glanzmann's thrombasthenia or associated with congenital disorders, e.g. heart disease).

BLEEDING DISORDERS

von Willebrand's disease

This is the most common congenital bleeding disorder. A prevalence of 1% of the population is a minimum estimate.

Von Willebrand factor is synthesised by endothelial cells and secreted directly into plasma; it is also made in megakaryocytes and subsequently stored in platelets. Circulating von Willebrand factor facilitates platelet adhesion to endothelium, while platelet activation causes release of stored von Willebrand factor for platelet aggregation. von Willebrand factor is the carrier protein for factor VIII in plasma and prevents its degradation.

There are more than 20 subtypes of von Willebrand disease, of which six are the most common and involve reduction in plasma levels, impaired formation (and therefore function), and failure to bind to factor VIII protein which is destroyed and produces mild haemophilia.

GP Overview 13.1 Bruising

Haematological causes

Low platelet count
- Leukaemia, drug induced, aplastic anaemia
- Congenital intrauterine infections (TORCH)
- Maternal ITP + maternal anti-platelet antibodies
- Haemolytic uraemic syndrome

Abnormal platelet function
Congenital, e.g. von Willebrand's
Drugs, e.g. aspirin
Uraemia
Liver disease

Capillary damage
- Henoch–Schönlein purpura
- Infection
- Mechanical, e.g. pertussis
- Inherited, e.g. Ehlers–Danlos

Coagulation disorder
- Inherited e.g. haemophilia, Christmas disease, von Willebrand's

Important features in history
- Family history
- Drug history/infections
- Trauma—accidental and NAI (explanation of bruising)

Examination
- Site, size, duration of bruises, associated findings, e.g. hepatosplenomegaly, lymphadenopathy
- Pattern bruising for NAI

Investigations
- FBC, platelet count, coagulation screen
- Autoantibody screen, bone marrow aspirate, factor VIII/IX/X/XI/XII levels
- TORCH screen

All forms are autosomal recessive (unlike haemophilia).

An increase in the activated partial thromboplastin time (APTT) may be suggestive of the disorder while platelet aggregation studies using ristocetin may identify the subgroup. The prothrombin time (PT) is normal.

Symptoms include epistaxis, menorrhagia, skin bruising and postoperative bleeding, especially after dental or tonsillar operations. Avoidance of trauma, e.g. body contact sport, should be carefully considered.

Several drugs increase circulating levels of von Willebrand factor but the most useful is DDAVP (des amino-D-arginine vasopressin). This releases endothelial von Willebrand factor and also stabilises the endothelium. It is used when bleeding is a problem and prior to surgery. Many drugs have anti-platelet effects and should be avoided; these include non-steroidals, cephalosporins, some antihistamines, caffeine and valproate.

Non-virus-treated cryoprecipitate is not used for frank bleeding; factor VIII concentrates which have been treated are an alternative.

Haemophilia

Haemophilia A is caused by reduced factor VIII activity, and haemophilia B (Christmas disease) by reduced factor IX. Both are transmitted on the X chromosome (sex-linked recessive). There are approximately 150 different mutations, and more than 95% of carriers can be detected by analysing intron 22 on the X chromosome.

As with von Willebrand disease the PT is normal and the APTT is prolonged. Tests of platelet function are normal. Factor VIII is reduced or absent depending on the severity of the condition.

Since factor VIII does not cross the placenta, bleeding may begin in the neonatal period, especially after injections. When the child becomes mobile, bleeding after minor injury may occur for many days. The major problem is bleeding into joints, especially the elbows, knees and ankles, which may appear to be spontaneous. Osteoporosis and limitation of joint movement follows repeated haemarthroses when the joint may become fixed.

Treatment was formerly limited to avoidance of trauma but blood transfusions were given and in the 1950s factor VIII concentrates were used. Transmission of hepatitis B and C then became a problem, and 55% of treated patients were infected with HIV. The factor VIII gene has now been cloned and genetically engineered pure clotting factor has become available for replacement.

The basis of treatment is the administration (by parents and later by the children themselves) of factor VIII at the first sign of symptoms. Factor VIII is not yet widely given prophylactically. DDAVP increases factor VIII levels and when given intravenously may produce a therapeutic rise within 45 minutes. The nasal spray works more slowly. Hyponatraemic fitting may occur if there is injudicious fluid administration with DDAVP.

Spontaneous mouth bleeding can be treated orally with drugs which prevent clot lysis (anti-fibrinolytic agents). Two are available, ε amino caproic acid and tranexamic acid, but both should be used in conjunction with standard treatment. One of the main problems of haemophilia treatment is the development of factor VIII or IX antibody when more frequent administration of high dose replacement is required.

Disseminated intravascular coagulation (DIC)

This is a consumptive coagulopathy which occurs most often in severely ill children following infection. It leads to bruising and bleeding, and coagulation tests confirm low platelets, raised fibrin degradation products and prolonged prothrombin time.

Management involves treating the primary problem and replacement of the coagulation factors with fresh frozen plasma and platelets. Heparin and antithrombin III may also be used.

APLASTIC ANAEMIA

This is caused by either reduction or absence of the cellular bone marrow elements and clinically is manifest as a pancytopenia. Two types are recognised: inherited (Fanconi anaemia) and acquired.

Fanconi anaemia

This is an autosomal recessive condition characterised by short stature, abnormal radii and thumbs, café-au-lait spots, renal abnormalities and developmental delay. Bone marrow failure occurs at school age and presents with bleeding and bruising and anaemia. Treatment with bone marrow transplantation has been used and there is an increased risk of leukaemia.

Acquired anaemia

This is a very uncommon condition; often no cause is found. Possible causes include:

- drugs—chloramphenicol, sulphonamides, gold, anti–thyroid drugs, organic solvents
- infections—hepatitis, EB virus.

Treatment

Bone marrow transplantation from an HLA identical sibling is best and is curative. Anti-human thymic globulin, steroids, cyclosporin and cytokines can produce a remission.

ONCOLOGY

ACUTE LEUKAEMIAS

Risk factors (Box 13.2)

Acute lymphoblastic leukaemia accounts for more than 30% of all childhood cancer and 80% of leukaemia in children (Table 13.2). The peak incidence is from 2–5 years; the prognosis is worse in boys and if the child's age falls outside this range.

Clinical presentation

Pallor and a tiredness which is not behavioural are the most common features on presentation. In the early stages there may be continuing fever from an apparent viral illness but then appropriate symptoms and signs appear as the leukaemia cells infiltrate tissues:

- The child may limp and the bones may be tender.
- Platelet production may be reduced resulting in petechiae, bruising or frank haemorrhage.
- Lymph nodes may become large and do not feel like those of chronic inflammation.
- The spleen and liver may be enlarged at presentation.
- Occasionally, raised intracranial pressure may give rise to intermittent headache and vomiting.

Diagnosis

The diagnosis can often be made on the blood film when blast cells are present and platelets are low. Sometimes the white cell count may be normal, but anaemia and a raised ESR usually indicate the need for bone marrow aspiration. Cell markers and classification of the type of leukaemia help in determining prognosis and treatment (Table 13.2).

Treatment

This should be undertaken in a recognised centre using a standard nationally approved regimen. The objective is to induce remission, i.e. to reduce the number of blast cells in bone marrow to less than 5%. This is usually achieved in about

---

Box 13.2	Risk factors for acute leukaemia

- Ionising radiation (pre- and postnatal X-rays)
- Very high birth weight
- Presence of the Philadelphia chromosome (22q–) (more commonly seen in chronic myeloid leukaemia)
- Down's syndrome
- Neurofibromatosis
- Schwachmann–Diamond syndrome
- Fanconi anaemia
- A sibling with leukaemia
- Several chromosomal translocations

Table 13.2 Leukaemias

Type	Classification
Acute lymphoblastic: > 80% of all childhood leukaemias	*Immunological* a. Non-T non-B cell. Best prognosis and most common b. T cell c. Null cell d. B cell. Worst prognosis and least common *French-American-British morphological classification of blast cells:* a. $FABL_1$. Best prognosis and most common b. $FABL_2$ c. $FABL_3$
Acute non-lymphocytic	a. myeloblastic b. myelomonocytic
Chronic myelocytic	
Chronic juvenile myelocytic	

95% of patients within 4 weeks. The protocols used involve vincristine, prednisolone and L-asparaginase, with the addition of daunorubicin for high risk patients in some centres.

The central nervous system may harbour leukaemic cells which are not removed by the standard induction regimens. Whilst preventive measures using intrathecal methotrexate and craniospinal irradiation may prevent CNS and subsequent systemic relapse, the growth changes and neuro-intellectual disturbances caused by irradiation are forcing the exploration of protocols that use chemotherapy alone. Blood transfusions are frequently required; allopurinol is also given to destroy the increased load of nuclear metabolites which damage the kidneys.

Induction is followed by early and then late intensification treatment, when pulses of cytotoxic drugs such as cytosine arabinoside, daunorubicin, vincristine, etoposide and thioguanine together with intrathecal methotrexate are given. Prednisolone, mercaptopurine and methotrexate with monthly vincristine is continued on a regular basis for two years.

Pneumocystis lung infection is always a concern; co-trimoxazole can be used. If there is relapse of the leukaemia, however, it may not be amenable to further treatment and bone marrow transplantation should be considered.

The role of the general practitioner in the overall management is important in terms of emotional support for the family, liaising with the oncology centre and helping with venepunctures. The early detection of infection and supervision of antibiotic treatment together with suspicion of relapse is, however, one of the principal objectives of all carers.

CHRONIC LEUKAEMIAS

These constitute only about 3% of all leukaemias.

Chronic myelocytic leukaemia. In this, the classic adult form, there are large numbers of all types of maturing granulocyte cells in the blood, bone marrow and sites of extramedullary haematopoiesis, e.g. liver and spleen. Reciprocal translocation between chromosome 9 and 22 produces the Philadelphia chromosome and is a specific marker. At first there are few symptoms and signs but anaemia and other features develop as the slowly expanding myeloid reservoir infiltrates organs. These features become marked in the later blast phase crises.

Drug treatment is with busulphan, and splenectomy may be helpful. Although the blast phase can be treated with vincristine and prednisolone the prognosis is poor.

Juvenile chronic myelocytic leukaemia presents in children younger than 2 years with an eczema-like rash, sometimes with café-au-lait marks, lymphadenopathy, hepatosplenomegaly and recurrent respiratory infections. Haematological indices show anaemia and thrombocytopenia, and the white cell count may be as high as $200 \times 10^9/l$.

The Philadelphia chromosome is absent and busulphan is ineffective.

LYMPHOMAS

Hodgkin's disease most frequently occurs in adolescent boys. The most common presentation is with enlarged lymph nodes, solitary or grouped, but usually in the supraclavicular region or axillae; there is no systemic illness. The glands feel firm, are painless and can be 'shotty' in the groins. Those of the upper cervical region are less commonly involved. The cell type is the Reed-Sternberg cell, which contains two nuclei. Nonspecific symptoms, including fatigue, pruritus and urticaria, are seen in 33% of cases.

Diagnosis is by histology, but treatment and prognosis depend on ascertaining the extent of internal involvement. Mediastinal spread occurs in 60% of cases and is shown on X-ray. CT scanning may detect abdominal spread but can miss glands in the coeliac axis and mesentery. Lymphangiography, where possible, is 95% accurate.

Treatment is based on age and stage related protocols using *m*ustine hydrochloride, *o*ncovocin, *p*rednisolone and *p*rocarbazine (MOPP) and other cytotoxic drugs. Radiotherapy to large masses can be successful. The overall prognosis is approximately 90% survival at 5 years.

Non-Hodgkin disease is the most common lymphoma, occurring mainly in children under

15 years old with a peak incidence in the under fives. The Epstein–Barr virus has been found in 95% of malignant cells in the Burkitt's lymphoma subgroup.

B and T cell markers form the basis of classification, which has some prognostic value. Unlike Hodgkin's disease there is no propensity for lymph node involvement. Both the upper and lower cervical glands are affected as well as lymphoid tissue in thymus, mediastinum, spleen, liver, mesentery and pelvis. Cells of the T cell line tend to affect the mediastinum, those of B cell line the abdomen and other sites, e.g. skin, bone, lung and CNS. The lymphoma is diagnosed by evaluating biopsy specimens.

Staging is required to plan treatment; it ranges from a single node and primary nodes with regional involvement, to extensive disease affecting the CNS.

Treatment is with a combination of agents including cyclophosphamide, cytosine arabinoside, total body irradiation and bone marrow transplantation.

SOLID TUMOURS

General information (Box 13.3)

Triggering of malignancy may be induced by chemicals or UV irradiation, both of which alter DNA structure. The result is that a tissue stem cell may proceed along a malignant pathway.

Proliferation may follow when external agents influence cell signal factors, or from the effect of

---

Box 13.3 Risk factors for neoplastic disease
Age   • Retinoblastoma and Wilms' tumour more common under 5 years   • Lymphomas and bone tumours most common around puberty   *Congenital abnormalities*   • Hemihypertrophy associated with renal, adrenal and liver tumours   • Absence of pectoralis major (Poland syndrome) associated with leukaemia   • Neurofibromatosis and tuberous sclerosis associated with nerve cell tumours

---

internal factors such as the pubertal growth spurt, which explains the high incidence of some tumours at this age.

Oncogenes induce neoplasia and are derived from normal genes which have either undergone insertion of viral material, translocation, localised mutation, or DNA sequence amplification. Burkitt's lymphoma commonly displays the *c-myc* oncogene, whilst the *ras* oncogenes— although sometimes found in childhood neuroblastoma and rhabdomyosarcoma—are more commonly associated with adult bowel cancers. The concept that some genetic material suppresses tumour formation is demonstrated in retinoblastoma, Wilms' tumour, neuroblastoma and rhabdomyosarcoma—conditions where specific loss of segments of DNA is found.

Spread of cancer cells may also be the result of oncogene and growth factor interaction whereby the immediate extracellular matrix of the cancer cell degrades to allow attachment and eventually locomotion of the malignant cells to distant sites.

Central nervous system tumours

CNS tumours account for 23% of cancers in children in the UK. They are mostly (60%) infratentorial gliomas, i.e. astrocytoma, glioblastoma and ependymoma, and are seen in children aged 2–10 years. Supratentorial tumours (40%) occur in infants and adolescents. Less common is the medulloblastoma, which consists of highly malignant undifferentiated round cells affecting the cerebellar vermis and fourth ventricle.

If the tumour is infratentorial the presentation is usually with headache, and sometimes morning vomiting which may be diagnosed as migraine. These symptoms can be deceptive by being intermittent. Altered behaviour or personality change is common; cerebellar ataxia and nystagmus must always be looked for.

If the tumour is supratentorial the presentation is with convulsions and focal neurological signs. Diagnosis is by CT or MR scan. Sudden release of intracranial pressure by lumbar puncture should not be undertaken because of the risk of coning.

Unfortunately the majority of tumours are malignant and not easily treated surgically.

Non-malignant astrocytomas have a good prognosis with surgery but those that are malignant have a poor outcome even with irradiation. Medulloblastomas have usually metastasised at diagnosis; even aggressive treatment with surgery, irradiation and chemotherapy only produces 50% survival at 5 years.

Craniopharyngioma is an uncommon developmental tumour arising from a remnant of Rathke's pouch. It is amenable to surgery but there is frequent visual loss because of its suprasellar position and replacement hormone treatment is required.

The aftercare of all tumours should take into account cognitive change, the psychological and direct sequelae of chemotherapy, endocrine disturbances and the ever present threat of deterioration owing to recurrence.

Wilms' tumour (nephroblastoma)

Wilms' tumour constitutes 8% of UK children's cancer. The tumour consists of a mix of undifferentiated cells together with embryonal structures such as tubules and glomeruli. There is an association with aniridia and deletion of material on chromosome 11p13, but multiple genes may be involved.

The tumour mainly presents in children aged between 2½ and 4 years and is rare after 10 years of age. Hemihypertrophy and the syndrome of large tongue, umbilical hernia and gigantism are frequent associations. The most common presentation is with an abdominal mass, haematuria and sometimes hypertension. 5% of cases are bilateral at presentation.

Diagnosis is by ultrasound; a chest X-ray will detect spread to the lungs, and CT scan elucidates CNS involvement.

Treatment is surgical and depends on the staging (Table 13.3). The 4-year survival in stages I and II is about 90%, that for stages III–V is about 50%.

Neuroblastoma

Neuroblastoma constitutes 7% of UK children's cancer. These tumours arise from neural crest tissue and consist of variably differentiated sympathetic ganglion cells; they may thus occur anywhere from the adrenal medulla to the thoracic or cervical sympathetic chain ganglia. Spontaneous involution is possible. They occur mainly in toddlers and are the most common extracranial tumours of childhood.

The presentation may be neurological, depending on the site of the tumour, but can vary from the vaguely unwell child who complains of limb pains and looks pale to the frankly ill child who has an abdominal mass and metastases to the eye and bone marrow causing profound anaemia. Diarrhoea may be an early feature.

Diagnosis is by ultrasound, plain X-ray, CT scan and associated biochemical tests such as raised urinary catecholamines (VMA), white cell count and ESR. Bone marrow biopsy may be the only positive test. Bone scan and MIBG (meta-iodo-benzyl-guanidine) scans are performed to detect metastases.

Treatment is not rewarding; because there are often metastases at diagnosis the survival rate at 5 years is less than 10%. The prognosis is much improved if surgery is possible, and chemotherapy with immunotherapy and cytokines may produce even better results in due course.

Table 13.3 Staging of Wilms' tumour

Stage	Treatment
I. Tumour restricted to kidney and completely excised	Vincristine and actinomycin D
II. Tumour extends beyond kidney but completely excised	Chemotherapy and irradiation
III. Local lymph node and abdominal spread but not completely excised	Multiple chemotherapeutic agents and irradiation
IV. Distant haematogenous spread	Multiple chemotherapeutic agents and irradiation
V. Bilateral renal disease	Multiple chemotherapeutic agents and irradiation

Bone tumours

These account for 6% of UK children's cancer.

Osteosarcoma is the most common. It occurs in the long bones of adolescents and is highly but locally malignant. The tumour has a pseudo-capsule and often there are adjacent but discrete 'skip metastases'. Distant haematogenous spread is very common, especially to lungs, but local node involvement is rare since there is no lymphatic system in bones.

The presentation is with pain at the site of the tumour in an otherwise well teenager. The neighbouring joint may be involved by a patho-logical fracture.

Diagnosis is by radiographic or other scanning technology, especially MRI.

Treatment is surgical and limb sparing, with the use of prostheses where possible. Preopera-tive combination chemotherapy is also required but its continuation after surgery is controversial.

Ewing's sarcoma is less common, may be familial and also occurs in the second decade when bone growth is maximal. The pelvis and femur are the bones most frequently affected. The tumour cells are divided by connective tissue sheets: this, together with periosteal reaction, produces an 'onion skin' appearance on X-ray.

Presentation is with localised pain, with or without swelling.

Treatment is by surgical excision and local irradiation for the primary lesion with systemic chemotherapy for eradication of micrometastases. The cure rate can be as high as 50%.

Rhabdomyosarcoma

5% of UK children's cancer is caused by rhabdo-myosarcoma. This tumour is of undifferentiated mesenchymal tissue and presents at around 4 years of age with a second peak at about 17 years.

It usually presents in the head and neck, where there may be a painful soft tissue swelling or obstruction of the upper airway channels in-cluding bloody nasal discharge, croupy voice changes, middle ear deafness and orbital pro-ptosis. The second most common presentation is genito-urinary, with haematuria, testicular swelling, vaginal bleeding or an abdominal mass.

Metastases to lung and bone occur; treatment, either surgical or with irradiation and chemo-therapy, is disappointing.

IMMUNOLOGY

The immune system in childhood is immature and this accounts for the increased frequency of 'intercurrent infections' in the first few years of life. Transplacental 'protection' lasts only a few months.

The following five components interact within the immune system:

1. The environment

The environment presents an antigen or allergen, consisting of either a chemical or a complex organism, to a target cell which may be injured or die. The immune system intervenes by recruiting cells, antibodies, complement and cytokines.

2. Cells

Phagocytes. These engulf the environmental agent, an act which is performed by mononuclear cells, neutrophils and eosinophils. They are mobilised by chemotactic factors from the complement system. Recognition of antigens is accomplished by CD (cluster differentiation) and HLA (human leukocyte antigen) markers, the latter being involved in recognising 'self' from 'non-self'. Impairment of this system results in autoimmune disease.

Phagocytosis (Box 13.4). Pluripotent stem cells found in bone marrow differentiate along different cell lines to produce erythrocytes, platelets or white cells which have a phagocytic function:

Neutrophils (granulocytes)
- Involved in acute inflammation and bacterial killing.
- Highly differentiated mature phagocytes.

Box 13.4 Mediators of phagocytosis

- Inflammatory releasing factors
- Chemotactic factors
- Opsonising factors
- Adhesive factors

Production of mature neutrophils (polymorphs) is stimulated by inflammatory mediators such as endotoxins and cytokines. Chemotactic factors attract the neurophils to the site of the inflammation where they adhere to the invading organism. The process of ingestion involves opsonising factors and degranulation of the phagocytic cell.

Monocytes

- Slow moving and involved in chronic bacterial infections (e.g. tuberculosis, parasites).
- Enter tissues and scavenge for fixed debris.

Eosinophils are active in allergic reactions, parasitic infections and some skin diseases.

Lymphocytes. These are either thymus derived (T cell) or 'Bursa of Fabricius derived' (B cell). The latter mature in bone marrow.

T cells are either helper or suppressor, and perform their function by producing effector and regulatory cytokines, or natural killer cells which destroy other cells displaying hostile antigens. The newborn infant has good T cell function and can respond, for instance, to BCG vaccination. Lymphocytes are not phagocytic.

B cells mature into plasma cells and, after antigen exposure, produce memory and other cell types which generate antibodies when rechallenged. Thus, at birth, B cell function is relatively poor and neonates are susceptible to infections, especially those caused by Gram-negative organisms.

3. Antibodies

Antibodies (immunoglobulins), produced by B cells, consist of two heavy (H) chains joined by a disulphide bridge to two light (L) chains.

IgM

- Does not cross the placenta because of its large size; hence its presence in the neonatal circulation is strong evidence of intrauterine infection, e.g. rubella and CMV.
- Production of IgM starts after a few days in response to the massive antigen challenge of the new environment (primary response).

IgG

- Is a small molecule which crosses the placenta and occurs in all body fluids.
- Maternally derived IgG antibodies protect the infant from a wide range of infections caused by Gram-positive bacteria and viruses.
- Cord blood concentration is similar to (or even greater than) maternal blood.
- The infant's production of IgG increases over the first 8 months of life as maternal IgG is eliminated.
- Adult levels are reached by approximately 8 years of age.
- There are four IgG subclasses which perform different functions and can be individually deficient, causing specific immunological disorders.
- IgG is the main antibody involved in secondary immune responses.

IgA

- The main antibody in external (gastro-intestinal, respiratory, urogenital) secretions.
- There are two subclasses.

IgD

- Present on the surface of B cells.
- Role unknown.

IgE

- Present in all body fluids.
- Important for immunological response to parasites.
- Mediates immediate allergic reactions.
- Receptors are on mast cells and basophils.

4. Complement

Complement, in contrast to cellular and immuno-globulin defence, is non-specific and is responsible for terminating early infection which then becomes subclinical. On the first encounter with an antigen, before antibodies are formed, the 'alternative complement pathway' attaches C3b to the antigen and in turn activates C5–C9 which have the capability to lyse bacterial membranes. C3b also prepares (opsonises) bacteria for phago-cytosis. The 'classical complement pathway' is activated by antigen–antibody complexes and stimulates production of mediators such as hista-mine, which increases vascular permeability and facilitates the passage of macrophages. Prosta-glandin mediators act as pyrogens, and leuko-trienes stimulate neutrophil motility.

5. Cytokines

These are produced by both lymphocytes (lym-phokines) and macrophages (monokines). There are four groups:

a. interferons
b. erythropoietin and associated interleukins
c. anti-cancer adjuvants (interleukin IL-1, 2, 4 and 6)
d. anti-inflammatory cytokines (tumour necrosis factor—TNF, transforming growth factor—TGF, and interleukins).

IMMUNODEFICIENCY DISEASES
Phagocytes

Chronic granulomatous disease is X-linked with moderate expression in female carriers. Bacteria are ingested by neutrophils as normal but are not killed because of failure of production of superoxide radicals and H_2O_2. Streptococci, pneumococci and *H. influenzae* which produce H_2O_2 are killed. Staphylococci, *Serratia marcescens* and fungi on the other hand are not and become severely pathogenic.

The symptoms are skin infections and inflam-mation of lymph nodes, bone and bowel. Pro-phylactic trimethoprim to prevent Pneumocystis disease is very valuable but otherwise treatment is based on aggressive anti-staphylococcal and anti-fungal measures.

Adhesion deficiency disorder presents with de-layed wound healing and recurrent surface infec-tions, which may spread to cause severe systemic infection. Treatment consists of aggressive use of antibiotics and meticulous hygiene.

Chediak–Higashi syndrome is an autosomal recessive disorder. Neutrophils are defective, leading to chronic mouth infections. Associated features are platelet dysfunction and later neurological symptoms. Death may be precipitated by Epstein–Barr virus infection.

Lymphocytes

T cell deficiency is usually combined with B cell deficiency and is found in the Di George syndrome when the 3rd and 4th pharyngeal pouches do not develop properly with consequent deficiency of thymus and parathyroids and abnormalities of the heart and great vessels. The genetic deletion is on the long arm of chromosome 22 (22q11). Hypocalcaemia and congenital heart defects are the major problems.

Severe combined immunodeficiency (SCID). The most common form is X-linked. T and B cell lines as well as immunoglobulins are deficient. The presentation is with severe infection and failure to thrive in the first few months; treatment is by bone marrow transplantation.

B cell deficiencies. The most common is agammaglobulinaemia, which is also X-linked and presents in the first months of life with pneumococcal, staphylococcal and *H. influenzae* related illnesses. Treatment is by intramuscular injection of immunoglobulin.

Immunoglobulins

Hyper IgM syndrome presents with recurrent pyogenic and Pneumocystis infections. The underlying defect is inability to produce IgA and IgG, which are very low, while the IgM may be normal or very high.

Selective IgA deficiency relates to secretory IgA which lines the respiratory and gastrointestinal systems; infections in these areas are consequently common. There is an association with SLE.

Hyper IgE (Job) syndrome is not infrequent and usually involves increased staphylococcal susceptibility.

Wiskott–Aldrich syndrome is associated with both high IgE and IgA and presents with eczema, recurrent infections and bleeding from thrombocytopenia. Its transmission is X-linked recessive.

Complement

C1q deficiency predisposes to meningococcal disease. Other complement deficiencies have a significant association with SLE as well as *Neisseria* infections, e.g. gonococcus.

Hereditary angioedema results when C1 inhibitor is not produced. Swelling can occur rapidly without pain after mild trauma, especially in the neck.

Cytokines

The interleukins and tumour necrosis factor are heavily involved in the control of T killer cells, B cells and particularly IgE, and are therefore involved in many disease processes.

ALLERGY

Allergy is a harmful physiological reaction mediated by an immunological mechanism.

Types of reaction

Type I (anaphylaxis)

Antigen-triggered cross-linking of IgE on the surface of mast cells and basophils initiates the early release of mediators (Box 13.5) which in turn cause vasodilatation and blood vessel permeability, an outpouring of mucus, and contraction of bronchial wall smooth muscle. They also facilitate mobilisation of eosinophils, neutrophils and monocytes. This early anaphylactic reaction occurs within one hour and settles shortly after. Rarely, the reaction may be life threatening because of laryngeal oedema, bronchospasm and shock after insect stings or food allergens.

Box 13.5   Mediators of immediate allergy

- Histamine
- Leukotrienes
- Prostaglandins
- Platelet activating factor
- Interleukins
- Tumour necrosis factor
- Eosinophil chemotactic factor

Type II

A second late phase response, which is associated with the infiltration of eosinophils, monocytes and T cells, occurs about two days after antigen exposure and is related to long-term allergic disease. IgG and IgM antibodies are formed which will combine with cellular antigens on subsequent challenge and activate the complement system. This is the mechanism of some drug reactions.

Type III (Arthus reaction)

IgG and IgM antibodies combine with circulating antigens to form antigen–antibody complexes which may be deposited in tissues and cause vascular damage. This is the mechanism of serum sickness.

Type IV

These are cell mediated reactions caused by T lymphocytes combining with and destroying specific antigens; examples are tuberculin skin tests and contact dermatitis.

Atopic diseases

These are the most common allergic disorders in children. They affect the skin and respiratory tract causing dermatitis, rhinitis and asthma. There is a strong familial predisposition and atopy is often associated with other allergic problems such as allergy to food and insect stings. The mechanism is an IgE mediated type I reaction.

Epidemiology

- Many cases do not present for medical care and so are not included in standard surveys. It is likely that approximately one third of the general population suffers from allergy.
- 12–15% of school children have asthma.
- Around 5% of pre-school children have atopic eczema.
- Food allergy occurs in around 8% of young children.

- Approximately 15% of the population have urticaria at some time in their life.
- Atopic diseases tend to present in early life, become more severe over the subsequent few years and then steadily resolve by adolescence.

Investigation

- History is most important. A diary of episodes may reveal patterns and triggers.
- Skin tests—a wide range of allergens are available in soluble form and can be 'pricked' into the skin. A specific trigger may be identified but some atopic children react to almost everything. The usual 'wheal and flare' response is suppressed by antihistamines and interpretation of results can be difficult. The risk of an anaphylactic reaction is remote but a resuscitation kit must be available.
- Elevated IgE and eosinophilia are non-specific evidence for allergic disease.
- Serology—radio allergosorbent tests (RASTs) measure allergen specific IgE antibody and so can identify specific triggers.

Management

Allergen avoidance is always the first line of treatment. If a specific trigger is identified it may be easily eliminated. Emotional consequences must be expected, however, if removal of the favourite household pet is required. House dust mites, which are the most common triggers of asthma and allergic rhinitis, are very difficult to eliminate but the concentration in the home can be reduced (see Chapter 5).

Drug treatment is necessary if the allergen cannot be avoided (e.g. pollen) or cannot be identified.

- Corticosteroids suppress inflammation and stabilise basophils and mast cells. They are best administered topically in very small doses to avoid the inevitable side-effects of systemic use.
- Sodium cromoglycate also stabilises mast cells and specifically inhibits the allergic response. It is given topically as a spray or drops.
- Antihistamine drugs block histamine receptors

and so prevent the adverse physiological effects of histamine released from mast cells and basophils. Their universal side-effect is drowsiness, which can interfere with educational and social functions. Non-sedative preparations are now available, e.g. loratadine, terfenadine.

- Adrenergic agonists cause bronchodilation and are used in asthma (β_2 adrenergic receptors are the most important).
- Hyposensitization (immunotherapy) is rarely used because it can only be performed if the specific allergen is known and because it is unreliable. There is a small (1%) risk of anaphylaxis.

Common food antigens are cow's milk protein, transferred both in utero and breast milk, components of formulae such as wheat and peanut as an addition to flour, and also fish and tree nuts. Viruses, house dust mite, animal furs especially cat, cockroach proteins and mould from damp are common respiratory allergens; seasonal pollens, particularly grasses, affect the upper respiratory tract and eyes. Food allergy diminishes over the first few years while sensitisation to inhaled allergens increases.

Most blood IgE protein is fixed to mast cells and basophils, thus diminishing the value of measuring circulating IgE, but specific IgE (RAST) tests can be particularly helpful if selective skin tests are also positive.

Anaphylaxis

The manifestations of an allergic reaction are organ specific:

- Vasodilation and vascular permeability of skin causes angio-oedema and urticaria.
- The intestine may suffer similarly and produce pain.
- Nasal and conjunctival mucosae become reddened with an outpouring of secretions causing hay fever; this, in combination with bronchospasm in the lungs, can present as fatal status asthmaticus.

An anaphylactic reaction occurs when the entire vascular bed is suddenly affected causing instantaneous hypotension and collapse.

Treatment is aimed at stabilising the mast cells with topical agents, e.g. cromoglycate and steroids. Once the reaction is underway specific treatment with bronchodilators, antihistamines, plasma volume expanders and, especially, adrenaline may be required. Airway support with intubation or tracheostomy may also be needed.

Peanut allergy

The widespread use of peanut as an addition to flour or to bulk marzipan or even to imitate other nuts by sculpturing and reflavouring has recently come to public attention.

Peanuts are one of the most common foods causing allergic and anaphylactic reactions in children. The prevalence is 0.3–7.5% and is more common in those with atopy; fatal reactions occur almost always in subjects with asthma. Sensitisation can occur in utero but is more likely from breast milk or inhalation. Contamination of food processing equipment during switch-over from peanut to other usage is also important.

Approximately 50% of people with peanut allergy are also allergic to other nuts, especially almonds.

The symptoms experienced range from urticaria and angio-oedema to laryngeal swelling, which is the most common cause of death, through asthma, rhinitis, itching, vomiting, diarrhoea and cardiac arrest. The onset may be a strange sensation in the mouth, and the reaction can occur within a few minutes of contact. Aspirin, alcohol and exercise may accelerate the reaction.

Skin prick tests are reliable in children and are positive in about 50–70% of patients confirmed to be allergic. They are negatively predictive, but are unreliable if positive. RAST testing is less sensitive but potentially serious allergic reactions should be considered when both RAST and skin prick are positive.

Direct oral challenge can be undertaken but parents are often reluctant to allow this. Challenge with peanut oil has been found to be safe but it should be remembered that there are reports of infants shown to be allergic to formulae and vitamin supplements which contain peanut oil and protein.

Treatment consists of avoidance; this can be reinforced by advice from a dietician. Most accidents occur in teenagers, particularly when they are away from home and parental control.

The value of prophylactic treatment with known mast-cell stabilisers and vaccination schedules is as yet unproven. The main drug which should be used is adrenaline by injection. Aerosolised adrenaline absorbed directly from the mucosa of the mouth may be helpful, but in the presence of impending anaphylaxis or other severe reaction adrenaline injected intramuscularly via a spring loaded pen (Epi-Pen) at 5–10-minute intervals can be life saving. While the dose should be adjusted for weight, to give too much or to give an extra dose can be safer than undertreatment, a very important consideration when school teachers are asked to carry the equipment.

Nut allergy is usually a lifelong condition and any suggested re-introductions should only be done under strictly supervised circumstances.

Insect stings

- These are usually relatively trivial but in approximately 1% of the population can cause severe anaphylactic reactions.
- In the UK the most common causative insects are bees and wasps.
- Treatment is as for anaphylaxis. After the first episode an Epi-Pen can be carried.
- Hyposensitisation is sometimes helpful.

Urticaria

- This can be caused by a wide range of allergens as well as systemic disease.
- The characteristic features are raised erythematous oedematous areas of skin which are usually intensely itchy.
- It is often associated with angio-oedema which causes non-pitting swelling of loose tissues, e.g. the periorbital and genital areas.
- Management is the same as for other allergic disorders. A course of oral antihistamines or corticosteroids can be helpful in some persistent cases.

FURTHER READING

Warner J O, Jackson W F 1994 Color atlas of pediatric allergy. Wolfe, London

Internet address

Haematology
http://edcenter. med.cornell.edu/CUMC_PathNotes/Hematopathology/Hematopathology.html

14

Rheumatology and orthopaedics

Richard Newton

MINOR PROBLEMS OF INFANCY AND EARLY CHILDHOOD

There are minor skeletal problems that cause considerable concern to parents but which are of no consequence to the child. Often these unusual patterns are related to the intrauterine development of the fetus leading to deformation. These congenital deformations can be contrasted with the congenital malformations which relate to embryogenesis and are more serious and of long-term significance.

Metatarsus varus (fore-foot varus, hook fore-foot)

This is the most common of the skeletal deformations. There is in-toeing of the foot with a degree of curvature of the medial border (Figure 14.1). It is usually easy to flex and abduct the hip and flex the knee to demonstrate the intrauterine position of the legs. The varus deformity can readily be corrected to produce a straight medial

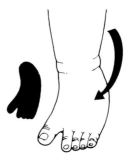

Fig. 14.1   Metatarsus varus.

border of the foot. The condition is frequently bilateral. The intrauterine position is taken up by the infant; thus the situation may be accentuated initially and certainly does not fully correct until the foot is weight-bearing. The pattern of growth then leads to gradual straightening of the foot.

Passive stretching is all that is required during the initial weeks, and the deformity will gradually correct.

Orthopaedic referral should be made if the degree of varus deformity is marked or progressive, particularly if a deep vertical crease is present at the mid-point of the medial border of the foot.

Talipes equinovarus (Figure 14.2)

Occasionally there is more severe deformity with gross degrees of the talipes and associated abnormality of the posterior part of the foot. The abnormal position of the foot cannot be corrected passively and orthopaedic referral is essential.

Talipes calcaneovalgus (Figure 14.2)

This is less commonly a significant problem. The foot is everted and dorsiflexed. The usual cause is intrauterine pressure and the condition resolves

during the first few months of life. Physiotherapy to the foot is all that is required.

Talipes may be associated with chromosomal abnormalities or, rarely, congenital neuromuscular disorders. There may be associated dysmorphic features. These infants require referral for paediatric and orthopaedic advice.

Deformation of the feet may reflect pressure on the hip joint, and it is particularly important to perform a careful examination for congenital dislocation of the hip in these children.

In-toeing (Figure 14.3)

This may be apparent before the child starts walking but is usually of concern once walking is established. It may be unilateral or bilateral. The gait of the child can be well balanced but appear very cumbersome; sometimes the in-toeing is severe enough to cause falling by tripping over the feet. The child needs to be examined both walking and on the couch.

When the child is examined supine the cause of the in-toeing may be shown to be partly related to the hip, because of femoral anteversion, or to the tibia from tibial torsion, or to the foot from fore-foot varus (described above) or a combination of these factors. The position at the hip is determined by the development of the femoral neck, femoral anteversion giving rise to the position of the leg. On examination, medial rotation of the hip can be fully achieved passively to give marked in-turning of the foot, but external

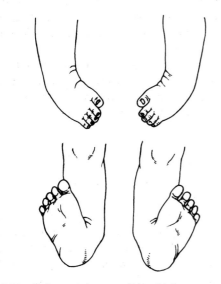
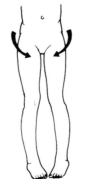

Fig. 14.2 Talipes equinovarus (A) and talipes calcaneovalgus (B).

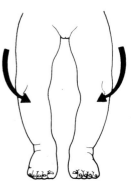

Fig. 14.3 In-toeing.

rotation is limited and may only be possible to just beyond the neutral position. Femoral anteversion improves with growth and development, usually resolving by the age of 8 years. Rarely improvement does not occur and there may then be a need for rotational osteotomy.

External rotation

This is less common and is caused by femoral retroversion. The child walks with the feet pointing outwards; on the couch there is limitation to passive medial rotation of the hip. Natural resolution occurs.

Genu varum (tibial bowing)

There is a varying degree of lateral bowing of the tibia in the infant. This also reflects the intra-uterine position during development. The degree may be marked but is usually moderate and the deformation corrects with time, particularly once the legs are weight-bearing. On rare occasions a more severe degree of progressive deformity may indicate a secondary cause such as rickets, chondrodysplasias, or infantile tibia vara (Blount's disease).

Genu valgum (knock-knees)

In this situation medial deviation of the knees gives rise to separation of the medial malleoli when the child is standing (Figure 14.4). Assess-

Fig 14.4   Genu valgum.

ment of the condition is best made with the child supine, the patellae facing vertically and the skin of the two knees just adjacent. Assessment is made with regard to the separation of the internal malleoli: referral should be made to the orthopaedic clinic if this distance is greater than 10 cm. Examination by this technique also allows serial measurements to be made to ensure that resolution is taking place.

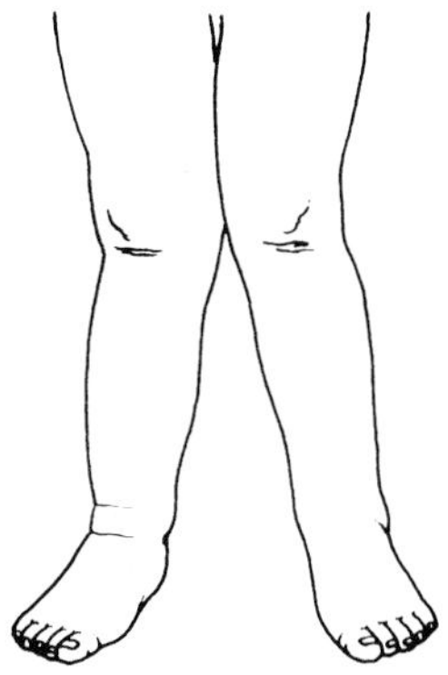

Tiptoe walking

Walking on tiptoe may indicate an underlying neurological disorder giving rise to tightness of the gastrocnemius muscles. Some children walk on tiptoe from habit; this in itself may also lead to contracture of the tendo Achilles. The condition needs to be carefully assessed by examination of the tendo Achilles, ensuring that when the child is lying supine it is possible to dorsiflex the ankles fully to at least 90°. The examination should also include assessment for other neuromuscular deficit. The child with muscular dystrophy may present with a tendency to walk on tiptoe because of muscular weakness and flexion at the hip. There may be delay in independent walking, a waddling gait and bulky appearance of the calf muscle. The classical Gower's sign (see Figure 9.5, p. 215) may be elicited by asking the child to rise from lying to standing, when the arms will be used to lever the trunk into the upright stance.

Tiptoe gait may be a sign of cerebral palsy.

If these additional signs are present or the tiptoe gait does not resolve promptly then referral to the paediatric clinic should be made.

Flat feet (pes planus—Figure 14.5)

The longitudinal arch of the infant and toddler is not well developed as a pad of fat is present in the arch. Walking with the feet flat on the ground is therefore normal in early childhood. There may also be a tendency for the foot to be everted. The situation resolves with time. The only advice which may be required is the wearing of firm fitting shoes with a heel.

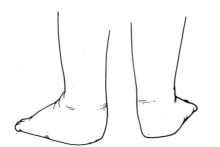

Fig. 14.5 Flat feet (pes planus).

Persistent flat feet may be associated with the hyperelasticity syndromes. Assessment of the foot in the older child can be performed by asking the child to stand on tiptoe or by passively dorsiflexing the big toe, when the longitudinal arch will become visible. Failure to produce an arch to the foot could indicate bony abnormality and orthopaedic referral is indicated.

CONGENITAL DISLOCATION OF THE HIP (Development dysplasia of the hip) – see page 52

INFANTILE CORTICAL HYPEROSTOSIS (CAFFEY'S DISEASE)

This rare condition occurs in early infancy. The infant is generally fractious and difficult to manage. On examination there may be soft tissue swellings which are tender and commonly overlie the mandible, clavicles and skull. Later there may be X-ray changes. The infant may fail to thrive because of the debilitating nature of the condition. The disease tends to be self limiting. Corticosteroids may be indicated in the treatment.

OSTEOCHONDRITIS

This is a destructive lesion which may affect various areas of bone growth. The cause is not known but its effect is an avascular necrosis, usually self limiting.

Perthes' disease

This is osteochondritis of the hip joint. It usually presents with a limp and affects children aged between 3 and 10 years, the peak incidence being in mid childhood. It occurs more commonly in boys and may be bilateral. On examination there is limitation of both active and passive movements of the hip joint with no systemic illness or fever.

X-ray of the hip demonstrates characteristic changes with widening of the joint space in association with necrosis of the epiphysis (Figure 14.6). The condition requires close orthopaedic supervision to achieve the best long-term result. The course of the osteochondritis is variable and may cause interruption of activity and schooling for up to three or four years.

The other osteochondroses tend to have a less profound effect on the child but can cause acute pain over variable intervals.

Sever's disease

The epiphysis of the calcaneum is affected. There is acute localised pain of the posterior aspect of the calcaneum with swelling and sometimes redness of the skin. This can interfere with walking and requires special attention to footwear with a raised heel. Spontaneous resolution occurs but may take 6–18 months.

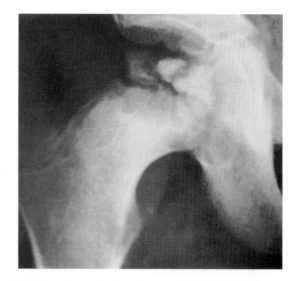

Fig. 14.6 Gross Perthes' disease of the femoral head.

Osgood–Schlatter disease

The tibial tuberosity may become affected in adolescence. There is acute pain on walking and tenderness of the tibial tuberosity. Treatment is symptomatic with resting of the leg and then graduated rehabilitation.

Scheuermann's disease

This is an osteochondritis affecting the vertebrae which may lead to a kyphosis. There may be minimal symptoms or a degree of backache. It is more common in boys. Management is with postural exercises.

SLIPPED FEMORAL EPIPHYSIS

This condition occurs in late childhood or early adolescence and is slightly more common in males, often associated with obesity. The presentation is usually with a limp, associated with pain referred to the knee. There may be sudden onset in association with an injury. There is limitation of movement of the affected hip with changes on X-ray. Careful orthopaedic management is essential to achieve the best outcome.

CHONDROMALACIA PATELLAE

This condition probably occurs secondary to muscular stress and is usually seen in adolescent girls. The symptom is pain related to the knee-cap, particularly on exercise. Characteristically the pain in the knee may be felt when sitting with knees flexed. On examination crepitus may be felt on flexion of the knee with pain on palpation. This condition is self limiting but is difficult to manage as the symptoms are variable in degree. Activities which exacerbate symptoms should be avoided, but physiotherapy directed to strengthening the quadriceps in particular and maintaining as much movement as possible is important.

It may be difficult to differentiate this condition from other problems of the knee that require intervention and orthopaedic referral.

SCOLIOSIS

This is a lateral curvature of the spine which may occur in the thoracic or lumbar regions and is described as being concave to left or right; it may be associated with vertebral rotation (Figure 14.7). It is important to differentiate a postural scoliosis which is readily correctable from a structural scoliosis which requires referral to the orthopaedic surgeon.

Structural scoliosis may be primary or secondary. Primary scoliosis may present during infancy or in mid childhood or adolescence. In the infant the scoliosis is usually in the thoracic region and concave to the right. There may be other signs of asymmetry such as plagiocephaly. Spontaneous resolution occurs in 50% during the first year but referral should be made as soon as the diagnosis

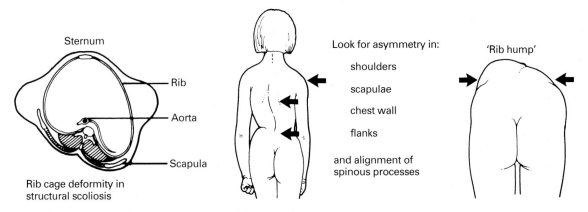

Fig. 14.7 Structural scoliosis, its anatomy and clinical detection.

is suspected as progression may be rapid. Treatment may be lengthy and involve placing the infant in a spinal brace or plaster jacket.

The scoliosis of adolescence is more common in girls, usually affects the mid-thoracic spine, and is concave to the right. Inspection of the spine should be part of the routine examination of the adolescent. It is important to expose the spine fully by removing top clothing in order to make the necessary assessment. A scoliosis, if present, becomes more marked on flexion of the trunk and is often associated with a prominence of the posterior rib cage, this being caused by spinal rotation. Again there should be prompt referral to the orthopaedic surgeon.

FRACTURES

Fractures are a common occurrence in childhood. Most result from accidents and present acutely requiring attendance at hospital for X-ray and orthopaedic management, however particular attention should be paid to fractures occurring during infancy and in the toddler age group.

Non-accidental injury continues to be a problem of diagnosis (see p. 360). Medical awareness of the condition, then termed the 'battered child syndrome', was raised in 1962 by the paediatrician Henry Kemp and radiologist John Caffey. A high index of suspicion is necessary to arrive at the diagnosis of non-accidental injury but it is also important to avoid an inquisitorial approach towards parents who, following a genuine accident to their child, are feeling guilty and are consequently vulnerable to further emotional distress. It is important to take time at presentation of the child with a physical injury to obtain a detailed history of the event and to assess the interval between injury and presentation for advice. If there is doubt about the type of injury and the history of the event or an unexplained delay in presentation then further paediatric assessment must be obtained. The younger the child the more urgent the need for close supervision, and there should be a low threshold for admitting children in the first year of life to allow calm and rational assessment of the situation.

Fractures in young children tend to be of the greenstick variety. Suspicion is raised by the finding of spiral fractures which may be related to twisting type injuries (Table 17.2). There may be an associated pattern of bruising which would point to ill-treatment of the child. Fractures of the skull require admission for observation. Significant head injury, whether or not there is a fracture of the skull, also requires supervision, very often in hospital, particularly if there is associated drowsiness or vomiting. The ready availability of CT imaging has made management of head injury considerably easier but the need for close clinical observation remains.

The child presenting with a limp or decreased use of the upper limb associated with pain may have sustained an injury, not necessarily witnessed by parents or related to maltreatment. Painful swinging of young children by the upper limb or forceful jerking of the upper limb may lead to subluxation of the head of the radius. There is likely to be pain at the time of injury although this may subside. There will be limitation of full extension of the elbow and supination of the forearm. X-ray may not be helpful. Reduction of the subluxation is usually easily accomplished and restores full movement to the forearm.

Stress fractures

Stress fractures do occur in children, particularly at adolescence in those pursuing strenuous physical activity. The most common site is the metatarsal, giving rise to pain on walking and a limb with localised tenderness.

CONGENITAL SKELETAL ANOMALIES

As individual problems these conditions are rare. As a group they are important because they give rise to long-term disability of varying degree and require attention, particularly during the child's school years.

Goldenhar's syndrome

In this condition there are:

• hemivertebrae, which may give rise to scoliosis

- abnormalities of the ear with absent external auditory canal, deformed pinna and deafness
- asymmetry of the face with poorly developed mandible
- absent radii with radial club hand in some cases.

Skeletal asymmetry

There may be hemidystrophy with relative impairment of growth of the upper and lower limbs in association with congenital hemiplegia. Hemihypertrophy is a feature of intrauterine growth retardation syndrome (Russell–Silver syndrome) and Beckwith–Wiedemann syndrome which may be associated with Wilms' tumour.

Hypochondroplasic syndromes may lead to short stature. There may be evidence of the condition on X-ray of the lumbar spine where the normally increasing interpedical distance between L1 and L5 is absent.

DISORDERS OF JOINT AND BONES

Conditions affecting the skeletal system usually present with pain on movement, difficulty with weight-bearing, swelling or deformity of the limb or joints, or a combination of these factors. There may be an associated systemic disturbance, particularly fever.

Acute infections

Septic arthritis

Septic arthritis may occur throughout childhood but it is most common below the age of 3 years. Any joint may be affected. Infection of the peripheral joints is more easily detected; infections of hips and spine may not be evident initially on presentation.

The earlier the diagnosis of a septic arthritis is made the better the outcome. The infection may arise following a penetrating injury but it is more usually blood borne and there is often no obvious precipitating cause. There may be a coincidental history of minor injury.

Clinical features. The onset of a septic arthritis is usually sudden and the child complains of pain which may be associated with restrictive movement and lack of weight-bearing. The affected joint is swollen and tender with markedly restricted movement and pain on passive movement. Septic arthritis of the hip may be more difficult to diagnose.

The most common infecting organisms are *Staphylococcus*, *Streptococcus* and *Haemophilus*; the *Salmonella* organisms are less common.

Assessment of the hip joint may be difficult, particularly in a young child. The leg may be held flexed at the hip and internally rotated. It may be difficult to extend the leg fully, but if this is possible then careful assessment of passive internal and external rotation of the hip joint is a sensitive test and may detect slight limitation of passive movement on comparison of the affected side with the normal side. The other large joints present with more obvious evidence of swelling, often accompanied by rubor and erythema.

Management. It is essential that early diagnosis is made. A full blood count may give evidence of a raised white cell count with neutrophilia; the erythrocyte sedimentation rate (ESR) and C-reactive protein (CRP) are also raised. Early referral for specialist opinion is required for investigation, including a blood culture, before embarking on appropriate antibiotic treatment. It may be necessary to aspirate or surgically explore the joint.

Osteomyelitis (Figure 14.8)

It may be difficult to differentiate a septic arthritis from osteomyelitis as the infection frequently occurs around the epiphysis. These conditions may have similar presenting features. On examination there is likely to be localised bony tenderness which may or may not be associated with swelling. There is usually an acute onset with fever and general malaise.

Early referral to hospital is indicated if osteomyelitis is suspected. Investigation may include exploration of the infected bone, and treatment by intravenous antibiotics may be necessary.

Radiological evidence of osteomyelitis is often not seen early in the condition; a normal X-ray

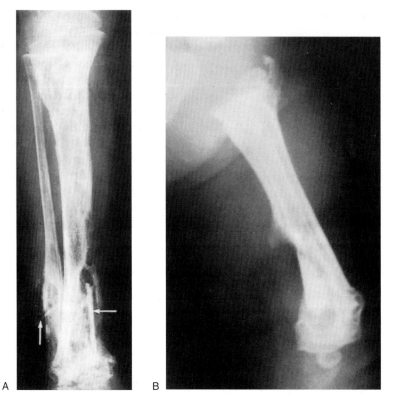

Fig. 14.8 A: Advanced osteomyelitis involving the whole of the right tibia and lower end of the fibula. Note sequestrum in tibia and further sequestrum being extruded from the fibula (arrows). B: Osteomyelitis of the femur and septic arthritis of the hip in a neonate.

therefore does not exclude the diagnosis, but bone scans may be helpful.

Irritable hip

This is an accepted but somewhat unsatisfactory term for a common symptom of childhood. The child starts to complain of pain on walking; this is often associated with a limp and reluctance to weight bear. A predisposing incident or unusual activity may not be recalled; there is no systemic disturbance. The pain may be located to the knee.

On examination there is likely to be an abnormality of gait with a greater or lesser degree of discomfort. On the couch the position of the leg may indicate spasm of the muscles around the hip joint. There may be relatively minor signs on formal examination of the hip joint but impairment of internal rotation is one of the more sensitive ways of assessing the joint. The most important differential diagnosis is that of septic arthritis; referral for an orthopaedic opinion is required in cases where there is any doubt.

The aetiology of the irritable hip syndrome has not been determined but it is likely to be a ligamentous or minor capsular injury. This condition usually resolves after a few days of bed rest. Initially the addition of leg traction is sometimes beneficial.

Reactive arthritis

This is a group of conditions in which there is arthralgia or arthritis associated with infection but the joints do not necessarily show any evidence of an infecting organism.

Rheumatic fever (see p. 111)

This is characteristically flitting in nature. The large joints—knees, ankles, elbows and wrists—are affected, the small joints being spared. The joints may be extremely painful with associated swelling and redness. Less frequently the joints are only minimally affected, giving rise to arthralgia and no abnormal signs. The joint may be affected for 2–3 days, and more than one joint may be affected at any one time.

Postviral arthritis

The most common arthritis/arthralgia as a single entity in childhood is non-specific postviral arthritis. It usually presents with pain affecting the main joints associated with soft tissue swelling. Both large and small joints may be affected, and a number of joints may be involved at any one time with variation of the degree of discomfort.

There is usually a definite history of a previous febrile illness, 10–14 days beforehand. Investigation may find evidence of a viral infection: parvovirus is an important cause and may give a remitting/relapsing pattern of joint symptoms over a number of months. Rubella, although now an uncommon condition with modern immunisation schedules, may also cause a postinfective arthritis. It is sometimes possible to obtain the virus from the joint effusion. Other organisms which may cause a reactive arthritis are enteric infections such as Salmonella (*typhimurium* or *enteritidis*), Campylobacter and Yersinia, or Mycoplasma infection.

Kawasaki's disease (mucocutaneous lymph node syndrome – see p. 112)

Lyme disease

Lyme disease is an infection caused by a spirochaete, *Borrelia burgdorferi*, which is carried by a tick (species of Ixodes). It was first reported from Lyme in America and has now been described in Australia and Europe. The condition is seasonal and geographical, the tick living on deer, cattle and rodents. The illness may occur at any age and is not confined to childhood. The initial phase is a rash with fever although the tick bite itself may go unnoticed. The history of the tick bite (if it can be obtained) is of a red area which expands over a week to produce an annular lesion—erythema chronicum migrans. At this stage there may be high fever and general malaise with lymphadenopathy, muscle and joint pains.

The arthritis of Lyme disease develops after two or three weeks and mainly affects the large joints, particularly the knee, elbows and shoulders. The arthritis may last a few weeks or have an intermittent relapsing remitting pattern.

There may be cardiac and neurological complications of this disease, but both are rare in childhood.

The diagnosis depends on obtaining the appropriate history supported by a positive immunofluorescence test.

The complications can be reduced or avoided by early treatment. The organism is sensitive to penicillin and erythromycin (tetracycline is probably the drug of choice but its use is contraindicated in children).

Henoch–Schönlein purpura

Schönlein described the association of purpura and arthritis, Henoch that of purpura and gastrointestinal disease. The more important association may be that of renal involvement. The condition is one of widespread vasculitis affecting the capillaries of the joints, skin, gastrointestinal tract and kidneys. The platelet count and clotting studies are normal.

Clinical features. Clinically the condition presents primarily with joint pain, skin rash or abdominal pain, or a combination of these symptoms. The arthritis commonly involves the large joints, often more than one at a time. The soft tissue around the joint is frequently swollen. The rash is not a true purpura, being slightly raised, and characteristically is prominent in the skin of the dependent areas, particularly the gluteal region and around the ankle joints (see Fig. 16.6, p. 351). The rash may also occur on the upper limbs. The abdominal pain may be severe and accompanied by gastrointestinal bleeding, giving rise to melaena or, less commonly, haematemesis; intussusception may be a further complication.

There is frequently involvement of the kidneys. This often results only in microscopic haematuria but it is vital that this aspect of the condition is identified and closely followed up to ensure complete resolution.

It may be possible to look after children with Henoch–Schönlein purpura at home, but investigation to exclude other causes of purpuric rash needs to be undertaken; this may involve a full blood count and renal function check with regular measurement of blood pressure, examination of urine for protein and blood and serum creatinine estimation. The degree of systemic illness and, in particular, abdominal pain is variable—some children have severe symptoms and these can be of variable intensity, giving fluctuations in the degree of illness. Severe symptoms and/or significant and persistent haematuria are indications for paediatric referral. Renal involvement with haematuria and proteinuria, in association with severe gastrointestinal symptoms which may give rise to further protein loss from the alimentary tract, can lead to hypoproteinaemia and consequent oedema.

Management. The condition is self limiting and the prognosis is good. Some children have a very difficult course with remissions and relapses, however, and in this situation considerable support is necessary for both child and family. It is essential to follow the condition until there has been complete resolution of symptoms, in particular microscopic haematuria. The child should be further assessed at 6 and 12 months after resolution of the haematuria, with measurement of blood pressure and confirmation that the haematuria and proteinuria have resolved.

Juvenile chronic arthritis (JCA)

This is a disease of childhood, by definition starting under the age of 16 years and giving rise to joint disease of longer than 3 months' duration. The aetiology is uncertain. There may be a history of injury but it is likely that this just brings the illness to attention. The principal symptom relates to the joints; characteristically the pain and stiffness is worse in the morning.

There are three main types. These have distinctive patterns but there is a degree of overlap of natural history.

Pauciarticular (oligoarticular)

This is the most common form of chronic arthritis of childhood. By definition four joints or fewer are affected. It accounts for approximately 50% of children with JCA and there are three subgroups:

Subgroup 1. This affects young children, usually under the age of 6 years, and is markedly more common in girls. The onset of the arthritis in this age group can be subtle with minimal signs and symptoms. The parent may notice joint swelling. There may be a limp. The joint most commonly affected is the knee, followed by the ankle, elbow and small joints of the hands. There are no systemic symptoms, and in particular no fever. On examination the affected joint has limited movement, often accompanied by discomfort with soft tissue swelling, but not necessarily an effusion. On careful examination other joints may show some soft tissue swelling.

This group of children have a high incidence of antinuclear antibody (ANA) and there is a strong association with iridocyclitis. The presentation of uveitis may be subtle and regular ophthalmic examination by slit lamp is essential to detect the early involvement of eye disease. The long-term outlook in this group is good and the joint disease gradually resolves in the majority of children. Iridocyclitis, if it develops, may persist longer than the joint disease.

Subgroup 2. This affects older children, usually over the age of 9 years, and is more common in boys. The knees and ankles are most frequently affected and there may be an associated plantar fasciitis or tendonitis, particularly involving the Achilles tendon. There is a strong possibility of later involvement of the sacro-iliac joint. These children have an increased incidence of tissue type HLA B27 and are negative for ANA.

Subgroup 3. This is uncommon, presents at any age, usually affects few joints asymmetrically and has a strong link with psoriasis, of which there may be a family history. The joint disease tends to be destructive and progressive.

Polyarticular

This affects about 20% of children with arthritis; by definition five or more joints are affected. The joints usually affected are knees, ankles and wrists and the metacarpal and proximal phalangeal joints in a symmetrical pattern. The cervical spine and temporo-mandibular joints may also be involved. The IgM rheumatoid factor differentiates polyarticular arthritis into two types; those who are negative for Rh factor have a more favourable outcome.

RhF positive polyarticular disease is more common in girls. The onset is usually later, after the age of 12 years, and the condition tends to present with involvement of the small joints of the hand. RhF positive polyarticular disease tends to be progressive and severe.

Polyarticular with systemic onset

This is the classical Still's disease; approximately 10% of children with JRA present in this manner.

Clinical features. Characteristically the illness presents with high fever (39.5°C or greater) which peaks daily, often in the evening. The child is generally very unwell, particularly during the febrile episodes, and is relatively improved during troughs of fever. There is lymphadenopathy, splenomegaly and frequently an erythematous rash which is fluctuating in extent, macular and mainly affects the trunk and proximal part of the limbs. There may be a pale rim to the discrete areas of the rash. The rash may show the characteristics of exacerbation on skin pressure (Koebner phenomenon).

The investigation of children with chronic arthritis is characterised by a high ESR. There is often an accompanying anaemia with a raised white count, and the platelet count may also be high. Serology has been mentioned above; see also Table 14.1. The differential diagnosis will include postinfective arthritis and, in the systemic disease, any condition giving rise to pyrexial illness lasting for two weeks or more.

Management. It is appropriate to refer the child for a specialist opinion. Further investigation is likely to be required and treatment may be long term.

The first line drug treatment is with nonsteroidal anti-inflammatory agents, in particular naproxen. The dosage is 10–15 mg/kg per day and may be administered 12-hourly. Ibuprofen can be tried if this is not successful. Aspirin, which was formerly used, has the disadvantages of gastric toxicity, its possible relationship with Reye's disease and the occasional problem of inducing an asthma attack.

Children with more aggressive joint disease may require treatment with penicillamine or long-term steroid or immunosuppressive drugs, of which methotrexate is probably the most effective and best tolerated in the long term.

Table 14.1 Differentiation of subgroups of juvenile chronic arthritis

	Age at onset	Joints	Uveitis	RhF	ANA
Systemic disease	Throughout childhood	Any	Rare	Negative	No
Polyarticular type 1	Throughout childhood, usually early	Any	Rare	Negative	25%
Polyarticular type 2	Late childhood	Small joints, later any	Rare	100%	50–75%
Pauciarticular group 1	Early childhood	Large joints	High risk, especially ANA positive	Negative—good prognosis Positive—severe disease	40–75%
Pauciarticular group 2	Late childhood	Large joints lower limbs	10–20% acute	Negative	No
Pauciarticular group 3	Childhood	Asymmetric large and small	10–20% chronic	Negative	15–50%

Supportive management is also extremely important for children with chronic arthritis. Pain and associated muscle spasm give rise to impaired movement of joints with a tendency to flexion spasm. This in turn leads to contractures of both capsule and tendons, disuse of the muscles and wasting and weakness—a self-perpetuating cycle. It is extremely important to try to alleviate pain and encourage physical activity; the role of the physiotherapist is essential. One also must take into account the effect of chronic disease on both child and family and the importance of supporting the emotional aspects of a fluctuating and possibly long-term illness. Encouragement is required to ensure consistent activity and physiotherapy. There may be a tendency for denial both from the child and the parents which leads to non-compliance with treatment. It is important to continue with analgesia and relieve pain so that physical activity ensures a full range of movement in the affected joints. Attention must also be paid to schooling, limiting the amount of time missed and ensuring appropriate support within the classroom with regard to seating and gross and fine motor skills, particularly hand writing.

Other systemic causes of joint disease include inflammatory bowel disease, haemophilia and sickle cell disease. It is also important to remember that limb pain referable to long bones or joints may be a presenting symptom of leukaemia.

NON-SPECIFIC LIMB PAINS OF CHILDHOOD

Children of all ages may complain of pain, usually related to thighs or shins, which commonly wakes them at night. The children have full activity by day with no other symptoms or signs on history or examination. Reassurance and advice to parents to avoid reinforcing attention seeking is all that is usually required. The pain is sometimes referred to as 'growing pains', an unsatisfactory term. The aetiology is unknown. Treatment consists of giving sympathy and massaging the limb with as brief an interaction between parent and child as possible.

Paracetamol or aspirin may be used in as low a dose as possible.

REFLEX SYMPATHETIC DYSTROPHY

This condition tends to affect the distal part of the limb, most commonly the upper limb, in school age children or young adolescents. There is complaint of continual pain affecting the limb, very often the hand, exacerbated by any movement. The problem may result in impaired writing and hence lack of progress at school.

On examination there are impaired active movements and pain on passive movements of the limb. There may be vascular changes with mottling of the skin and subcutaneous puffiness. Lack of movement of the limb exacerbates the problems, giving rise to a vicious circle which may lead to emotional benefit to the child and associated 'belle indifference'.

Management consists of a firm explanation that the problem is secondary to lack of movement; graduated physical activity is required, and it is very often better initiated under the supervision of a physiotherapist. Analgesia is helpful during the recovery.

SYSTEMIC LUPUS ERYTHEMATOSUS (SLE)

This condition is rare in childhood; the peak incidence is in adolescence. There is a markedly increased frequency in females, particularly after puberty when the ratio is 10:1. Clinically presentation is characterised by an episodic pattern and involvement of variable and multiple organ systems. The onset may be as a generalised illness with fever of uncertain origin associated with arthritis, arthralgia or myalgia, and involvement of the lungs, heart, kidneys, central nervous system or skin. There are a variety of skin rashes mainly involving the hands, feet and nail folds. Raynaud's phenomenon and the butterfly rash seen in adults occur less often in childhood.

Investigations are likely to show a moderate anaemia, possibly autoimmune in nature, with a raised ESR; leukopenia and thrombocytopenia may occur. Serological investigation will help in diagnosis: IgM rheumatoid factor is often positive but the most usual finding is that of a positive antinuclear antibody titre (ANA), without which the diagnosis would be doubtful. Antibody to single strand DNA is often present. Treatment is difficult and complicated and requires referral to a specialist unit.

FURTHER READING

Weiner D S 1993 Pediatric orthopedics. Churchill Livingstone, New York

15

Paediatric surgery

S. Capps

PROBLEMS OF THE NEWBORN

Diaphragmatic hernia

Congenital diaphragmatic hernias occur at the oesophageal hiatus, posterolaterally (Bochdalek hernia) and retrosternally (Morgagni hernia). The most common type is the posterolateral hernia; it results from a partial or complete absence of the diaphragm which occurs on the left side in 85% of cases. Abdominal viscera herniate into the chest and there is associated pulmonary hypoplasia. Diaphragmatic hernia is commonly diagnosed antenatally by maternal ultrasound.

Diagnosis

Respiratory distress and cyanosis occur at a variable time after birth. The more severe cases present at birth, but some may not be noticed for months. The abdomen is scaphoid and there is mediastinal displacement away from the side of the hernia. There is an absence of breath sounds on the side of the hernia. The diagnosis is confirmed by chest X-ray.

Differential diagnosis:

- Congenital lung malformations
- Cyst adenomatoid malformation of the lung.

Management

Following resuscitation, which includes ventilation, paralysis and the passage of a nasogastric tube, the infant should be transferred to a regional unit. It may take several days for a child to become stable, and stability should be achieved before surgical intervention is undertaken. The diaphragmatic defect is closed directly or, if large, is repaired using a prosthetic patch. Non-rotation of the gut is common, and after the intestines have been returned to the abdominal cavity the base of the mesentery is widened, placing the small bowel on the right side of the abdomen and the colon on the left. In spite of advances in neonatal ventilation and resuscitation, mortality remains high, mainly because of pulmonary hypoplasia and pulmonary hypertension. Approximately 60% of babies survive.

Oesophageal atresia

Oesophageal atresia has an incidence of 1 in 3000 live births. A history of maternal polyhydramnios is common. The newborn baby presents with excess mucus and mild respiratory distress. The most common form of oesophageal atresia (Figure 15.1) has an associated distal trachea–oesophageal fistula (85%).

Diagnosis

Confirmation of the suspected diagnosis is made by attempting to pass an 8F oesophageal tube, which is seen to curl up in the proximal oesophageal pouch on a chest X-ray. The presence of air in the stomach and small bowel confirms the presence of a fistula. Fluid aspirated through the tube will not be acidic when tested with litmus paper.

Management

The neonate should be nursed head up to pool secretions in the upper blind-ending oesophageal pouch, which is kept empty by continuous low pressure suction, thus minimising the risks of aspiration of saliva. Minimal handling and the avoidance of bagging via a face mask will reduce the problems of stomach distension and splinting of the diaphragm caused by air entering the distal oesophagus via a trachea–oesophageal fistula.

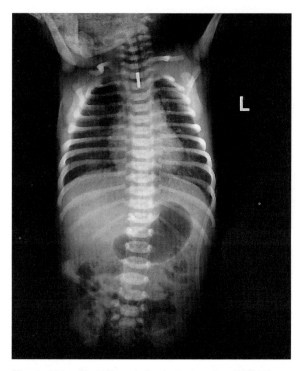

Figure 15.1 Chest X-ray in tracheo–oesophageal fistula showing nasogastric tube in blind upper oesophageal sac and air in stomach confirming fistula between distal oesophagus and trachea.

Associated anomalies

These are common and include anorectal malformations, hemivertebrae, radial dysplasia, and renal and heart abnormalities.

Treatment

When the infant is stable, and following transfer to a regional unit, a right posterolateral thoracotomy and extrapleural approach is made to divide the fistula and perform a primary oesophageal anastomosis. If the oesophageal gap is large, a delayed primary repair or oesophageal replacement is necessary.

Complications

After oesophageal repair in the neonatal period, stricture formation at the site of anastomosis occurs in approximately 25% of cases and requires oesophageal dilatation. Abnormal peristalsis at the site of atresia is also common; food needs to be liquidised, chewed well or accompanied by frequent drinks during meals.

Neonatal bowel obstruction

There may be a history of maternal polyhydramnios. Antenatal ultrasound scans show dilated bowel.

Causes

- Atresia
- Malrotation and midgut volvulus
- Meconium ileus
- Hirschsprung's disease.

Clinical features

Bile-stained vomiting should always alert the clinician to the possibility of bowel obstruction. The condition should be investigated urgently and, in the absence of sepsis, considered to be bowel obstruction until proved otherwise. Abdominal distension may occur and is usually confined to the upper abdomen in cases of duodenal atresia. Delay in passage of meconium beyond the first 24 hours may be secondary to Hirschsprung's disease. Infants with anorectal anomalies may pass meconium via the urethra or vaginal introitus or through a cutaneous fistula in the perineum.

Investigation

Abdominal X-ray shows distended bowel and fluid levels. The classical appearance in duodenal atresia is a double bubble from dilatation of the stomach and proximal duodenum. Two or three loops of distended bowel may indicate jejunal atresia. Where there are many dilated loops of bowel, this may be from ileal atresia. Calcification is sometimes seen following antenatal perforation of the gut causing meconium peritonitis, and is seen in complicated meconium ileus and in some cases of atresia. Free gas in the peritoneal cavity indicates postnatal perforation. Absence

of gas beyond the proximal duodenum may suggest volvulus of the midgut secondary to malrotation; this condition can be confirmed by upper gastrointestinal contrast studies.

Management

When the diagnosis of neonatal bowel obstruction has been confirmed, the stomach should be decompressed using an 8F nasogastric tube. Fluid and air is aspirated from the stomach and the tube left on free drainage. An intravenous dextrose infusion should be started and the child transferred to a specialist unit.

Meconium ileus

Approximately 10% of babies with cystic fibrosis present with meconium ileus. There is distal ileal obstruction caused by inspissated bowel contents, with a foamy appearance in the right lower abdomen. A barium enema shows an unused or microcolon. Gastrografin enemas administered in a specialist unit are used to dislodge the sticky inspissated meconium and thus relieve bowel obstruction without the need for surgery. Complicated meconium ileus may be suspected by the finding of calcification on X-rays or the presence of free gas in the peritoneum. Surgery is required in these cases. The diagnosis of cystic fibrosis is confirmed by raised serum immunoreactive trypsin (IRT) and a sweat test.

Hirschsprung's disease

This condition is characterised by an aganglionic segment of bowel which extends from the anus through the rectum and into the sigmoid colon (Figure 15.2). It has an incidence of 1 in 5000 live births. In 10% of cases, the condition may affect all of the colon. There is delayed passage of meconium beyond 24 hours; the differential diagnosis includes functional obstruction, seen in premature babies and following birth asphyxia, and the meconium plug syndrome. The condition is confirmed by rectal suction biopsy in a specialist unit, and the pathologist assesses the rectal mucosa and submucosa for the presence of

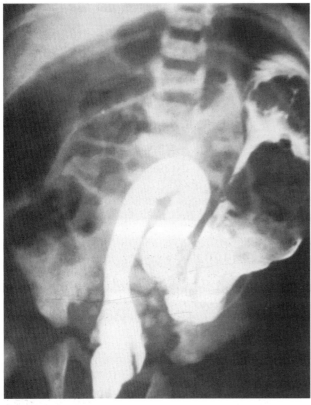

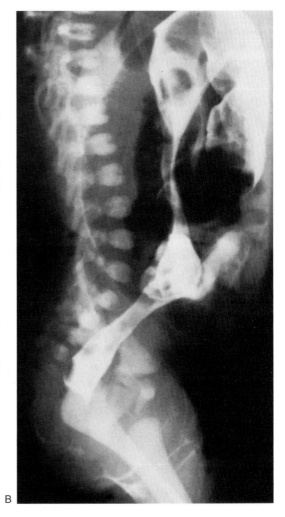

Figure 15.2 A,B: Hirschsprung's disease. There is a fairly long aganglionic segment. B: Lateral view.

ganglia and abnormal nerve trunks. Following confirmation of the diagnosis, treatment consists of excising the abnormal aganglionic bowel and anastomosing bowel which has normal innervation to the anal canal. This procedure is increasingly carried out as a primary procedure in the neonatal period.

Malrotation

In malrotation the base of the mesentery is narrow, the caecum being close to the retroperitoneal attachment of the duodenum, and the duodenal jejunal flexure is to the right of the midline. The midgut is liable to twist on this narrow mesentery, causing volvulus and subsequent ischaemia from the second part of the duodenum to the mid transverse colon. Bile-stained vomiting is caused by occlusion of the duodenum at the base of the twisted bowel. In older children vomiting is often accompanied by intermittent abdominal pain and pallor. Urgent surgical intervention is required to untwist the bowel and widen the base of the mesentery.

Anorectal anomalies

The anus does not open in the correct position. In high (supralevator) anomalies, it opens into the urethra in the male, or into the vagina in the female. In low anomalies, the bowel may end in an anocutaneous fistula. A single perineal opening occurs in a cloacal anomaly, when bladder, vagina and rectum emerge together.

Associated anomalies include:

- oesophageal atresia
- abnormalities of the renal tract (40%)
- vertebral (sacral) agenesis
- congenital heart disease.

Low anomalies can be treated by a perineal operation in the first few days of life. High and intermediate anomalies usually require a preliminary colostomy which relieves the bowel obstruction and allows the bowel to resume a normal size, followed by a pull-through operation such as a posterior sagittal ano-rectoplasty (PSARP) at the age of a few months. In the long term patients may have problems with faecal incontinence and constipation.

Necrotising enterocolitis (NEC)

Necrotising enterocolitis occurs most commonly in premature babies and is often associated with hypoxia or prolonged periods of hypotension. The aetiology of NEC is unknown, but poor gut perfusion leading to areas of necrosis and secondary bacterial infection affects the bowel wall over a variable length. Full thickness necrosis of the bowel wall may cause perforation.

Diagnosis

The neonate appears sick and there are often signs of sepsis with temperature instability, poor peripheral perfusion, a distended abdomen and increasing volumes of gastric aspirate, which may become bile stained. Later blood is seen in the stools and a plain abdominal X-ray reveals the characteristic sign of intramural bowel gas (Figure 15.3). If perforation of the bowel occurs, free gas may be seen above the liver or outlining the ligamentum teres.

Management

Following initial resuscitation using intravenous fluids including colloids, antibiotics such as

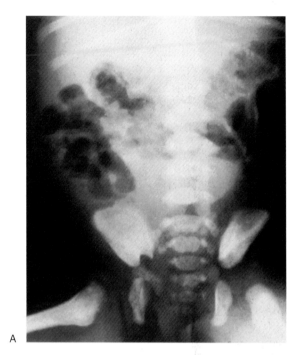

A

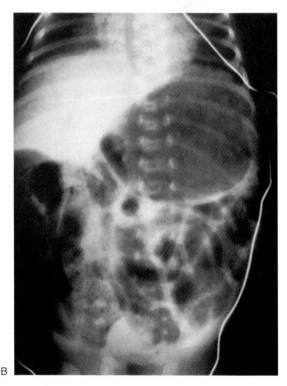

B

Figure 15.3 A,B: Necrotising enterocolitis. A: Note the appearance of the faeces in the gut and air in the bowel wall. B: There is gas in the portal tracts in the liver.

gentamicin, penicillin and metronidazole, and the passage of a nasogastric tube, enteral feeding is stopped for 10 days and nutrition is given intravenously. Most neonates respond to medical management; surgery is considered in those who fail to improve or develop a perforation or a mass causing bowel obstruction which fails to resolve. Stricture formation in the affected bowel, particularly the colon, occurs in 20% of cases.

ABDOMINAL WALL DEFECTS

These conditions are particularly amenable to antenatal diagnosis during maternal ultrasound examination. Antenatal counselling for the parents as well as planned delivery in a specialist centre is possible in these cases. Caesarean section is not usually necessary.

Associated anomalies include:

- congenital heart disease
- renal malformations
- Beckwith–Wiedemann syndrome.

Exomphalos

This is a congenital herniation of abdominal viscera into the base of the umbilical cord. The exomphalos consists of a sac of amniotic membrane and peritoneum covering the enclosed viscera.

Gastroschisis

The abdominal wall defect is to the right of the umbilicus and is usually small. There is no sac. The bowel loops are thickened and matted, having been in contact with amniotic fluid which contains urine. Pressure necrosis of the emerging bowel and its mesentery at the base of the defect may cause an atresia.

Management

The exposed bowel should be wrapped in clingfilm to minimise heat and fluid losses. The film is best wrapped around the body with the bowel supported on the anterior surface of the abdomen to optimise venous and lymphatic drainage of the exposed gut. Following the passage of a nasogastric tube and the setting up of an intravenous infusion, the child is prepared for surgical closure of the defect as soon as possible. In cases where primary abdominal wall closure is not possible because of the small scaphoid abdomen and the dilated thick-walled gut, a temporary silo is constructed to accommodate the bowel. Delayed secondary closure of the abdomen is usually possible within 1 week.

The umbilicus

An *umbilical polyp* is most often caused by a granuloma and can be treated with silver nitrate or, if large and pedunculated, by simple ligation.

Persistence of the *vitello-intestinal duct* may cause an umbilical discharge of small bowel content. The bowel mucosa at the umbilicus has a bright red velvety appearance and does not respond to the local treatment used for a granuloma. The vitello-intestinal duct is in continuity with the terminal ileum and should be excised.

A *urachal fistula* is an abnormal connection between the urachus at the fundus of the bladder and the umbilicus. It is an unusual abnormality and is sometimes associated with bladder outlet obstruction such as posterior urethral valves.

Umbilical hernias are common, especially in children of African and West Indian ancestry. There is a defect in the linea alba underlying the umbilical cicatrix which may be several centimetres in diameter. Most umbilical hernias resolve spontaneously in the first 3–4 years, and surgical closure should be reserved for those that persist after this age. They seldom cause any discomfort and strangulation is rare. Parental anxiety can normally be alleviated by a careful explanation of the natural history of the condition.

Supra-umbilical hernias, like epigastric hernias, occur through a defect in the linea alba above the umbilicus and do not close spontaneously. They sometimes cause pain when extraperitoneal fat becomes trapped in the narrow neck of the linea alba defect; this is relieved by surgical repair.

NEURAL TUBE DEFECTS (see also p. 65)

These include spina bifida (defect of the vertebral neural arch), anencephaly, encephalocele and hydrocephalus. They are becoming less common with improvements in nutrition and antenatal screening.

Spina bifida occulta is a defect in the bony arch with no meningeal or skin involvement, and is most often an incidental finding seen on X-rays of the lumbosacral spine.

A *meningocele* is a skin-covered lesion with cystic protrusion of the meninges but without underlying neurological involvement. In cases of lipoma of the cauda equina, fatty tissue surrounds the cord and nerve roots and may cause tethering of the nerves during growth. There may be a primary neurological defect which becomes worse because of traction on the cord and nerve roots.

In *meningomyelocele* the cord is abnormal and adherent to a plaque of tissue on the surface of the back. The neurological deficit depends upon the level and nature of the lesion and ranges from pure sacral lesions with only bladder and anal involvement, to total paralysis caudal to a thoracic defect.

Approximately 70% of cases of meningomyelocele develop *hydrocephalus* secondary to an associated Arnold–Chiari malformation, where there is displacement of the hindbrain and fourth ventricle through the foramen magnum into the vertebral canal. Hydrocephalus is also caused by other obstructions of the cerebrospinal fluid pathway, or occurs secondary to intracranial bleeding or meningitis. Hydrocephalus is managed by the insertion of a valve system and ventriculo-atrial or ventriculoperitoneal shunting.

Most cases of meningomyelocele are referred to a surgical centre for closure of the defect within 48 hours of birth to minimise the risk of infection. In cases where the defect is large, extending over several vertebral bodies and high in the thoraco-lumbar region leading to severe paralysis of the lower limbs, or in the presence of other associated major abnormalities, extensive counselling and discussion between the parents and attending clinicians is necessary.

Orthopaedic assessment is often best done by an experienced physiotherapist who will record lower limb movement and tone and supervise passive manipulation of fixed deformities. The urinary tract is investigated using ultrasound scans; attention should be directed towards making sure that the bladder empties, if necessary by introducing clean intermittent catheterisation at an early stage.

Shunt complications include blockage and infection. The signs and symptoms of blockage are headache, vomiting, altered level of consciousness, squint, increased tension in the anterior fontanelle and papilloedema. Acute blockage requires urgent referral to a specialist unit for revision of the shunt. Infection of a shunt system is most commonly caused by *Staphylococcus epidermidis* and presents with malaise and low grade fever.

Urological management

Abnormal bladder function leads to urinary tract infections which, in the presence of reflux, may cause renal damage. Urinary incontinence is also a common complication of bladder and bladder sphincter dysfunction. Annual ultrasound scans are used to assess renal growth and bladder emptying. Isotope renograms can detect renal scars (DMSA). Urodynamics are the most useful method of assessing bladder function and demonstrate vesico-ureteric reflux and bladder outflow obstruction. Overactive detrusor contractions are most often treated using the anticholinergic oxybutinin. Incomplete bladder emptying is managed by clean intermittent catheterisation which can be done by the patient if there is sufficient manual dexterity.

INGUINO-SCROTAL PROBLEMS

The testis descends to the scrotum during the final trimester. The peritoneal protrusion from the abdomen through the inguinal canal and into the scrotum normally obliterates. If this processus vaginalis persists, allowing peritoneal fluid to pass into the scrotum, a communicating hydrocele will form. If the processus vaginalis is wide, bowel will move towards the scrotum and produce a hernia.

Hydroceles. These are common. Most resolve spontaneously by the age of 18 months and surgery is therefore not required unless they persist after this age.

Inguinal hernia. These never resolve spontaneously and should be treated surgically as soon as possible after detection to minimise the risks of bowel incarceration and damage to the testis.

Clinical assessment

Hydroceles are often lax; when they are confined to the scrotum, the spermatic cord can be felt above the swelling. They are painless and there is no impulse on crying. In toddlers and older boys the swelling tends to enlarge later in the day, and hydroceles are also more noticeable during viral illnesses when the volume of intra-peritoneal fluid may increase.

An inguinal hernia often takes the form of an intermittent swelling extending from the inguinal region towards the scrotum. Only large hernias reach the scrotum. Inguinal hernias can be reduced by gently squeezing the hernia in line with the inguinal canal, as if trying to push a sponge through a key hole. The bowel can be felt and sometimes heard to gurgle as it slips back into the abdominal cavity. If the hernia will not reduce and it is tense and tender, urgent surgical referral is indicated.

Incarcerated or strangulated inguinal hernia

This is most common in the first 2 years of life and is a surgical emergency. Pressure on the testicular vessels produced by the incarcerated bowel within the confined inguinal canal may cause testicular necrosis and subsequent atrophy. If a hernia remains irreducible, the resulting bowel obstruction causes abdominal distension and vomiting.

The differential diagnosis of inguinal swelling includes:

• encysted hydrocele—non-tender, not inflamed and without signs of bowel obstruction

• lymphadenitis lateral to external inguinal ring.

The treatment of incarcerated hernias is reduction under sedation and analgesia.

Treatment of inguinal hernia

Infants with inguinal hernias should have a herniotomy as soon as possible, preferably in a specialist centre where skill and expertise minimise the risks associated with anaesthesia and surgery. In premature infants, especially those born before 32 weeks' gestation, the incidence of contralateral hernia is significant and exploration of both sides under one anaesthetic should be considered. In girls, the inguinal sac may contain the ovary and fallopian tube.

Varicocele

This occurs in early puberty and is caused by dilatation of the pampiniform plexus of veins in the spermatic chord. It is usually left sided. Most varicoceles are asymptomatic but some produce a dull ache which may be worse after exercise. A varicocele may affect spermatogenesis as the testis is kept warmer than normal. Varicoceles may rarely be caused by obstruction of the testicular veins by tumours such as Wilms'. A renal ultrasound scan should be requested. The patient is best examined standing up and the appearance and feel of the dilated veins has often been described as being like a bag of worms.

No treatment is required if the varicocele is asymptomatic, and if the testis is normal in size and shows no signs of atrophy. Untreated cases may result in infertility. Treatment is by high ligation of the testicular veins, either by an open procedure or laparoscopically.

Cryptorchidism

The testis requires to be 2 or 3°C cooler than the body for spermatogenesis to occur. The testis may be arrested in its descent at any point between its origin within the abdomen and the scrotum. In full-term boys the incidence of undescended testes is approximately 2.5%; the condition is more common in the premature, rising to 20% in those born at 30 weeks' gestation. Most of these testes will descend in the first year of life, giving an incidence of 0.9% at one year. Occasionally a testis may be ectopic, when it has strayed from its normal line of descent. The optimal time for surgical treatment is in the second year of life; after this time morphological changes occur in the germ cells.

Examination for undescended testis should be done with the child lying comfortably on a couch in a warm room. One hand should be placed in the iliac fossa and gently but firmly moved in the line of the inguinal canal, thus milking an undescended testis towards the scrotum. The other hand should attempt to palpate the testis and pull it down into the scrotum. The testis should reach the bottom of the scrotum. Retractile testes can be manipulated to the bottom of the scrotum, but are pulled up towards the inguinal region by the cremaster muscle.

Testicular torsion

Torsion occurs suddenly and is painful. The testis and epididymis twist on the spermatic cord, usually within the tunica vaginalis (intravaginal); this is usually associated with an abnormal attachment of the tunica (clapperbell testis) or an undescended testis. Urgent surgical intervention is required within a few hours to prevent irreversible ischaemic damage to the testis. At exploration a gangrenous testis should be excised, but a congested and purple looking testis may improve when the torsion is reduced. The affected testis and the contralateral normal testis should be fixed in the scrotum to prevent recurrence.

Torsion of a testicular appendage (hydatid of Morgagni) presents with more localised pain, and a tender dark nodule may be seen or felt on the upper pole of the testis. Epididymitis in the absence of a urinary tract abnormality such as neuropathic bladder or vesico-ureteric reflux is uncommon in young boys, and a swollen, tender testis and hemiscrotum should be assumed to be caused by torsion until proved otherwise.

Idiopathic scrotal oedema

Redness and oedema of the scrotum extends onto the adjacent perineum and inguinal region. The cause is unknown but there is often a raised eosinophil count. It subsides spontaneously within 2–3 days.

Testicular tumours

These include teratomas, rhabdomyosarcomas, yolk sac tumours and orchioblastomas; they present as painless testicular swellings. They are all rare and the child should be referred urgently to a specialist centre.

THE HEAD AND NECK
Inclusion dermoids

These cysts occur at fusion lines, have a yellow-white appearance and contain keratinized epithelial cells. The most common is the external angular dermoid at the lateral end of the eyebrow. Other common sites for inclusion cysts are the anterior and posterior fontanelles, the bridge of the nose and the midline in the neck. These cysts continue to enlarge as the child grows and should be excised.

Pre-auricular sinuses

These are often seen as a small opening on the front of the helix of the ear. If the sinus becomes infected, antibiotics are required followed by complete excision of the sinus, which may extend some distance in front of the ear.

Cervical abscess

Cervical lymphadenitis often results from upper respiratory tract or ear infections. Occasionally the lymph nodes become overwhelmed by infection, resulting in abscess formation. The lesion is red, fluctuant and tender. Antibiotics can prolong the process and produce induration. Once an abscess has localised and begun to point, it should be incised and drained under general anaesthesia. These lesions are most often caused by common bacterial infections but occasionally result from non-tuberculous mycobacterial infections. The latter are most often seen in pre-school children and cause purple or dark red discolouration of the skin. Treatment is by excision of the infected lymph nodes, which are then sent for culture and histology.

Thyroglossal cyst

Midline cervical swellings may be caused by:

- submental lymph nodes—associated with infection in the mouth
- dermoid cysts—slow growing and subcutaneous
- thyroglossal cysts—attached to the hyoid bone
- ectopic thyroid
- goitre—at site of normal thyroid.

Thyroglossal cysts arise from the thyroglossal duct, which may persist following development of the thyroid gland at the base of the tongue (foramen caecum) and its migration into the neck. Thyroglossal cysts often become inflamed because of the connection with the mouth via the thyroglossal duct. Thyroglossal cysts move with the tongue and on swallowing. The cyst and its tract must be excised; because the tract is closely applied to the hyoid bone, the body of the hyoid bone is also excised. Recurrence is likely if the body of the hyoid bone is not excised.

Branchial fistulae/remnants

Persistence of the second branchial cleft may give rise to a blind-ending sinus or a fistula between the tonsillar fossa and the skin overlying the anterior border of the sternomastoid muscle, at the junction of its lower and middle thirds. There may be a discharge of mucus from such fistulae and occasionally they become infected.

Second branchial arch remnants appear as skin tags with underlying cartilage over the lower third of the sternomastoid muscle. Branchial cysts often do not become apparent until later in childhood and are deep to the sternomastoid muscle. Treatment is by excision at any time after the first 6 months of life.

Cystic hygroma

This is a developmental swelling containing lymphatic tissue and may occur in the neck, lips, tongue and axilla and groin. Treatment is usually surgical.

PENIS

Problems with the foreskin are perhaps the most common conditions referred to paediatric surgeons. Preputial adhesions to the glans are normal in early childhood and prevent the foreskin from being fully retractile. Provided there is an adequate opening, no attempt to retract the foreskin should be made before the age of 5. The opening is best assessed by lifting the foreskin away from the pubis (chimney sign). Smegma (desquamated epithelium) accumulates below the adhesions and may cause irritation or be misdiagnosed as a dermoid or sebaceous cyst. Smegma is released as the preputial adhesions separate, and occasionally is mistaken for an infection with a discharge of pus.

Phimosis

Phimosis is a narrowing of the non-retractile foreskin and is physiological in pre-school boys. Circumcision is rarely required for medical reasons before the age of 5. In pathological phimosis, the tip of the foreskin is scarred, white and non-retractile, and surgery is usually required.

Paraphimosis

Paraphimosis occurs when a slightly tight foreskin becomes stuck in the coronal groove following retraction over the glans. The prepuce and glans become swollen, oedematous and painful. Urgent surgical referral is required if the foreskin cannot be advanced over the swollen glans.

Hypospadias

Hypospadias occurs in approximately 1 in 300 boys. The urethra opens on the ventral surface of the penis. The external urethral meatus may be in any position from the perineum to the base of the glans. In the most common type of hypospadias, the meatus is at the corona. Ventral curvature of the erect penis is called chordee. In association with an abnormally sited urethral meatus, there is the typical appearance of excess dorsal foreskin and a deficiency of the ventral foreskin. Ultrasound examination of the renal tract, looking for upper urinary tract anomalies, is only indicated in the more severe forms of hypospadias. Circumcision should be avoided until the urethral defect has been rectified.

The best time to carry out operations for correction of hypospadias is between the ages of 12 and 18 months or, in some more complex cases, after the age of 3. It is often wise to avoid subjecting boys to penile surgery when they are 2 years old and being potty trained. The aim of surgery is to produce a straight penis with a urethral opening on the glans, from which a good, straight, single stream of urine is passed in a forward direction.

Circumcision

The indications are shown in Box 15.1. Children of all ages feel pain and therefore should have adequate analgesia. Neonates may have abnormal coagulation, increasing the risk of haemorrhage following circumcision.

Complications

The most common complications following circumcision include haemorrhage, discomfort and infection. Infection is not as common as is generally thought; crusting, which occurs on the glans where the foreskin has been peeled off

---

Box 15.1 Indications for circumcision
• Pathological phimosis (scarred prepuce) • Recurrent balanitis • Structural anomalies of the urinary tract at risk of ascending infections, i.e. vesico-ureteric reflux • Religious—non-medical

---

whilst separating the preputial adhesions, can be misdiagnosed as infection. Meatal stenosis and injury to the glans or urethra are less common complications.

Epispadias and ectopia vesicae

Epispadias and ectopia vesicae occurs in both sexes and often involves deficiencies in the bladder neck. These are rare conditions, occurring in 1:25 000 births. In the female the clitoris is bifid and the urethral opening is wide, leading to problems with urinary continence. In the male the urethral opening is on the dorsal surface of the penis; in its most severe form, the penis is cleft throughout its length and the bladder is exposed on the surface of the body with separation of the pubic symphysis (ectopia vesicae).

Early closure of the bladder and approximation of the pubic bones should be carried out in a specialist centre.

BREAST LESIONS

Neonatal breast hypertrophy caused by maternal hormonal influence is common and resolves spontaneously. Inflammation in these cases is usually caused by a staphylococcus and should be treated with flucloxacillin. If a fluctuant abscess forms, it requires drainage via a small circumareolar incision.

Prepubertal mastitis occurs in both sexes; one or both breast discs become enlarged and painful. The condition usually settles without treatment, and surgery is best avoided so as not to damage the developing breast tissue. Male gynaecomastia is seen at puberty and often causes embarrassment. Most cases regress but mastectomy may be necessary if the condition persists.

Precocious breast development under 7 years of age should be investigated to exclude the various causes of precocious puberty.

Cosmetic excision of accessory nipples may be requested.

Breast tumours are exceptionally rare before puberty.

THE ABDOMEN

Appendicitis

Appendicitis is the most common surgical cause of abdominal pain after 1 year of age. The differential diagnosis includes:

- gastroenteritis
- non-specific abdominal pain (NSAP) (including mesenteric adenitis)
- ovarian causes in adolescent girls
- viral infection
- urinary tract infection
- pneumonia.

Clinical features

The child presents with peri-umbilical pain which later moves to the right iliac fossa. Vomiting is common, as is a low grade fever. Young patients may develop high temperatures. Local peritonitis causes increased tone in the anterior abdominal wall, and the child guards against deep palpation. Rebound tenderness is not a useful sign and causes distress if attempts are made to elicit rebound. It is often better to ask if the pain is worse when travelling over bumps in a car, or asking the patient to jump. Percussion tenderness is often present. In cases of retrocaecal or pelvic appendicitis, the diagnosis may be more difficult and there is less tenderness. Appendicitis is uncommon under the age of 5.

Rectal examination is not helpful in most cases, but may help in difficult cases or when a pelvic abscess is suspected. The latter can be assessed using ultrasound scans. Lower abdominal pain is rarely caused by urinary tract infections in the absence of any urinary symptoms.

In cases where the diagnosis is uncertain, regular review, preferably by the same clinician, should occur at intervals of a few hours. In such cases, a white blood cell count with a polymorph leukocytosis confirms an acute pyogenic infection, and an abdominal X-ray may show signs of oedematous bowel, localised fluid levels or the presence of a calcified faecolith. The process of active observation will soon differentiate between those patients who have appendicitis, requiring surgery, and those with other conditions such as gastroenteritis or non-specific abdominal pain.

Management

The treatment of acute uncomplicated appendicitis is appendicectomy. If a mass is found in the right iliac fossa during clinical examination or on ultrasound, conservative treatment with antibiotics may be advisable. When an abscess has formed this should be drained and antibiotics given, followed by 'interval' appendicectomy 6–8 weeks later.

Pyloric stenosis

Gastric outlet obstruction is caused by hypertrophy of the circular muscle of the pylorus (Figure 15.4). It occurs in 7 per 1000 live births and has a 6:1 male preponderance. It usually presents between the ages of 3 and 6 weeks with progressive, non-bile-stained, forceful vomiting following which the child is hungry. The differential diagnosis includes overfeeding, gastro-oesophageal reflux and sepsis. In the latter case the child is not keen to feed and is lethargic.

On examination there may be signs of dehydration and weight loss with loose skin over the upper thighs. Visible peristalsis is often seen in the left hypochondrium, and a pyloric tumour is palpable between the umbilicus and right costal margin at the edge of the right rectus muscle. The child is best examined from the left

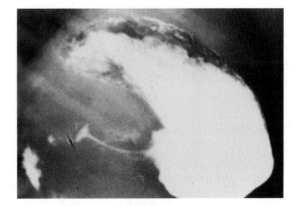

Figure 15.4 Congenital pyloric stenosis.

side using the index and middle fingers of the left hand. It is helpful to relax the baby by allowing it to feed during the examination. If the first test feed is inconclusive, a reassessment should be made a few hours later; if doubt remains, an ultrasound scan will reveal the thickness of the pyloric muscle.

Prior to surgical treatment, correction of the metabolic alkalosis and rehydration is required using half normal saline and 5% dextrose. The treatment of choice is pyloromyotomy (Ramstedt's operation).

Oral feeds can be recommenced the day after surgery; an occasional vomit in the first 24–48 hours is not unusual. Postoperative wound infections are more common than in other surgical procedures in infancy and are probably secondary to malnourishment.

Meckel's diverticulum

A Meckel's diverticulum occurs in 2% of the population and usually causes no problems. It arises from the antimesenteric border of the terminal ileum and is a persistence of the intestinal end of the vitello-intestinal duct. The diverticulum or adjacent ileum occasionally contains gastric mucosa, and the acid produced from this ectopic mucosa causes ulceration and painless rectal bleeding which may be severe and presents most often in infancy. A technetium-99 pertechnetate scan will show a hot spot at the site of the ectopic mucosa. The diverticulum and adjacent small bowel should be excised in such cases. Other complications of Meckel's diverticulum include intussusception, where the diverticulum acts as a lead point, and volvulus of the gut around a band leading from the diverticulum to nearby structures.

Intussusception

A segment of bowel (usually ileum) becomes invaginated into the distal adjacent bowel, and is propelled by peristalsis so that the small bowel enters the colon (ileo-colic intussusception). The condition occurs most often between 4 and 18 months of age with a peak incidence at 5–7 months. The lead point is usually an oedematous and swollen area of gut wall (Peyer's patch). Older children are more likely to have a pathological lead point such as a polyp or Meckel's diverticulum. They present with episodic colicky abdominal pain, pallor, drawing up of the legs and vomiting. Late in the history, blood may appear from the rectum and the child becomes listless and lethargic. A longitudinal mass is often palpable in the line of the colon. Diagnostic delay is common; the classical presentation of pain, drawing up of the legs and redcurrant jelly stools is not always present, and the diagnosis should be considered in any child who presents with colicky abdominal pain and pallor. Ultrasound is useful in cases where a mass is not palpable.

Management

An intravenous infusion is commenced, and resuscitation using colloid or crystalloid is required. Following initial resuscitation, the child should be sedated and given analgesia before a diagnostic and therapeutic enema is carried out. Air enemas are safer than barium and are best carried out by an experienced radiologist in a centre where surgical expertise is immediately available. The success rate following a therapeutic air enema with good sedation is in the region of 85%.

Intussusception recurs in approximately 10% of cases; in this event a second enema may be attempted. Further recurrence should be treated by open surgery; in these cases a pathological lead point is likely to be present. Indications for surgery in intussusception include signs of peritonitis, septicaemia and failure of the air enema.

THE ANUS

Anal fissure is very common in children and is the cause of red blood on the surface of the stools and pain on defecation. The differential diagnosis is listed in Box 15.2.

> **Box 15.2** Differential diagnosis of rectal bleeding in children
>
> *Neonates*
> • Necrotising enterocolitis
> • Midgut volvulus
> • Haemorrhagic disease of the newborn
> • Anal fissure
> • Swallowed maternal blood.
>
> *Bright red bleeding in a well child—surface of stool*
> • Anal fissure
> • Polyps
> • Rectal prolapse
>
> *Larger blood losses*
> • Meckel's diverticulum
> • Peptic ulcer
> • Oesophageal varices
>
> *Sick child*
> • Intussusception
> • Gastroenteritis
> • Henoch–Schönlein purpura
> • Crohn's disease
> • Ulcerative colitis

Anal fissure

The passage of large, hard stool splits the anal mucosa, causing bleeding. There is pain on defecation with bright red blood on the surface of the stool. The condition can be treated by using stool softeners such as lactulose, but anal dilatation under a general anaesthetic is required in persistent cases where pain is a dominant feature.

Rectal polyp

These are not painful. They cause blood on the surface of the stool. Investigation by sigmoidoscopy will reveal the polyp; these are almost always benign in children.

Rectal prolapse

The idiopathic form of rectal prolapse is common in toddlers but is also associated with cystic fibrosis and myelomeningocele. Management of rectal prolapse includes treatment for constipation and limiting the time spent sitting on the toilet. If the prolapse becomes troublesome with bleeding and ulceration of the rectal mucosa, the condition may be treated by submucosal injection of 5% phenol in almond oil.

Perianal abscess

This condition is common in young children and results from infection of an anal gland. An abscess appears adjacent to the anus. A perianal fistula occasionally develops between the opening of the abscess on the perineal surface and the anal valve in the anal canal. Treatment consists of laying open the fistula tract under general anaesthesia.

FURTHER READING

Spitz L, Steiner G M, Zachary R B 1989 A colour atlas of paediatric surgical diagnosis. Wolfe Medical, London

Internet address

http://home.coqui.net/titolugo/index.htm

16

Infectious diseases, immunisation and dermatology

Andrew Raffles

INFECTIOUS DISEASES

Pyrexia of unknown origin (PUO)

It is relatively rare for a child to present with a fever greater than 38°C lasting for more than 1 week in whom no source of infection declares itself. Investigation is necessary as the child may be in the early stages of a disease which is serious for him or her, or for others. There is a very long list of possible causes, including infections, neoplastic disease, connective tissue disease, malingering and Munchhausen's syndrome by proxy (see GP Overviews 16.1, 16.2).

Notifiable diseases
(Box 16.1 and Table 16.1)

Doctors in England and Wales have a statutory duty to notify a 'Proper Officer' of the local authority (usually the Consultant in Communicable Diseases in the Health Authority) of cases of certain infectious diseases. These notifications should be made on clinical evidence and need not be microbiologically confirmed. The aim is to alert the authorities at local and national levels to outbreaks so that investigation and control measures can be undertaken.

GP Overview 16.1 Fever

Common causes

Upper respiratory
- Coryza
- Pharyngitis
- Adenitis
- Croup
- Sinusitis
- Otitis media
- Tonsillitis

Lower respiratory
- Bronchiolitis
- Pneumonia

Gastrointestinal
- Diarrhoea/vomiting

Oral
- Dental abscess
- Herpangina
- Herpetic gingivitis
- Mumps

Central nervous system
- Viral/bacterial meningitis

Genitourinary
- Urinary tract infection
- Salpingitis

Musculoskeletal
- Septic arthritis
- Osteomyelitis

Systemic + rash
- Cellulitis
- Scarlet fever
- Meningococcal

Serious causes

Upper respiratory
- Epiglottitis
- Croup
- Retropharyngeal abscess

Lower respiratory
- Pneumonia
- Bronchiolitis

Gastrointestinal
- Diarrhoea/vomiting
- Appendicitis
- Peritonitis

Central nervous system
- Meningitis
- Encephalitis
- Cerebral abscess

Cardiac
- Myocarditis
- Endocarditis
- Pericarditis

Systemic
- Meningococcal
- Toxic shock

Collagen/vascular
- SLE
- PAN
- Rheumatic fever
- Kawasaki's disease
- Stevens–Johnson syndrome

Miscellaneous
- Malignancy
- Renal
- Reticulosis
- Poisoning

GP Overview 16.2 Pyrexia of unknown origin (PUO)

Present for longer than 1 week and greater than 38.0°C

Causes
- Normal variation
- Dehydration/overheating
- Malingering
- Munchausen's syndrome by proxy
- Child abuse
- Infection, e.g. tuberculosis, typhoid, congenital infection, Toxocara
- Absorption of blood–post-trauma or post-surgical
- Juvenile arthritis
- Drugs/poisons

Rarer causes
- Collagen disorders
- Malignancy
- Granulomatous, e.g. sarcoid
- Kawasaki's disease
- Crohn's disease, ulcerative colitis
- Liver disease
- Subdural haematoma
- Riley–Day syndrome, agammaglobulinaemia

Suggested tests
FBC
Thick film (if malaria possible)
Blood cultures
ESR
CRP
Biochemistry screen
MSU
Stool + ova, cysts, parasites
Chest X-ray

Follow-up tests
- Viral studies/bacteriology screening
- Serology + torch screen
- Monospot
- RA/ANF
- Autoantibodies
- Tuberculin test
- X-rays/ultrasound
- CT/MRI scans

Box 16.1	Notifiable diseases

Acute encephalitis
Acute poliomyelitis
Anthrax
Cholera
Diphtheria
Dysentery
Food poisoning
Leptospirosis
Malaria
Measles
Meningitis
Meningococcal septicaemia
Mumps
Ophthalmia neonatorum
Paratyphoid fever
Plague
Rabies
Relapsing fever
Rubella
Scarlet fever
Smallpox
Tetanus
Tuberculosis
Typhoid fever
Typhus
Viral haemorrhagic fever
Viral hepatitis
Whooping cough
Yellow fever

Exanthemata

Details of the classical features of exanthemata caused by infectious diseases are given in Table 16.2.

SPECIFIC INFECTIONS

Congenital infection

The major period of organogenesis is during the first trimester of pregnancy. Maternal infection during this time (even if subclinical) may cause embryopathy by transplacental transmission of virus and result in structural malformations (Table 16.3).

The diagnosis of most congenital infections is made on the history and clinical findings, confirmed by finding specific IgM in cord or neonatal blood.

Herpes simplex virus (HSV)/Human herpes virus (HHV)

Neonatal herpes infection

Most cases are caused by HSV type 2 and result from direct contact during delivery with maternal genital herpes lesions.

Table 16.1 Notifications (deaths) in England and Wales (all ages)

	1993	1994	1995	1996	1997
Diphtheria	6 (0)	9 (2)	12 (1)	11 (0)	22 (0)
Encephalitis	18	30	37	25	33
Malaria	1198 (4)	1139 (11)	1300 (4)	1659 (11)	1476 (12)
Measles	9612 (4)	16 375 (1)	7477 (1)	5614 (0)	3962 (3)
Meningitis	2082 (218)	1800 (170)	2285 (209)	2686 (245)	2345 (224)
Meningococcal	1053 (35)	938 (19)	1146 (31)	1164 (44)	1220 (47)
Pneumococcal	239 (66)	220 (47)	241 (56)	297 (83)	300 (68)
H. influenzae	168 (6)	52 (1)	51 (0)	57 (0)	38 (1)
Meningococcal septicaemia	398 (122)	430 (111)	707 (154)	1129 (182)	1440 (182)
Poliomyelitis	1	0	1	1	2
Mumps	2153 (0)	2494 (0)	1936 (0)	1747 (0)	1914 (0)
Rubella	9724 (0)	6326 (0)	6196 (0)	9081 (0)	3260 (0)
Congenital	3 (13*)	7 (4*)	1 (5*)	12 (9*)	no data
Scarlet fever	5855	6193	5296	4873	3569
Tetanus	8 (3)	3 (0)	6 (1)	7 (0)	7 (2)
Tuberculosis	5921 (423)	5591 (418)	5608 (447)	5654 (416)	5859 (385)
Whooping cough	4091 (0)	3964 (3)	1869 (2)	2387 (2)	2988 (1)

*Terminations

Table 16.2 Exanthemata caused by infectious diseases

	Measles	Rubella	Chickenpox (varicella)	Roseola infantum (exanthem subitum)	Fifth disease (erythema infectiosum)	Hand, foot and mouth disease	Glandular fever (infectious mononucleosis)	Scarlet fever	Toxic shock syndrome
Epidemiology	Incidence declining in UK but major cause of mortality in developing countries	Endemic—incidence declining since MMR	Highly infectious—most children infected by school age	Most children infected by 2 years	Endemic outbreak every 4 years	Endemic Prevalence of specific antibodies directly related to age	Endemic	Epidemic	May occur in menstruating girls
Peak season	Spring and winter	Spring and winter	Spring and winter	All seasons	Spring and winter	Summer and autumn	Non-seasonal	Non-seasonal	Non-seasonal
Peak age	1–4 years	97% cases < 17 years	5–10 years	7–18 months	5–10 years	10 months– 3 years	Increases with age	5–15 years	15–25 years
Aetiology	Measles virus (RNA)	Rubella virus (RNA)	Herpes varicella zoster virus (DNA)	Human herpesvirus 6 and 7 (DNA)	Parvovirus 19 (DNA)	Coxsackie A16, A19 (RNA) Enterovirus 71 (RNA)	Epstein–Barr virus (DNA)	Erythrogenic *Streptococcus pyogenes*	Exotoxin-producing *Staphylococcus aureus*
Incubation	8–12 days	15–21 days	14–21 days	5–15 days	7–17 days	4–7 days	24–49 days	3–4 days	Abrupt
Prodrome	Yes—fever, cough, coryza, conjunctivitis	Yes—mild symptoms 1–5 days prior to rash	Yes— malaise, fever 5–6 days	No	Yes—headache, malaise for 2–3 days followed by asymptomatic phase for 7 days	Yes—fever, malaise, headache	Asymptomatic or mild URTI symptoms	No	No
Classical features	Koplik's spots, otitis media, rash starts behind ears (Figs 16.1, 16.2)	Fever, malaise Rash starts on face, spreads onto trunk and extremities Posterior cervical lymph-adenopathy	Crops of lesions that go through stages of macules, papules, vesicles and crusting	Fever lasting 3–5 days with maculopapular rash appearing over neck, trunk and face as fever subsides	Rash starts on face (slapped cheek appearance) and spreading to trunk and limbs Maculopapular evolving to a lace-like reticular pattern	Pharyngitis Vesicular lesions on hands and feet including palms and soles	Asymptomatic in infants and young children Fever, lymphadenopathy, tonsillitis, headache, malaise, myalgia, splenomegaly, petechiae on soft palate Rash may be macular, maculopapular, urticarial or erythema multiforme-like More vivid if ampicillin was administered	Fever, pharyngitis, cervical lymphadenitis, headache, vomiting, fine maculopapular rash over trunk and proximal extremities (Fig. 16.3) Circumoral pallor Strawberry tongue Desquamation occurs towards end of first week	High fever, hypotension, abdominal pain, diarrhoea, vomiting, myalgia Rash—diffuse, maculopapular Desquamation occurs 1–2 weeks after onset
Duration of symptoms	Variable 5–7 days	3–5 days	8–10 days	2–3 days	7–21 days	3–7 days	Weeks to months	10–14 days	

Table 16.2 (contd)

	Measles	Rubella	Chickenpox (varicella)	Roseola infantum (exanthem subitum)	Fifth disease (erythema infectiosum)	Hand, foot and mouth disease	Glandular fever (infectious mononucleosis)	Scarlet fever	Toxic shock syndrome
Diagnosis	Salivary antibodies	Salivary IgM	VZV specific IgM; EM of vesicular fluid; IF for antigens	Seroconversion; plasma viral DNA isolation in acute phase	Parvovirus IgM seroconversion; plasma viral DNA isolation in acute phase	Seroconversion; Inoculate subcutaneously and intracerebrally in suckling mice and observe for paralysis	Paul–Bunnell test; EBV specific IgM; Seroconversion	Bacterial cultures; ASOT	Bacterial cultures; Toxin identification
Differential diagnosis	Rubella; Roseola infantum (HHV6); Fifth disease (Parvo B19)	Roseola infantum (HHV6); Fifth disease (Parvo B19); Measles	Herpes simplex; Coxsackie A16	Measles; Rubella; Fifth disease	Chickenpox; Herpes simplex	Chickenpox; Herpes simplex	CMV infection, rubella, viral hepatitis	Measles; Rubella; Glandular fever; Toxic shock syndrome	Kawasaki's disease, scarlet fever, toxic epidermal necrosis; Group A streptococcal septicaemia
Sequelae/ complications	Pneumonia; Deafness; Encephalitis; SSPE	Embryopathy; Deafness	Encephalo-myelitis; Haemorrhagic varicella; Pneumonia; Embryopathy	Meningo-encephalitis; Seizures	Arthralgia; Aplastic crisis in those with underlying chronic haemolytic anaemias; Aseptic meningitis; Thrombo-cytopenia; Hydrops fetalis	Chronic or recurring skin lesions	Splenic rupture, upper airway obstruction, seizure, ataxia, VIth nerve palsy, Guillain–Barré syndrome, aplastic anaemia, myocarditis, interstitial pneumonia, Burkitt's lymphoma, nasopharyngeal carcinoma	Sinusitis, otitis media, mastoiditis, retropharyngeal abscess, broncho-pneumonia, rheumatic fever, glomerulo-nephritis	Multisystem failure, disseminated intravascular coagulation
Treatment	Symptomatic; Antibiotics for pneumonia and otitis media	Symptomatic	Symptomatic; Aciclovir in immuno-compromised	Symptomatic	Symptomatic	Symptomatic	Symptomatic	Antibiotics	Antibiotics and supportive
% Immunised	94% 1995	94% 1995 (MMR campaign) 80% 1998 because of autism scare	N/A	N/A	N/A	N/A	N/A	N/A	N/A

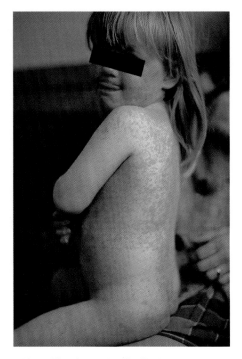

Figure 16.1 Measles rash—distribution.

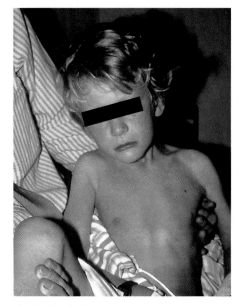

Figure 16.3 Scarlet fever.

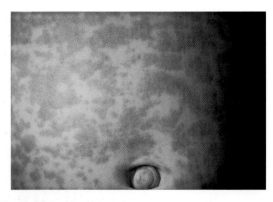

Figure 16.2 Measles rash.

Clinical features. Vesicles on skin or mucous membranes are the only lesions in approximately two thirds of cases. One third progress to systemic infection with encephalitis, pneumonia or hepatitis

Management consists of intravenous aciclovir.

Childhood herpes infection

Infection in childhood is caused by HSV type 1.

Clinical features. Primary infection may be asymptomatic or cause gingivo-stomatitis which can be very painful and interfere with feeding and drinking. Other children get conjunctivitis (dendritic ulcers can cause corneal scarring especially if treated with steroid eye drops), encephalitis or whitlows. Secondary reactivation may intermittently cause painful vesicles on the mucocutaneous border of the lips (cold sores).

Management. Topical aciclovir may offer some benefit for cold sores or stomatitis. Intravenous aciclovir should be started as soon as possible if encephalitis is suspected. Whitlows should be covered and kissing prevented in the presence of cold sores.

Cytomegalovirus (CMV)

Transmission. CMV is contained in all body fluids. It may be transmitted to children via saliva or breast milk.

Clinical features. Congenital infections are listed in Table 16.3.

Table 16.3 Congenital infections

Organism	Clinical features	Notes
Rubella	Sensorineural deafness 80% Heart disease 50% Learning difficulties 50% Cataracts + visual impairment 40%	Ensure rubella immune state for all women before pregnancy
Cytomegalovirus	Intrauterine growth retardation Jaundice and hepatosplenomegaly Thrombocytopenia Sensorineural deafness Learning difficulties Cerebral palsy	May result from maternal reactivated infection so immunisation not effective
Toxoplasmosis	Intracranial calcification Chorioretinitis Hydrocephalus Learning difficulties	May be progressive Maternal treatment with spiramycin reduces transmission
Herpes simplex	Skin lesions Chorioretinitis Microphthalmia Microcephaly Learning difficulties	90% of neonatal herpes infections are transmitted during delivery and cause skin lesions and secondary systemic infection
Varicella	Intrauterine growth retardation Limb anomalies Brain malformation Eye lesions	Severe neonatal illness can result from maternal infection in the last 3 weeks of pregnancy

Acquired infection is often asymptomatic (50% of pregnant women are seropositive). Immunocompromised children may develop severe systemic disease (hepatitis, pneumonia, retinitis).

Management. CMV is a herpes virus but antiviral drugs do not help. The virus is excreted in urine for several years, so toilet hygiene is important.

Toxoplasmosis

The causative organism is *Toxoplasma gondii*. Infection occurs world-wide and 50% of adults are immune. Transmission occurs by ingestion of oocysts from faeces of infected cats or eating infected meat.

Clinical features. Congenital infections are shown in Table 16.3. Acquired infection may be asymptomatic or cause mild symptoms, e.g. lympha-denopathy, sore throat and myalgia. Symptoms can be severe in immunocompromised children.

Management. Antibiotics—spiramycin, pyrimethamine and sulphadiazine.

Poliomyelitis

Poliomyelitis is caused by an enterovirus—antigen types 1, 2 and 3 as wild or attenuated vaccine virus. It is endemic in developing countries. Humans are the only host. Transmission occurs by the faecal–oral route.

Clinical features. The majority of cases are subclinical or cause mild non-specific illness. The virus is neurotropic and invades the central nervous system, causing aseptic meningitis or, rarely, paralytic polio from anterior horn cell damage.

Prognosis. The child's condition often improves but there may be some permanent lower motor neurone paralysis. Poliomyelitis rarely causes death through respiratory failure.

Diphtheria, tetanus and pertussis

Features of these three diseases are listed in Table 16.4.

Table 16.4 Diphtheria, tetanus and pertussis

	Diphtheria	Tetanus	Pertussis (see p. 121)
Organism	*Corynebacterium diphtheriae*	*Clostridium tetani*	*Bordetella pertussis*
Epidemiology	Rare in countries which immunise Humans are the only host	Spores are widely distributed in soil	World-wide, especially in temperate climates Humans are the only host
Transmission	Respiratory droplets	Direct contact with open wound (e.g. umbilical stump)	Repiratory droplets highly infectious
Incubation	2–5 days	0.5–4 weeks	7–10 days
Clinical features	Nasopharyngitis or laryngotracheitis with thick, grey adherent membrane	Exotoxin causes severe muscle spasm	Coryzal phase Paroxysmal phase—persistent bouts of coughing with cyanosis and vomiting Whoop often absent in young children Lasts up to 3 months
Complications	Respiratory obstruction Exotoxin causes myocarditis and motor neuropathy		Subconjunctival haemorrhage Encephalopathy Family exhaustion
Diagnosis	Culture DNA studies after PCR	Clinical	Lymphocytosis Culture of pernasal swab
Management	Specific antitoxin Intravenous penicillin/erythromycin	Tetanus toxoid booster if last dose > 10 years ago Surgical wound toilet Human tetanus immunoglobulin	Erythromycin in coryzal stage limits infectivity
Prognosis	Mortality 5–10%	Mortality high (> 50%) in neonates	Mortality approximately 1:1000 children aged < 6 months

Meningococcal septicaemia

Pathology

Meningococcus is carried in the nasopharynx by up to 25% of the well population. For unknown reasons the organism causes invasive disease in some contacts (but only 1% of carriers). Factors increasing susceptibility include concurrent infection, reduced immunity and smoking. The meningococci localise in the meninges and cause meningitis in approximately 15% of cases, but in approximately 60% the organisms multiply in the blood stream and secrete a potent endotoxin which causes septic shock. The remaining 25% have a combination of meningitis and septicaemia. Other foci of infection include endocarditis, osteomyelitis and arthritis.

Clinical features

Meningococcal septicaemia progresses quickly and can be fulminant, causing circulatory failure with intense peripheral vasoconstriction and autonomic breakdown. Diagnosis is easy because of the widespread purpuric rash (Fig. 16.4) in a very ill shocked child. Once septic shock has started because of massive endotoxin release, the prognosis is very poor and coma and death usually ensue within a few hours. Antibiotic therapy makes little difference at this stage but still must be given to limit further bacterial multiplication as some patients will survive.

Management

- Antibiotics (i.v. penicillin)
- Transfer to paediatric intensive care unit (PICU)

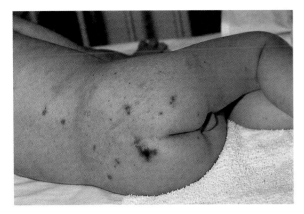

Figure 16.4   Meningococcal rash.

- Treat shock:
  —albumin/plasma infusion
  —i.v. normal saline
  —consider inotropic drugs (dopamine/
    dobutamine/adrenaline)
  —monitor central venous pressure (CVP)
- Ventilation–anticipate respiratory failure
- Blood/platelet transfusion for coagulation
  disorder—disseminated intravascular
  coagulation (DIC)
- Corticosteroid use is controversial.

Prognosis

The outcome for children who present with fulminating meningococcal septicaemia with a history of less than 8 hours is very poor. The prognosis is better if the evolution of the disease is slower, either because the natural course of the illness is less aggressive or because there is more time for treatment to work.

The overall mortality is approximately 30%; the majority of survivors make a full recovery.

Human immunodeficiency virus (HIV)

HIV occurs world-wide but is most frequent in mid-Africa. In developed countries it is associated with homosexuality and injected drug abuse.

In children the most common route of viral transmission is vertical from an infected mother via blood or breast milk. The virus is rarely contracted through infected blood transfusions (this is more likely in developing countries).

Clinical features. The virus compromises T4 lymphocytes and thus causes immunodeficiency. It may take up to 1 year for symptoms of acquired immunodeficiency syndrome (AIDS) to develop. These include opportunistic infections (*Pneumocystis carinii* pneumonia and CMV), recurrent bacterial infections, failure to thrive, encephalopathy and malignancy.

Diagnosis. Serology is unhelpful until the age of 18 months when maternal antibody has disappeared. Over the age of 18 months HIV antibody is diagnostic. A diagnosis can be made earlier by PCR technology.

Management:

- antibiotics for infection
- immunoglobulin
- routine immunisations except BCG
- anti-retroviral drugs
- no restriction of social or educational activities
- normal hygiene measures for body fluids.

Prevention of vertical transmission from HIV positive mothers. Caesarean section may reduce the risk from delivery. The mother must not breast feed. The results of maternal anti-retroviral therapy during pregnancy are at present unknown.

Enterovirus infection (excluding poliomyelitis)

The causative organisms are Coxsackie A and B and echoviruses. They have a world-wide distribution and cases of infection peak in the summer months.

Transmission occurs by the faecal–oral route and from respiratory droplets.

Clinical features:

- aseptic meningitis (especially in the late neonatal period and early childhood)
- rash
- gastroenteritis
- respiratory disease
- myocarditis

- pericarditis
- herpangina.

Diagnosis:

- viral culture of CSF, pharyngeal scraping, urine, stool
- serology
- DNA identification using polymerase chain reaction (PCR) technology.

Treatment is symptomatic.

Tuberculosis (TB)

Myobacterium tuberculosis is a slow-growing organism which is easily identified microscopically after Ziehl–Neelsen staining as acid-fast bacilli. Humans are the only host although *M. bovis* from infected cows rarely causes tuberculoid disease in humans.

It is estimated that approximately one third of the world's population is, or has been, infected by *M. tuberculosis*; the incidence, even in developed countries, has been increasing over the last decade. The highest rates are in families from India, Pakistan and Bangladesh, though West Indian children also have a higher risk than British children. In Africa the increased incidence of TB is associated with HIV infection.

Clinical features. The majority of TB infections cause minimal symptoms and are contained within the primary focus. This eventually calcifies and can be seen on chest X-ray. If immunity is suppressed (e.g. by chemotherapy, HIV infection) the primary infection may spread to cause systemic disease. Some *M. tuberculosis* organisms often remain dormant in the primary focus for many years and can be reactivated.

Pulmonary TB. See page 125.

Extrapulmonary TB. In approximately 2% of cases tubercle bacilli spread via the blood stream to seed in other parts of the body.

Miliary TB:

- rare in children
- multiple foci in many organs
- miliary shadowing in lungs may be seen on chest X-ray

- retinal tubercles may be seen on fundoscopy
- cerebral foci (tuberculoma) can cause neurological symptoms.

Tuberculous meningitis (TBM):

- caused by spread from brain seedlings
- causes increasing apathy and occasionally seizures
- CSF contains sparse tubercle bacilli and a lymphocytic pleocytosis
- if CSF is sterile diagnosis may depend on positive tuberculin test and identification of TB organisms from other sites; tuberculous antigen may be detectable on PCR
- urgent treatment with rifampicin or isoniazid plus pyrazinamide is needed
- steroids should also be given
- prognosis is poor; the recovery rate is approximately 20%.

TB in other sites causes osteomyelitis, pericarditis and nephritis.

TROPICAL DISEASES

Micro-organisms can now travel across the globe within 24 hours, and imported diseases are becoming more common.

Malaria

Malaria is caused by bites from a mosquito infected with the Plasmodium protozoan parasite (*P. falciparum, P. vivax, P. ovale, P. malariae*). The disease is endemic in most tropical and some subtropical countries below an altitude of 1500 metres.

Clinical features

Most cases present within 1 month of being infected but onset can be delayed for up to a year. A child with a fever who has travelled from a malarial area should be assumed to have malaria until proved otherwise.

The symptoms are very variable and may be mild or severe. They include headache, myalgia, cough, diarrhoea, vomiting, abdominal pain, rigors and drowsiness. Signs include anaemia, jaundice, splenomegaly, hepatomegaly and dehydration.

Complications include:

- cerebral malaria
- hypoglycaemia
- renal failure (blackwater fever)
- Gram-negative septicaemia
- anaemia.

Diagnosis

The parasites can be demonstrated on thick blood films taken during a fever.

Management

Drug treatment is determined by the species of malaria parasite and the country of infection (beware resistance). The choice of medication usually requires advice from a specialist tropical diseases unit. Chloroquine, quinine, primaquine and mefloquine are available drugs. Pyrimethamine and sulfadoxine are also used in *P. falciparum* malaria (beware G6PD deficiency).

Prophylaxis

Travellers to Africa, South Asia and the Pacific islands must be advised how to avoid mosquito bites (long clothes, mosquito nets, insect repellents) and to take chemoprophylaxis (mefloquine, chloroquine, proguanil, pyrimethamine and dapsone, depending on the area to be visited). Up to date advice can be obtained from an accredited travel health centre, a local Public Health Laboratory Service (PHLS) centre, or the Communicable Disease Surveillance Centre (CDSC) in London (Tel. 0208 200 6868).

Other tropical diseases

Table 16.5 lists some tropical diseases that are occasionally seen in the UK. Except for leishmaniasis, they cause a predominantly gastrointestinal illness. The most common serious disease is dysentery (passage of diarrhoea with pus), followed by typhoid (and milder paratyphoid) fever and cholera. Some types are caused by protozoa (Entamoeba, Giardia and Leishmania) and others by bacteria (Shigella, Vibrio and Salmonella).

WORMS

The most common infestation in the UK is threadworms (pinworms), experienced by most children at some time. The infestations listed in Table 16.6 are endemic in many parts of the world but may be brought here by travellers.

Some worms may invade the viscera and cause symptoms related to the particular affected organ (Table 16.7). Toxocariasis is the only one that can be contracted in the UK.

The Infectious Diseases section was written with the help of Dr Peter Chow.

Table 16.5 Tropical diseases

	Amoebic dysentery	Shigella dysentery	Giardiasis	Cholera	Typhoid fever	Leishmaniasis
Organism	Entamoeba histolytica	S. sonnei* S. flexneri* S. dysenteriae S. boydii (* found in UK)	Giardia lamblia	Vibrio cholerae	Salmonella typhi	L. donovani (visceral) L. major L. tropica L. brasiliensis L. mexicani (cutaneous)
Transmission	Faecal–oral or ingestion of contaminated water	Faecal–oral	Faecal–oral	Faecal–oral Contaminated water and food especially shellfish	Faecal–oral	Bite by infected sandfly
Epidemiology	World-wide	World-wide	World-wide	World-wide	World-wide	Tropical and subtropical
Clinical features	Asymptomatic mild gastrointestinal disturbance	Mild–severe diarrhoea May be watery and bloody	Asymptomatic or vomiting and diarrhoea	Asymptomatic or sudden severe diarrhoea and vomiting	Asymptomatic or diarrhoea and vomiting Systemic illness Rash in 20%	Visceral (kala-azar) • malaise • lymphadenopathy • hepatosplenomegaly • cutaneous red nodules
Complications	Severe abdominal pain, bloody diarrhoea Peritonitis Liver abscess	Dehydration Peritonitis	Steatorrhoea Malabsorption Failure to thrive	Dehydration Hypovolaemic shock Toxaemia Renal failure	Peritonitis Arthritis and osteitis	Visceral-reticulo-endothelial failure Cutaneous—skin ulceration and satellite lesions
Diagnosis	Stool microscopy Ultrasound for liver abscess	Stool microscopy	Microscopy of stool or duodenal aspirate or biopsy	Clinical and stool microscopy	Culture of organism from stool, blood or urine	Microscopy of biopsy or skin scraping
Treatment	Rehydration Metronidazole	Rehydration Antibiotics (ampicillin or co-trimoxazole) if systemic illness	Metronidazole	Rehydration Co-trimoxazole	Rehydration Antibiotics (ampicillin, trimethoprim, chloramphenicol)	Pentamidine

Table 16.6 Worm infestations

	Threadworms	Roundworms	Hookworms	Whipworms
Organism	*Enterobius vermicularis*	*Ascaris lumbricoides*	*Acyclostoma duodenale*	*Trichuris trichiura*
Transmission	Faecal–oral	Faecal–oral	Skin penetration	Faecal–oral
Epidemiology	World-wide very common	Tropical and temperate areas	Tropical areas	Tropical/subtropical damp areas
Clinical features	Perianal itching/vulvo-vaginitis	Worms in stools	Skin rash Iron deficiency anaemia Cough	Abdominal pain Diarrhoea
Complications		Larval pneumonitis (Löffler's syndrome)	Bloody diarrhoea	Rectal prolapse Iron deficiency anaemia
Diagnosis	Stool microscopy Sellotape test	Larvae in stool Eosinophilia	Stool microscopy	Stool microscopy
Treatment	Mebendazole for whole family	Piperazine or mebendazole	Mebendazole or thiabendazole	Mebendazole

Table 16.7 Invasive helminthiasis

	Schistosomiasis (bilharzia)	Strongyloidiasis	Cysticercosis	Hydatid disease	Trichinosis	Toxocariasis
Organism	*Schistosoma* species	*Strongyloides stercoralis*	*Taenia solium*	*Echinococcus granulosus*	*Trichinella spiralis*	*T. canis* *T. catis*
Transmission	Larvae from snails in infected water penetrate skin	Larvae from stool or soil penetrate skin	Faecal–oral	Ingestion of dog faeces	Ingestion of poorly cooked infected pork	Ingestion of dog or cat faeces
Epidemiology	Tropical/subtropical	Tropical	Tropical	World-wide, esp. temperate sheep-raising areas	World-wide	World-wide
Organs involved	Large bowel, liver, urinary tract	Gastro-intestinal tract, lungs Multi-system in immuno-compromised	Cysts in any organ especially brain, muscle, eye	Liver, lung, bone, brain, muscle	Intestine, muscle, lung	Visceral larva migrans Eyes
Diagnosis	Stool/urine microscopy Rectal biopsy	Stool microscopy Duodenal aspirate	X-ray, MRI scan Stool Histology of surgically removed cyst	Imaging—ultra sound, MRI Microscopy of cyst fluid (surgical)	Clinical muscle biopsy	Larva migrans—clinical + eosinophilia Fundoscopy Serology
Treatment	Praziquantel Niridazole	Thiabendazole	Albendazole Praziquantel	Albendazole, occasionally surgery	Steroids if severe	Thiabendazole Diethyl-carbamazine

IMMUNISATION

(This section is adapted from the *Hertfordshire Community Paediatric Guide* by Dr A Raffles and Dr J Heckmatt.)

Introduction

In 1796 Dr Edward Jenner, a country practitioner, initiated the process that has evolved into the present-day comprehensive immunisation programme (Table 16.8).

By 1991 in the USA, highly effective vaccines had caused the reported number of cases of diphtheria, measles, mumps, pertussis, poliomyelitis, rubella and tetanus to decline by 97% or more (the effect is probably currently even greater in the UK). The impact of vaccination on the health of the world's people is hard to exaggerate. With the exception of safe water, no other modality, not even antibiotics, has had such a major effect on mortality reduction and population growth.

Smallpox has now been eliminated worldwide and the eventual elimination of other diseases, such as polio and measles, would be possible with greater world political stability. Vaccination is the single most cost effective health measure, for example the MMR vaccine programme in the USA is estimated to have a cost–benefit ratio of 1:14.4. Although they are not completely devoid of adverse effects, the excellent safety record of vaccines contributes to their high benefit–cost ratios (Table 16.9).

Immunisation is a central feature of the care of children. The topic encompasses epidemiology, health education and promotion, and is important in the care of all children, especially the child with multiple problems. There are also many controversies and myths.

Handling of vaccines in the community

Ordering

A named person in each treatment centre is responsible for ordering the month-by-month supply of vaccine and ensuring that stocks are up to date.

Transport

World-wide, one of the greatest threats to successful vaccination is the failure to maintain the vaccines at their optimum storage temperature. Maintaining the cold chain (Box 16.2) is essential, and considerable effort and resources are required to ensure this.

Table 16.8 Schedule of routine immunisation

Age	Vaccine	Comments
2 months—first dose 3 months—second dose 4 months—third dose	DTP + Hib and oral polio	Primary course
12–15 months	MMR (measles, mumps, rubella)	Can be given at any age over 12 months
3–5 years	Booster DT and oral polio MMR second dose	Three years after completion of primary course
10–14 years (or infancy)	BCG	Only after a tuberculin skin test (except infants up to 3 months old without known recent contact with TB)
13–18 years	Booster tetanus/diphtheria (Td) and oral polio Give MMR to those missed in the 1994 MR campaign	The tetanus component must be omitted if the child has already had 5 doses

Key:
DTP = diphtheria/tetanus/pertussis (d = low dose diphtheria)
Hib = *Haemophilus influenzae* b
BCG = Bacillus Calmette–Guérin (for tuberculosis)
MMR = measles, mumps, rubella

Table 16.9   Immunisation and diseases prevented

Vaccine	Diseases prevented or incidence reduced
Diphtheria/pertussis/tetanus (DPT)	Acute diphtheria with cardiotoxicity, respiratory obstruction and paralysis Whooping cough ('the cough of a hundred days'), lung damage, anoxic brain damage. Before 1970s mortality 1:1000 Tetanus often fatal
Haemophilus influenzae type b	Meningitis, epiglottitis, cellulitis, osteitis, septic arthritis and pericarditis
Polio	Paralysis (permanent), respiratory failure (acute and chronic), encephalitis
MMR	Measles encephalomyelitis (1:1000–1:5000, 10% die, 15% handicapped), slow brain infection (SSPE) (*subacute sclerosing panencephalitis*), pneumonitis. otitis. Congenital rubella 70 cases/year before immunisation programme. Incidence of congenital rubella in UK now very low and most affected infants are born to non-vaccinated women who came to the UK as adults Mumps (CNS infection, sensori-neural deafness, orchitis, pancreatitis)
BCG	Does not prevent TB infection, but prevents miliary spread, meningitis and death, and secondary pulmonary disease Most useful in areas of low incidence
Meningococcus Group C	40% of meningococcal infections

> **Box 16.2**   The cold chain
>
> - Maintain vaccine at 2–8°C
> - Store vaccine in a special refrigerator, which should:
>   - —be specifically for medicinal products (not domestic)
>   - —have an uninterruptable electricity supply
>   - —have a max–min thermometer
>   - —not be used for food storage
>   - —have a temperature log book kept close by
>   - —be regularly defrosted (place vaccine in another fridge)
> - When using for a session, store vaccine in a cold-bag with ice pack (but do not let the vaccine freeze)
> - One staff member should be educated about correct vaccine storage and nominated to monitor the refrigerator's temperature and adjust the thermostat accordingly

Handling vaccine

- Check expiry date.
- Protect from light.
- Discard contents of multidose vials at the end of each session.
- Do not squirt live vaccine!
- Exercise care when administering oral polio from a 10-dose vial. Use disposable spoons.
- If you clean the skin, let any solvent dry. Solvent will denature live vaccine.

Disposal

- Place syringes, needles and reconstituted live vaccine in a sharps box.
- Return unused vaccine to the fridge immediately, at the front so it is used first next time.
- Return unused expired vaccine to the district pharmacy in a sealed envelope marked 'expired vaccine'.

Recording

In order to interpret any adverse reaction that might occur, always routinely record:

- batch number
- site of injection if two sites have been used
- expiry date
- signature and printed name of person giving the immunisation.

Anaphylaxis (see also p. 295)

An anaphylaxis pack with adrenaline 1:1000 (Table 16.10), 1 ml syringes, 25 gauge needles and a selection of airways must be available at every immunisation session.

In the event of any reaction occurring up to 72 hours characterised by difficulty breathing,

Table 16.10 Doses of adrenaline 1:1000 in case of anaphylaxis

Age	Adrenaline dose 1:1000
< 1 year	0.05 ml
1 year	0.1 ml
2 years	0.2 ml
3–4 years	0.3 ml
5 years	0.4 ml
6–10 years	0.5 ml
> 10 years	0.5–1 ml

swelling of the face, hoarseness, stridor, chest tightness, leading to pallor, limpness, apnoea and hypotension with tachycardia:

- Give *subcutaneous adrenaline*.
- If there is severe collapse, give *intramuscular adrenaline*.
- If there is no improvement in the patient's condition repeat the dose in 5–10 minutes, up to three times.
- Refer any patient with anaphylaxis to hospital for assessment and further treatment as necessary. All patients should be observed for 6 hours, in case of delayed reaction.

Report any adverse reaction to the doctor who administered the vaccine and also report on a yellow card.

Faint

In the first hour following a vaccination some school aged children may faint. There is pallor but *no* difficulty breathing. A strong vasovagal response is characterised by transient jerking movements or eye rolling. Lie the child down for 10 minutes.

This type of reaction relates to the pain and fear of injection and not specifically to the vaccine. Simple fainting is unusual in a young child, and sudden loss of consciousness is more likely to be due to anaphylaxis if a central pulse (carotid) cannot be felt.

Consent

The parents' consent, written or verbal, must be obtained before vaccination. Bringing the child to the vaccination, after invitation, is usually taken as consent by the parents so long as:

1. the nature of vaccination has been fully explained
2. the child is assessed as suitable
3. the parents feel their questions have been fully and sensitively answered
4. they have not expressed reservations.

Immunisation notes

The DHSS recommends that pre-school children should be vaccinated against:

- diphtheria
- tetanus
- whooping cough/pertussis
- *Haemophilus influenzae* type B
- poliomyelitis
- mumps
- measles
- rubella
- tuberculosis—neonatal BCG for selected cases.

Notes:

- There is now a combined vaccine for the first 4 diseases—ACT-Hib DTP.
- Inject DTP and Hib at separate sites if not given as the tetravalent injection (ACT-Hib DTP).
- Allow an interval of at least 3 weeks between injections of two live vaccines (e.g. polio, BCG). The *exception* is polio and MMR as part of the pre-school booster.
- Allow an interval of at least 3 years between the completion of the primary course and the pre-school booster.
- Immunise pre-term babies according to chronological age, not EDD.
- There is no lower weight limit for immunisation.

Common myths

Where ignorance exists, myths flourish. Wild stories used to depict the supposed dangers of cowpox vaccine: 'a child ran about on all fours like a beast, bellowing like a cow, and butting with its head like a bull'. While that myth can now be easily laughed off, new vaccines produce new myths. The media are happy to put about these myths uncritically with the potential of discrediting the whole vaccination programme. In the late 1970s and early 1980s the whooping cough scare was so profound that even doctors would advise that the vaccine was not very effective and might carry a distinct risk of encephalopathy. The fact of the matter is that the pertussis vaccine used in the UK is highly effective and carries no risk or a very much lower risk of brain damage (1 case per 300 000 doses) than the actual disease.

Current myths include the belief that (1) homeopathy is as effective as immunisation, (2) good housing, food and hygiene will protect the child, and (3) MMR vaccine causes autism. Whether or not homeopathic practitioners themselves support vaccination (a matter of dispute) is less important than the fact that, unlike current vaccines, homeopathic products have never been subjected to rigorous scientific scrutiny as potential prophylactics for some of the most dangerous infectious diseases known to afflict mankind.

The myth about the protective effect of modern living is completely misguided as modern living causes the average age of infection to rise, leading to an increase in severe symptomatic viral infections in older children and adults. The polio epidemics of the 1940s and 1950s are a likely example of this effect. Viral infections tend to be more severe with increasing age.

Parents have been frightened by scare stories concerning the MMR booster immunisation and have needed long discussions with their doctor. The worries are that measles could predispose to Crohn's disease and that MMR vaccination is a source of brain damage and autism. These arose following a report of finding measles virus in the intestine in Crohn's disease and a subsequent suggestion that measles vaccination may be a cause. Similar bowel changes were subsequently found in a small group of autistic children and a causal link to MMR vaccine was postulated. Critics stated that the epidemiological aspects of the study had serious methodological defects and also argued that the underlying biological premise was weak as the presence of measles virus in diseased bowel tissue had not subsequently been confirmed by other workers. Furthermore, the rise in the incidence of Crohn's disease antedated the introduction of measles vaccine by 20 years, and autism was first described in 1943, long before the introduction of MMR. The first signs of autism often appear around the age of 2 years, so there is a temporal association with vaccination. 100 000 000 doses of MMR have been given in the US but the American Institute of Medicine has not been able to establish any link.

Common questions (see also Box 16.3)

- Postpone immunisation if the child has a systemic febrile illness (not for 'snuffles', or a 'bit of a cough', etc. without general illness).
- Taking an antibiotic is not a contraindication, as long as the child is well.
- Allergy, including asthma, is not a contraindication, except for some specific allergies, mentioned under specific vaccines.
- Eczema is not a contraindication. (It was for smallpox vaccine.)
- A mother's pregnancy is not a contraindication. For oral polio, give advice about careful hygiene. For MMR, the subsequent feverish illness is not infectious.

Immunisation and immunosuppression

HIV infection

- Asymptomatic HIV positive individuals can be vaccinated as appropriate with the regular childhood vaccines, except for BCG which may disseminate. (Yellow fever vaccine is also contraindicated.)
- Symptomatic HIV positive individuals should not receive live vaccines.
- Polio virus may be excreted for longer than usual.
- Give human varicella zoster immunoglobulin (VZIG) following contact with the varicella

Box 16.3 Common questions about immunisation	
The child is adopted	The child should receive all immunisations appropriate for age. If there is any suggestion of maternal HIV, consult the adoption agency
The child came from abroad	Assume the child has received only those vaccines for which there has been documentary evidence
A course of vaccinations has been interrupted	Do not restart the course, give the remaining doses at appropriate time intervals
The risk of polio from swimming pools	Not in the UK. There may be a risk in developing countries
The child has already had the disease	With one exception (TB, see below), the child should still be vaccinated. No harm will come from vaccinating a child against a disease he has already had. The history of a disease is often inaccurate (particularly rubella) and many infections do not confer as good protection as the vaccination (e.g. polio, tetanus and Hib). TB is the one exception to this rule; the Heaf test must precede BCG vaccination.
The manufacturer's literature differs from the DoH recommendation	The former will be based on the original product licence, the latter on documented experience in the field. Follow the DoH guidelines
A nodule develops at the site of DTP injection	This is a common reaction when the dose is given superficially and is not a contraindication to completion of the course. Take care over the subsequent injection

zoster virus in symptomatic HIV positive individuals (consider it also if the CD4 count is low).

- Consider human normal immune globulin (HNIG) after exposure to measles, even if previously vaccinated, as vaccine efficiency may be reduced.

Other immunocompromised individuals

Patients receiving chemotherapy for malignancy or immunosuppression for autoimmune disease and following transplantation should not receive live vaccine. They should be re-vaccinated with DT 6 months after completion of chemotherapy and MMR 1 year after completion.

Give varicella zoster immune globulin (VZIG) and human normal immune globulin (HNIG) following human varicella virus or measles contact respectively as recommended.

Notes on individual vaccines

DTP vaccine

Combined Hib and DTP vaccine for a single injection is now available; the comments relating to DTP (see Table 16.11) generally apply. This

vaccine is given as the primary course at 2, 3 and 4 months.

DT vaccine

DT is given as the pre-school booster with the polio and MMR vaccines.

Low dose diphtheria vaccines

Tetanus and low dose diphtheria vaccine (Td) is the new booster for school leavers instead of single antigen tetanus. When the school leaver has already had 5 doses of tetanus vaccine, give low dose diphtheria (d).

Do not give paediatric strength diphtheria vaccine (D) to anyone over 10 years old.

N.B. The method of packaging of DT and Td does not clearly indicate that the two preparations have different applications.

Tetanus vaccine

The main indication for adsorbed tetanus vaccine is the treatment of patients with tetanus-prone wounds, see Table 16.12. A strong local reaction to tetanus is likely if vaccination is given within

Table 16.11 DTP vaccine

No contraindication to DTP (+Hib) vaccination if:	Comment
Positive family history of febrile convulsion	Give advice on prevention of fever
Positive family history of epilepsy	Give advice on prevention of fever
Cerebral damage in newborn period	Give vaccination unless evolving neurological abnormality
Immunisation after 6 months of age (particularly third dose)	Increased risk of fever + convulsion Prevent fever with paracetamol and tepid sponging
HIV positive individuals	DTP + Hib all inactivated
Modify DTP (+Hib) vaccination course if:	
Acute (febrile) illness	Advice Defer until child recovered
Primary course of DT started and parent wishes pertussis added later	Give DTP for subsequent doses of DT followed by acellular pertussis vaccine to complete the 3 doses of P at monthly intervals
A febrile convulsion or other severe general reaction has occurred after a previous dose of DTP	Seek specialist advice
A severe local reaction has occurred to a previous dose	Give DT and acellular pertussis vaccine
Child has an evolving neurological disorder or frequent seizures	Seek specialist advice

Table 16.12 Tetanus vaccine

Immunisation status	Clean wound	Dirty wound
Last of 3-dose course within last 10 years	Do not give	Give human tetanus immunoglobulin (HTI) if very high risk
Last of 3 dose course given over 10 years ago	Give tetanus vaccine	Give tetanus vaccine + HTI
Not immunised	A full 3-dose course of tetanus vaccine	Full course of tetanus vaccine + 1 dose HTI in a different site

10 years of a 3-dose course or if a total of 5 doses have already been given.

Haemophilus influenzae *type B vaccine (Hib)*

This vaccine is now given as part of the primary course and when mixed with DTP has not caused an increase in adverse reactions. It is now known that Hib vaccines produced by different manufacturers are antigenically interchangeable.

Children under 1 year old should have all three doses of Hib (at monthly intervals) even when they have had their DTP vaccinations. Unimmunised children between 13 and 48 months should be given a single dose of Hib (this can be with the MMR).

Poliomyelitis vaccine

- There are two forms: Sabin live oral vaccine (OPV) and Salk inactivated, injectable vaccine (IPV).
- A course started with one form can be completed with the other. The vaccine is given as part of the primary course and all three doses are essential for immunity.
- Breast feeding does not affect the efficiency of the vaccine.
- Unimmunised adults can be immunised at the same time as their children.
- Babies in special care can be given IPV until discharge, when the course can be completed with OPV.
- Recently immunised children can be taken swimming.

- Defer immunisation if the child has a diarrhoeal illness.
- OPV is contraindicated in immunosuppressed individuals (see above).
- Faecal excretion of virus lasts for up to 6 weeks and may lead to infection of an unimmunised contact, which is a danger in the rare instance that the contact is immunosuppressed (see above).
- The incidence of vaccine associated poliomyelitis following live OPV is 1 in 2 400 000 doses, but is highest for the first dose at a rate of 1 in 750 000 doses. It may occur in the recipient or in the contact case, the latter usually being incompletely vaccinated. *Contacts of vaccinated children must observe strict personal hygiene* (washing the hands after nappy changing).

Mumps/measles/rubella vaccine (MMR)

- MMR should be given at 13 months and again with the pre-school booster.
- MMR can be given with OPV as part of the pre-school booster. If the child missed the first dose of MMR, give a second dose 3 months later.
- Recall children who missed the measles/rubella (MR) campaign of 1994 and who have already had their pre-school boosters without MMR. Offer MMR to school leavers who missed the MR campaign (which can be given with Td and OPV).
- Give advice on reducing fever, particularly when there is a history of convulsions (Table 16.13).
- MMR can be used as prophylaxis to prevent a measles outbreak.

- A history of measles, mumps or rubella is *not* a contraindication.
- Non-authenticated complications include encephalitis and Guillain–Barré syndrome (i.e. incidence is no more frequent than background).

Contraindications to MMR

- These are live vaccines and should not be given to immunocompromised individuals or those with malignant disease (see above).
- Do not give within 3 weeks of BCG.
- Allergies to neomycin or kanamycin.
- Do not give within 3 months of injection of immunoglobulin.
- Pregnancy should be avoided for 1 month after immunisation.
- Egg allergy, even anaphylaxis, seems to confer little risk. If in doubt, give vaccine as a day case in hospital.

Bacillus Calmette–Guérin (BCG) vaccine

BCG is given to:

- Newborn babies or children of immigrants from countries with a high prevalence of TB: most countries in South East Asia and the Indian subcontinent (except Sri Lanka), Djibouti and Yemen in the Middle East, and most African countries. There is a wide variation in BCG immunisation policy in different areas of the UK.
- School children between 13 and 18 years. This is subject to local reviews.

Babies up to 3 months old are immunised without a prior skin test. All others *must* have a tuberculin skin test (usually the Heaf) before immunisation (see Figure 16.5 and Table 16.14).

Table 16.13 Complications of MMR

Complication	Time interval after vaccination	Incidence
Fever, malaise	1 week, lasting 2–3 days	Not given
Febrile convulsion	6–11 days	1 in 1000
Parotid swelling	3 weeks	1%
Mumps meningitis	3 weeks	Not with current vaccine
Thrombocytopenia	Not stated	1 in 24 000 after dose 1 at 13 months

Table 16.14 Interpretation of the Heaf reaction

Grade 0	No induration
Grade 1	Discrete induration at 4 or more needle sites
Grade 2	Induration around all 6 needle sites, merging but leaving a clear centre
Grade 3	Solid area of induration 5–10 mm wide
Grade 4	Solid induration over 10 mm wide. Vesiculation or ulceration may occur

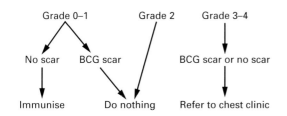

Figure 16.5 Decision tree after reading Heaf.

There are two preparations of BCG:

- intradermal—for routine intradermal administration
- percutaneous—only used in a multiple puncture technique.

Make sure you have the correct preparation.

What's new?

New introductions into current practice include:

- Acellular pertussis vaccine (APV). This monovalent preparation is available on a 'named patient' basis. It cannot be used for routine immunisation. Local reactions and pyrexias occur less often with APV than after the routine whole cell vaccine, especially when the immunisation is given after 6 months of age.
- Recent guidance from the United States Centers for Disease Control and Prevention now suggests the use of Salk (killed) vaccine for the first two doses at 2 and 4 months, followed by the oral (live) Sabin vaccine at the age of 12–18 months and again at 4–6 years. The rationale for this is that in the US there is a relatively high incidence of vaccine induced poliomyelitis compared with natural cases.
- From 1996 a second dose of MMR vaccine is recommended, to be given with the pre-school boosters. Children who have already had their pre-school boosters and missed the 1994 MR campaign should be recalled and given a second dose of MMR vaccine.
- A low dose diphtheria booster for school leavers (Td) in place of single antigen tetanus. *Make sure you have the correct diphtheria/tetanus preparation as the packaging does not clearly differentiate the purpose of the two vaccines.*
- A combined DTP and Hib vaccine.
- Meningococcal vaccines for Group C is available from 1999 for infants and school-leavers. Type B vaccine is under development.

DERMATOLOGY OF CHILDHOOD

Introduction

Paediatric diseases commonly present by changes noticed in the child's skin. These changes are easily seen by parents, grandparents and carers alike and can cause significant degrees of anxiety. The skin is the largest 'organ' in the body; in children, with their relatively large surface area, it is a useful window through which a diagnosis can be made, and often missed!

Rashes and other changes noted in the skin and mucous membranes may be disorders of the skin itself, e.g. ringworm, birthmarks, or signs of systemic disease, e.g. chickenpox, hand, foot and mouth disease, Kawasaki's disease, etc.

The examination of the skin is approached in a similar way to any other examination, namely by the taking of a thorough history and clinical examination.

History

- Present at birth?
- Any associated factors, e.g. fever?
- Any relieving factors, e.g. dietary avoidance?
- Associated symptoms:
  —itch
  —mucosal surface involvement
  —bleeding
  —joint involvement
  —abdominal pain
  —respiratory symptoms.
- Use of drugs/medicines.
- Recent immunisations.
- Allergies.

- Pets.
- Travel.
- Family history, e.g. eczema or, more rarely, psoriasis.

A family history may suggest an inherited or contagious process and the clinician may need to examine other members of the family. This is especially important in conditions such as scabies.

Examination

- Child well or unwell?
- Distribution of rash—scalp, nappy area, flexural, sun exposed sites, clothing protected sites, extremities, face or trunk or intertriginous areas.
- Any mucosal surface involvement, e.g. Kawasaki's disease, erythema multiforme, Behçet's syndrome?
- Local distribution/organisation, e.g. lesions diffusely scattered or clustered, linear, serpiginous, annular or dermatomal (Table 16.15).

Primary skin lesions:

- macule—a small flat lesion showing an alteration in colour
- papule—sharply circumscribed, slightly elevated
- nodule—soft or solid mass on or below the skin surface
- tumour—localised, palpable mass of varied size and consistency
- vesicle—a blister containing transparent free fluid
- bulla—a large blister
- pustule—a sharply circumscribed lesion containing free pus

Table 16.15 Organisation of lesions

Linear	Dermatomal	Serpiginous	Annular
Epidermal naevi	Herpes zoster	Psoriasis	Ringworm
Lichen striatus	Vitiligo	Erythema marginatum	Granuloma annulare
Contact dermatitis	Café-au-lait spot		Lupus
Warts	Port wine stain		Atopic dermatitis (eczema)
Ichthyosis	Pityriasis rosea		
Psoriasis	Drug reactions		
Incontinentia pigmenti			

Box 16.4 Features of secondary lesions

- Scale—dry and greasy fragment of dead skin
- Crust—a mass of exudate from inflammatory lesions consisting of serum, dry blood, scales and dry pus
- Ulcer—clearly defined deep erosion of the epidermis cutis
- Scar—a permanent skin change resulting in a new formation of connective tissue after destruction of the epidermis cutis
- Excoriation—any scratch mark on the surface of the skin
- Fissure—any linear crack in the skin, usually accompanied by inflammation and pain

---

- weal—an oedematous erythematous circumscribed elevated lesion that appears and disappears quickly.

Secondary lesions (Box 16.4). These evolve from the primary lesions listed above or result from the patient's manipulation of primary lesions or treatment.

Examination should also include the nails, hair, mucous membranes and the conjunctiva. These are all visible parts of the body that may be important in giving diagnostic clues.

THE NEWBORN

A number of innocent rashes occur in infants; they are usually temporary but may be quite dramatic and cause a significant degree of parental and family anxiety. Early recognition by general practitioners and paediatricians is important in order to provide appropriate support to families and to distinguish the common self limiting conditions from more serious disorders, which are rare.

Acrocyanosis and cutis marmorata

In these conditions changes in vascular tone result in variable colour change, particularly in the hands and feet and around the peripheries of the face. In acrocyanosis the condition principally affects the hands and feet, which become variably blue in colour without oedema or any other changes. Cutis marmorata is identified by bluish

purple mottling of the skin, particularly over the extremities. Both conditions are usually entirely harmless and disappear when the skin is warmed. They tend to resolve by 1 month of age, although in certain conditions, e.g. Down's syndrome, they may persist for much longer. The peripheral cyanosis is not associated with any central abnormality.

A more vivid variant is *harlequin colour change* when the infant shows a marked difference in coloration—bright red on one half of the body and blue on the other half. This recurs frequently until the infant is about 1 month of age and then resolves.

Milia

Milia are very superficial vesicles appearing on non-inflamed skin when the duct is blocked by sebaceous material. The lesions tend to occur in crops and resolve quickly.

Acne

Mild acne may develop in up to 20% of newborn infants. It usually consists of red papules and pustules, particularly over the nose and cheeks, and tends to clear without any specific treatment by 3 months of age.

Subcutaneous fat necrosis

Minor trauma to the skin, especially after forceps delivery, very commonly results in discrete nodules, particularly over the cheeks, back, buttocks, arms and thighs. The nodules are usually painless and resolve over the first 2–3 months of life. The lesions heal without any scarring but occasionally cause concern to families, particularly when they are readily palpable as nodules under the skin.

Newborns with scaly rashes

After delivery the skin is usually smooth and velvety. Desquamation may begin very quickly in post-mature infants and peeling may be present within hours of birth. Excessive desquamation,

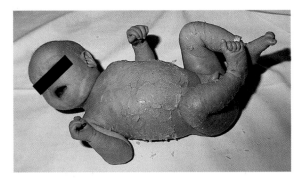

Figure 16.6   Collodion baby.

particularly within the first 24 hours of life, should however be considered abnormal and suggests an ichthyotic condition. The differential diagnosis consists of ichthyosis, which is in fact a group of scaly disorders; sophisticated tests are required to differentiate them. Collodion baby (Figure 16.6) is a example of an extreme form of ichthyosis. Mild scaly rashes usually respond well to emollients, although keratolytics may also be required.

Nappy rash (ammoniacal dermatitis)

Nappy rash is one of the most common skin disorders of infancy. It is in fact an irritant contact dermatitis and affects the nappy area because it is bathed in urine and faeces. The red skin rash with occasional ulcers is confined to the convex surfaces of the perineum, lower abdomen, buttocks and proximal thighs. The intertriginous areas are invariably spared, in contrast to candidiasis.

Nappy rash is occasionally complicated by secondary staphylococcal infection; this may occur in epidemics, particularly on postnatal wards.

Treatment is with barrier creams, regular nappy changing, and occasionally dietary manipulations to reduce the frequency of passage of loose stools.

Candidiasis

This is usually a fiercer eruption than nappy rash with sharper borders, red papules and pustules. Characteristically there are satellite lesions. The lesions typically occur in the skin creases and may be associated with oral thrush. Treatment is with topical (clotrimazole/miconazole, nystatin) and oral (nystatin) anti-fungal agents.

Seborrhoeic dermatitis (cradle cap)

This is characterised by salmon coloured patches with a greasy yellow scale, also beginning in the intertriginous areas such as the nappy and axilla, and on the scalp. A thick adherent scale on the scalp is referred to as 'cradle cap'. Post-inflammatory hypopigmentation may be quite marked, particularly in pigmented skins.

The cause of seborrhoeic dermatitis is unknown although infection has been postulated. It usually clears without treatment but often persists until the child is about 1 year of age and may be treated with emollients, low potency steroids and reassurance.

The differential diagnosis is wide but includes rare disorders such as histiocytosis X (Langerhans giant cell abnormality).

Pustular dermatoses of neonates

These are relatively rare conditions in the neonatal period and are usually innocent. Although they do not cause any upset in the infant they can be dramatic and cause quite a lot of parental and professional anxiety. It is important to distinguish these benign disorders from more serious disorders and to provide appropriate treatment and reassurance.

Benign pustular dermatoses. There are several benign pustular rashes which are common in infants.

Erythema toxicum neonatorum is the most common and can occur in a large proportion of full-term healthy infants. The condition usually presents within the first 2 or 3 days of life and continues for 2–3 weeks.

Transient neonatal pustular melanosis occurs in a smaller proportion (less than 5%) of infants and is usually noted particularly in black male infants. The lesions are usually present at birth as small, 2–5 mm pustules on a non-erythematous base, usually on the upper body. These lesions tend to develop a central crust which desquamates and then leaves a macule.

Acropustulosis of infancy occurs later in the newborn period, i.e. at the end of the first month. The pustules tend to appear on the peripheries. This condition tends to be more chronic and can continue for the first 2–3 years of life.

The differential diagnosis includes herpes simplex and varicella zoster (chickenpox), both of which produce vesiculo-pustular eruptions. The main concern is that in neonates there is a high risk of dissemination of herpes. Varicella is less common. The lesions normally present as small blisters, or in clusters of red papules and vesicles, and commonly occur over the scalp after a cephalic delivery. If herpes is suspected, treatment should be commenced with systemic anti-viral agents as there is a risk of herpes encephalitis with type 1 or type 2 virus.

Varicella zoster (chickenpox) immunoglobulin and aciclovir may be of value in suspected chickenpox.

Bacterial infection, particularly with staphylococci, may also present with vesicular pustular eruptions. The important diagnosis is the staphylococcal scalded skin syndrome (SSSS) which needs urgent treatment. SSSS may be a component of toxic shock syndrome in which systemic disturbances and shock predominate.

Bullous lesions

This is a large group of disorders characterised as the blistering dermatoses, of which *epidermolysis bullosa* is the most typical. There are several subtypes which usually present in early life with trauma induced blisters and separation of skin layers. Definitive diagnosis requires skin biopsy and electron microscopy. Treatment consists of minimising skin contact. The prognosis is poor as scarring and nutritional problems often occur.

Naevi

Naevus is a term used to describe a lesion that is either apparent at birth or that appears within the first few weeks of life. Naevi may be considered under the following headings:

Vascular naevi. The most common vascular naevus is the salmon patch (birth stork mark), visible over the nape of the neck and over the eyelids in healthy term babies. This tends to disappear within the first year of life.

Port wine stains. These tend to be present at birth but are relatively rare, being found in 0.2–0.3% of newborns. They tend to persist unchanged during childhood and may be associated with underlying vascular malformations, e.g. Sturge–Weber syndrome. Treatment includes the early use of laser therapy; urgent referral to a dermatologist or plastic surgeon skilled in the use of this therapy is important.

Haemangiomata. These are rarely present at birth but may occur in up to 10% of infants by 4 weeks of age. They tend to be more common in pre-term infants. The lesions begin as barely visible red macules which rapidly grow to form bright red compressible capillary haemangiomata (strawberry haemangiomata). They usually stop growing by 6–12 months of age; early signs of involution then occur (central pallor is an early sign) with full involution occurring by 3–4 years of age in 80% of cases. Treatment is indicated if they interfere with the orbit. Rarely they may be associated with heart failure (Kasabach–Merritt syndrome). Laser therapy has been used, as have other therapies such as interferon.

Epidermal naevi. These are a common paediatric finding; they present as localised, linear, warty, hyperpigmented papules.

Congenital pigmented naevi. These are pigmented macules which are occasionally associated with hair growth noticed at birth or within the first few months of life.

They may vary from a very bluish discoloration, commonly called 'Mongolian blue spot', to giant congenital pigmented (melanocytic) naevi covering a large percentage of the skin. The majority, however, are small and rarely cause any problem although they may arouse a high degree of parental anxiety. There is a small risk (5%) of malignant change after puberty in giant naevi.

ATOPIC DERMATITIS (ECZEMA)

This is a common condition of infancy and childhood with an incidence of approximately 3–5%

between 6 months and 10 years of age; 60% of patients can be expected to have the diagnosis made (or missed) by their first birthday. A further 30% develop the disease between 1 and 5 years of age. Over 75% of children with atopic dermatitis improve by the age of 10–14 years although the remainder may go on to develop chronic adult disease. There is commonly a family history of atopy, and inheritance may well be maternal.

Atopic dermatitis is referred to as eczema but is best described by its appearance, i.e. erythema, scaling, vesicles and crusts with associated lichenification and pigmented changes in chronic conditions. Itch is one of the principal symptoms. The distribution is diagnostic, see Table 16.16.

Typically the rash is made up of red itchy papules and plaque. The lesions are symmetrically distributed over the face, scalp, trunk, and extensor surfaces of the extremities in infancy, with more circumscribed lesions on the flexural surfaces in older children and adolescents. Atopic dermatitis (eczema) may take several forms. *Discoid eczema* describes discrete coin-shaped red patches seen in many patients with atopic dermatitis. This form may be particularly itchy and is also very difficult to treat. *Papular eczema* may be the only manifestation of atopic dermatitis and tends to be noticed over the extensor surfaces of the arms and legs, particularly in toddlers.

In infancy the greatest difficulty is controlling the symptom of itch. Children commonly go to bed with unaffected skin only to wake the following morning with torn, excoriated skin with bleeding. This is distressing to parents and to the sufferer alike. Chronic itching leads to lichenification and scaling. If the hands and feet are affected, they can be very difficult areas to treat.

Complications are those of sleep disturbance because of itching, and secondary infection. This may be staphylococcal or herpetic and may lead to staphylococcal scalded skin syndrome or eczema herpeticum and Kaposi varicelliform eruption in more severe cases.

Treatment is by use of emollients, an allergen avoidance diet which may help in a few cases, and steroid therapy, e.g. 1% hydrocortisone. The use of occlusive dressings (wet wrapping) with steroid therapy may also be beneficial. Liberal use of antihistamines to discourage itching is often extremely effective. In very severe cases admission to hospital may be required.

PSORIASIS

This is a relatively uncommon diagnosis of childhood. It is characterised by red, well demarcated plaques of dry thick silvery scale.

It is a multifactorial disorder, and allergy is not a feature. In childhood the first presentation may in fact be a psoriatic arthopathy which may pre-date the classical lesions. Psoriasis may be precipitated by upper respiratory tract infection (guttate psoriasis) and the lesions are often induced in areas of local injury, such as scratches, surgical scars or sunburn (Koebner phenomenon).

The course of psoriasis is chronic and unpredictable. Treatment may be with emollients, corticosteroids, tar products and keratolytics. The use of ultra-violet light therapy with psoralen photosensitisers is often beneficial. Children with psoriasis require an expert paediatric dermatologist opinion.

CONTACT DERMATITIS

This is a relatively common disorder in childhood. In its most common form irritant contact dermatitis results in blistering, erythema and itchiness of the skin. A typical example of this occurs on contact with poison ivy and rhus. Another common cause of contact dermatitis is photocontact, either from direct sunlight or photosensitisers. Juvenile spring eruption, characterised by blistering lesions on the hands, feet and ears, is an example of this photosensitivity.

Sometimes the cause of the contact dermatitis is obvious, as in plant secretions or nickel-containing jewellery. Other common contact

Table 16.16 Distribution of eczema

Age	Distribution
Infancy	Trunk, face and limbs
Childhood	Flexural surfaces, ankles and neck
Adolescence	Flexural surfaces, hands and feet

allergens include rubber and glues or dyes in shoes; an example is 'trainer foot' which usually presents as blistering of the soles of the feet when sweaty feet are in contact with synthetic materials in training shoes.

Treatment consists of allergen avoidance and short-term steroids with emollients. Oral steroids may be indicated in severe cases. The differential diagnosis includes tinea pedis.

PITYRIASIS ROSEA

Pityriasis rosea is a common innocent self limiting disorder which can occur at any age. There is often a prodrome of malaise prior to the rash. There is usually a herald patch, which is a 3–5 cm isolated oval scaly pink patch anywhere on the body. This then clears and within a fortnight many small lesions appear on the trunk, usually in a distribution running parallel to dermatomes and giving a typical 'Christmas tree' pattern. Occasionally inflammation is intense, causing blistering. The rash tends to reach a peak in several weeks and fade over 6–12 weeks. Ultraviolet light may hasten improvement. Post-inflammatory hyper- and hypopigmentation may occur. The cause is unknown but the peak incidence is in late winter. The differential diagnosis includes pustular psoriasis, viral exanthemata (e.g. roseola), drug rashes and tinea.

INFECTIONS
Viral infections

Herpes simplex is a common cause of mouth ulcers in toddlers and school aged children. Primary herpetic gingivostomatitis is common in infants and toddlers; spread may occur to the areas of the skin around the mouth, as well as to the hands. Treatment is symptomatic as the symptoms improve over 7–10 days.

If the hard palate is involved then enteroviral infections are a more likely cause, and if there is no diffuse inflammation associated with the lesions they are more likely to be aphthous ulcers.

Primary herpes simplex can involve any cutaneous or mucous membrane surface. Most infections are caused by HSV type 1. HSV type 2 is more commonly found in the genital area, however it may also be found in non-genital areas and type I may spread to genital sites.

Recurrence of herpes simplex infections is triggered by respiratory infection or stress and manifests as cold sores. Superadded infection with Streptococcus may occur, particularly on the hands and face. Impetigo caused by Streptococcus and Staphylococcus may mimic herpes; the bullae, however, tend to be larger.

Varicella zoster (chickenpox)

This is usually a mild self limiting infection in most children. It has an incubation period of 14–21 days. The lesions tend to consist of small papules with central umbilication which then blister and crust. New papules and vesicles continue to appear for 3–4 days and can occur anywhere over the skin and mucous membranes (Figure 16.7).

Complications occur if the child has severe eczema (varicelliform eczema). Re-activation of chickenpox virus in the sensory ganglia leads to shingles. The rash may have clusters of red papular vesicles corresponding to a dermatome. Symptoms are variable: there may be no

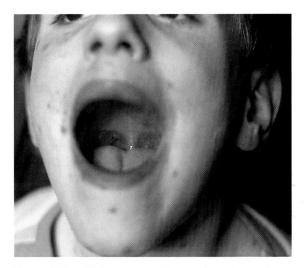

Figure 16.7 Chickenpox—vesicle on palate.

symptoms or localised itching and burning may occur.

There is a danger of spread to contacts, especially to the elderly, pregnant women and immuno-compromised children and adults.

Herpes zoster and Herpes simplex

These may be difficult to differentiate, particularly when there are only a few lesions. Management is usually by treatment of symptoms only, but in immunocompromised children, i.e. those who have HIV or lymphoreticular malignancy, treatment with high dose aciclovir may be essential. Prophylaxis is unnecessary unless the child is immunocompromised. It should be noted that shingles is infectious; children with shingles should be isolated from children who are susceptible to chickenpox.

Hand, foot and mouth disease

This is a viral eruption caused by Coxsackie A16. It is highly infectious and has its peak incidence in the late summer and autumn. The incubation period is 4–7 days, and there is a 1–2-day pro-drome of fever, anorexia and sore throat followed by the development of 3–6 mm thin-walled vesicles on a red or non-inflamed base. Lesions most commonly occur on the palms, soles, and sides of the hands and feet (Figure 16.8). This rash is characterised by vesicles which rapidly ulcerate. There may be associated systemic symptoms such as diarrhoea, fever, sore throat and cervical adenopathy. The illness clears in less than a week.

Acquired immune deficiency syndrome (AIDS)

The prevalence of HIV in children is relatively low. There are a number of classical skin lesions. In children under 1 year of age chronic oral thrush and intertriginous candidiasis are common. Other important opportunistic infections may occur, including mycobacterial infection of the skin and impetigo. Persistent nappy rash and oral candidiasis are a clue to diagnosis. Widespread recurrent herpes gingivostomatitis and

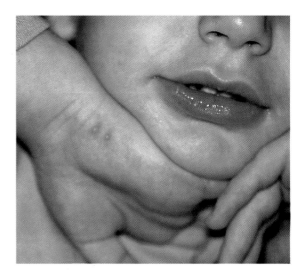

Figure 16.8 Hand, foot and mouth disease.

disseminated herpes simplex are a frequent problem, as are chronic herpes infections.

Molluscum contagiosum caused by the pox virus may be the first sign of AIDS in an otherwise healthy child. Disseminated deep fungal infections with cutaneous involvement are seen in more advanced cases.

Scabies infestation may be widespread because of immunodeficiency. Other cutaneous findings in children with AIDS include bruising from idiopathic thrombocytopenic purpura and vasculitis. Cutaneous Kaposi's sarcoma is rare.

Warts and molluscum contagiosum

Warts are benign epidermal tumours produced by human papilloma virus infection. The incubation period is variable and most lesions disappear within 3–5 years. Warts on the soles of the feet are called verrucae. Warts can be found on the trunk, oral mucosa and conjunctiva; warts occurring in the ano-genital area are called condylomata acuminata.

Molluscum contagiosum is caused by a large pox virus. Lesions are characterised by sharply circumscribed single or multiple superficial pearly papules. Most are umbilicated. Molluscum is endemic in young children and can involve any area of the body.

Both warts and molluscum are spread by trauma (Koebner effect) and are contagious. Treatment tends to be limited to the use of topical irritants or excision with electrocautery or freezing.

Warts are usually a nuisance rather than a major problem but they may present a serious management problem in children with immunodeficiency or those who are receiving chemotherapy.

Bacterial infections

Impetigo

This is a skin infection caused by Streptococcus and Staphylococcus. It is usually a self limiting illness but it may spread to family members and classmates. Lesions tend to be doughnut shaped with a central crust and satellite lesions. Bullous lesions may occur. Impetigo pustules over the hands and feet are painful. Treatment is with appropriate antibiotic therapy. Children do not need to be excluded from school if the lesions are covered.

Staphylococcal scalded skin syndrome (SSSS)

This is related to primary staphylococcal infection with toxin production. The skin tends to be tender and erythematous; minimal forces will produce sloughing of the skin or blister formation (Nikolsky sign).

Healthy children respond well to anti-staphylococcal antibiotics (e.g. flucloxacillin). These should be given parenterally in severely ill children or those who are immunocompromised.

Staphylococcal infection

This is a common problem in older children. Children tend to develop recurrent pustules with occasional deep-seated abscess or carbuncles involving the hair follicle. There may be associated cellulitis. This condition is often associated with severe acne. Treatment should be symptomatic, with antibiotics if indicated.

Fungal infections

Two types of fungal organisms, dermatophytes and yeasts, produce clinical dermatological disorders.

Dermatophyte infection

The dermatophytes include tinea or ringworm fungi which can infect the skin, nails and hair.

Tinea corporis is usually a superficial fungal infection of non-hairy skin and has been called ringworm because of its characteristic shape. Tinea corporis can occur in any age group and is usually acquired from an infected domestic animal or direct human contact. It is diagnosed by scraping the skin and demonstrating hyphae in potassium hydroxide solution. Treatment is with local or systemic anti-fungal agents.

Tinea pedis (athlete's foot) is a fungal infection of the web space of the feet. It is usually acquired from contaminated floor space and can be very irritating. If treated with topical steroids as eczema it will spread. Treatment is by local and occasionally systemic anti-fungal agents.

Yeast infection

The most common yeast infection of the skin is **candidiasis**, which infects the intertriginous areas (see p. 348). It may also occur around the mouth.

Tinea versicolor. This is a common skin lesion characterised by multiple small oval scaly patches with a guttate (raindrop) distribution on the upper chest, back and proximal upper extremities. Tinea versicolor is caused by a yeast, Pityrosporum, and is often associated with hyper- and hypopigmentation. The pigmentary changes may take many months to clear, particularly on dark-skinned patients.

INFESTATIONS
Scabies

Scabies is a common infectious dermatosis produced by the Sarcoptes mite. The pregnant female burrows through the outer epidermis to deposit her eggs and this leaves an itchy linear burrow, found particularly on the finger webs, wrists, elbows, genitalia and axillae. Secondary infection of the burrows with the production of pustules, crusting and cellulitis is frequent.

The diagnosis should be considered in any infant with a widespread papular rash which involves the palms and soles, particularly if other members of the family are infected. Parents often have lesions on the chest, acquired from holding infected children.

Treatment is with malathion or permethrin as determined by local consultation with the pharmacists, as each health district has its own policy as to which treatment should be used because of resistance.

Nits

Nits or headlice are frequently encountered and may present in the clinical examination. They are commonly found on the scalp, eye lashes and pubic area. Lice are 6-legged insects visible to the unaided eye. Lice are identified close to the skin under the short hairs at the sides and back of the scalp; the eggs are identified by their attachment to the hair. The eggs or nits can be removed by fine tooth combing after applying shampoo and conditioner ('bug-busting'). Medication is with carbaryl, malathion or pyrethroids as determined by local prescribing policy.

SUPERFICIAL SKIN TUMOURS

Granuloma annulare

This is an annular eruption, usually beginning as a papule which then spreads. The lesions are most common over the extensor surface of the lower limbs, feet, fingers and hands but other areas can be involved. Their origin is unclear but they appear to be associated with trauma or infection. There is a particular association with diabetes mellitus in adults. Steroid cream may be effective in reducing them.

Xanthomas

These are yellow dermal tumours composed of lipid-laden histiocytes. They tend to occur on the extremities and over the insertion of tendons. They are usually associated with elevation of triglyceride.

Keloids and scars

If the skin is damaged there is a proliferation of fibroblasts in the dermis. This lays down collagen and may lead to the formation of a scar. A hypertrophic scar is referred to as a keloid. Keloids are occasionally associated with connective tissue disorders such as Ehlers–Danlos syndrome and are more common in Negro races.

Neurofibroma

Neurofibromas are the most common tumours of neural origin, and may present to the paediatrician. They occur in neurofibromatosis and are usually soft, compressible skin coloured tumours arising in the dermis, often following the line of cutaneous nerves. There may also be café-au-lait spots.

PETECHIAL/PURPURIC LESIONS

Bleeding into the skin which does not blanch when pressure is applied is called a petechia. When it occurs in pinpoint areas and large confluent areas these are referred to as ecchymoses or bruises respectively. The most common cause of purpura is traumatic bruising. Petechiae are only occasionally seen in healthy children, particularly on the upper part of the neck and face after vigorous coughing or vomiting.

Idiopathic thrombocytopenic purpura

Haemorrhage into the skin with purpura and petechiae is common in children with low platelet counts resulting from idiopathic thrombocytopenia purpura. The differential diagnosis includes other causes of thrombobocytopenia such as leukaemia.

Disseminated intravascular coagulation

Bacterial sepsis, particularly meningococcal sepsis (see Figure 16.4), leads to disseminated intravascular coagulation with widespread bleeding into the skin and viscera. Petechiae progress rapidly to ecchymoses and massive areas of purpura.

Purpura fulminans is a specific form of this, in which widespread haemorrhage into the skin leading to necrosis. Protein C deficiency and other causes of thromobophilia may lead to similar skin rashes.

Henoch–Schönlein purpura (HSP)
(anaphylactoid purpura or allergic vasculitis)
(see also p. 305)

This is one of the most common forms of inflammatory vasculitis leading to purpuric lesions. The purpura is often palpable and may be associated with urticaria. Scalp oedema and periarticular swelling (Schönlein's purpura) and abdominal colic with melaena (Henoch's purpura) may occur during or after the appearance of the rash. The rash is characteristically on the buttocks and the extensor surface of the arms and legs (Figure 16.9). The rash may occur episodically for 2–4 weeks, with each group of lesions lasting 3–5 days.

Vasculitis may involve the kidneys (see Chapter 14, p. 305). Diagnostic tests include the demonstration of low complement C3.

KAWASAKI'S DISEASE (see p. 112)

Kawasaki's disease is characterised by high fever lasting 10–14 days, associated with conjunctivitis, pharyngitis, erythema and oedema of the hands and feet. A morbilliform, scarlatiniform or urticarial rash is commonly seen in the groin and axillae. During the resolution of the illness, there may be erythema and fissuring of the lips and desquamation of the palmar and plantar skin.

ERYTHEMA MULTIFORME

This is a distinctive acute hypersensitivity syndrome that can be triggered by numerous drugs, viruses and bacterial infections, and may follow

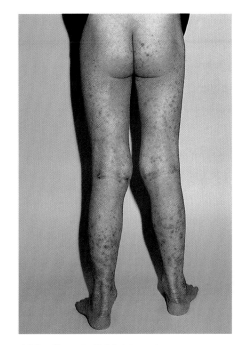

Figure 16.9   Henoch–Schönlein rash.

immunisation. Lesions may occur anywhere on the body but involvement of the palms and soles is common. Target lesions with dusky red macules and weals are common and have an annular shape. The eruption may continue with crops of lesions and last from 1–3 weeks. It is of note that the mucous membranes are spared.

Toxic epidermal necrolysis (Stevens–Johnson syndrome)

This represents the most severe end of the erythema multiforme spectrum. It is a severe reaction affecting the skin and mucous membranes in association with drug hypersensitivity (especially sulphonamides) and following viral infection. The children are systemically unwell and a generalised painful erythema develops with blistering, which may be haemorrhagic, and sloughing of large areas of skin. Mucosal surfaces such as the mouth and conjunctivae are often also affected. This is a potentially lethal condition in the most severe cases and needs to be differentiated from SSSS. Treatment is symptomatic with steroids and antibiotics.

URTICARIA (see also p. 296)

This is the sudden appearance of transient well demarcated weals that are usually itchy and have a peripheral flare. The individual lesions may last for several minutes and move quickly around the body. Acute urticaria, which usually lasts for less than 6 weeks, is caused by hypersensitivity reactions to drugs, food, insect bites or acute infections, both bacterial and viral. The process may continue as a chronic urticaria which lasts from 6 weeks to many years. Treatment is often by exclusion of drugs and foods known to cause the condition. The most severe versions of this condition are idiopathic angiooedema and dermatographism.

ERYTHEMA ANNULARE

This urticaria-like reaction is triggered by the same events that trigger urticaria and erythema multiforme.

ERYTHEMA CHRONICUM MIGRANS

This condition is associated with Lyme disease which is caused by a bite from a tick carrying *Borrelia burgdorferi*. There may be associated systemic upset and meningo-encephalitis. Treatment is with antibiotics, particularly amoxycillin. The lesion usually starts 3–30 days after the tick bite as a single papule which then spreads.

PANNICULITIS

Panniculitis is an inflammatory process involving the fat as well as the skin.

Erythema nodosum

Erythema nodosum is the most typical form of panniculitis. Affected children, particularly teenagers, present with painful red subcutaneous nodules which evolve like bruises, usually over the shins, although the lesions may involve the arms and thighs. The lesions usually fade over several weeks but recurrences are frequent.

The most well known association is with tuberculosis but erythema nodosum can be associated with other infections, including viral pharyngitis, streptococcal pharyngitis, infectious inflammatory bowel conditions and drugs, e.g. sulphonamides and phenytoin. It is usually self limiting. Treatment, if necessary, can include oral steroids.

Cold panniculitis

Cold injury is not uncommon in children. In its most severe form it produces sclerema, with woody induration of the skin and a severely sick child. When the condition affects the toes, it is called chilblains.

FACTITIOUS CONDITIONS

Conditions of the skin and hair not usually caused by a natural process are considered under this heading; examples include loss of hair from traction injury (trichotillomania), skin bruising from rubbing with a coin, blistering from the application of caustic irritants, picking of acne spots, and bruising from non-accidental injury.

The skin may also be the site of psychophysiological disorders, i.e. stress aggravating a skin condition such as eczema.

FURTHER READING

Cohen B 1993 Atlas of paediatric dermatology. Wolfe, St Louis
Davies E G, Elliman D A C, Hart C A, Nicoll A, Rudd P T 1996 Manual of childhood infections. W B Saunders, London

Raffles A, Taylor S 1997 Diagnosis in colour, paediatrics. Mosby-Wolfe, London
Salisbury D, Begg N (eds) 1996 Immunisation against infectious diseases. Department of Health/HMSO, London

Internet addresses

UK infectious disease statistics
http://www.phls.co.uk

Infectious disease
http://hopkins-id.edu

17

Child protection

Jane Wynne

INTRODUCTION

It is not known how many children in the UK are abused each year. The National Society for the Prevention of Cruelty to Children (NSPCC) estimated that 1.5–2% of all children have been physically abused by the age of 17 years. These data were based on information from Child Protection Conferences and are almost certainly an underestimate, as is the quoted figure of 200–230 non-accidental deaths annually.

Studies of the incidence of child sexual abuse (CSA) indicate that 10–30% of girls and 5–15% of boys have been abused (the spectrum ranging from 'exposure' to rape).

Emotional abuse and neglect are probably the most widespread form of abuse and may be seen in conjunction with CSA and/or physical abuse. A harsh, criticised, loveless childhood is the most damaging in terms of long-term adult adjustment and competence.

Recognition of abuse

The recognition of abuse has increased (especially CSA), and the incidence has apparently risen by over 20 times in the last 20 years. There is debate about whether there is a real rise in the incidence of childhood abuse in the UK; there is some evidence of this in the case of severe physical injury.

- There were 35 200 children on Child Protection Registers (CPRs) in 1995 in the UK: 40% were registered as physical injury, 24% as

CSA, 30% as neglect and 6% as emotional abuse.

- CSA is more likely to be recognised in girls, while boys are more likely to be the victim of severe physical injury.
- Deaths usually result from head injury; the majority occur during infancy, and few after 5 years of age.
- Abuse continues throughout childhood but the majority of physically abused children seen are under 5 years.
- The firstborn is at greater risk of physical abuse than later-born siblings.
- Children with disabilities are more abused than their peers; this abuse includes CSA.
- Partner violence is commonly associated with physical abuse and sexual abuse of children.

Box 17.1 Child factors which are associated with child abuse

Pre-term
- Ill
- Parental anxiety
- Difficulty in relating to infant attached to 'machines'
- Will he/she die?

Low birth weight
- Difficult to care for
- Frequent feeds, slow/difficult to feed
- Night feeds, cries a lot
- Physical ill health

Feeding problem
- Slow
- Poor weight gain
- Provokes feelings of inadequacy/anger in carer
- Clumsy, messy feeding
- Screaming, tense, poor sleep pattern—as in drug withdrawal

Developmental delay (physical, learning, sensory)
Behavioural
- Overactive
- Aggressive

Emotional
- Wetting
- Soiling

Previous abuse
- Physical abuse—one third re-abused
- CSA—one third re-abused
- Neglect—one third also physical abuse
- Physical abuse—one third neglect, one sixth CSA
- All abuse is associated with emotional abuse to variable degree
- Unwanted pregnancy

The perpetrator of abuse

- Is usually the child's carer, a member of the family, or a friend.
- Is usually an adult.
- Men are responsible for most CSA and deaths; women are involved equally in other abuses.
- Children are infrequently the abuser, but teenagers are involved as the perpetrator in 25% of recognised cases of CSA and some physical abuse.

The majority of perpetrators do not have major mental health problems. Carers who abuse drugs are more likely to harm their children because of the physiological effects of the drug in utero and their lifestyle. Most of the 'recreational drugs' (opiates, amphetamines, barbiturates) may cause fetal damage if used regularly, and this is a preventable cause of disability.

Box 17.2 Family and social factors associated with child abuse

Socially disadvantaged families
- Poverty
- Poor housing
- Unemployment
- Homeless/hostel/bed and breakfast accommodation

Parents
- Young
- Lone
- Drug/substance abuse (increasing)
- Too many children
- Mental health problems
- Learning problem
- Physical disability
- Poor education
- Poor employment record—lack of necessary skills/training
- History of abuse in childhood: emotional abuse/harsh neglectful childhood especially damaging and may lead to permanent emotional impairment/conduct disorder/criminality
- History of disrupted childhood/foster care/children's home/secure accommodation

Social isolation
- No friends/family
- Lack of supportive extended family
- Impoverished locality lacking 'community' support

Partner violence (physical, sexual, verbal)
- Violent older siblings/baby sitter
- Carer is Schedule 1 offender

Parents who have been abused themselves may have difficulty in parenting and, in particular, meeting their child's emotional needs. Paradoxically, the mother who has been sexually abused may not be able to protect her child from abuse (in CSA 30–40% of the mothers were also victims of CSA). Nevertheless, the majority of parents who have been abused can parent adequately.

Parents with significant learning problems may be able to parent 'well enough' with support but regular review of the child's progress is essential.

It has been recognised in the last decade that abuse is endemic in many institutions: children's homes, schools (mainly residential) and foster homes.

Poverty makes parenting more difficult. The combination of social disadvantage and young, isolated, ill educated, inexperienced parents is the background to a significant amount of abuse.

Presentation

Whilst primary prevention of abuse is a long-term aim, early recognition of maltreatment is important to minimise its damaging effects (secondary prevention). Any doctor who works with children and families should be prepared to recognise child abuse or neglect. The presentation is very variable (see Box 17.3).

The initial assessment by the general practitioner should indicate whether there are grounds for referral to a paediatrician with an interest in child abuse or direct referral to social services, or whether further follow-up in the practice is the best option.

Diagnosis

History and examination

- Take details of the present complaint, relevant past medical and family history.
- Observe the child's demeanour.
- Weigh and measure and plot on growth chart.
- Make sketches of any injuries—describe the colour of the bruises and measure the lesions in centimetres.
- Is the child's developmental age appropriate?

Box 17.3 Presentation of child abuse

Questions

a During a routine health surveillance appointment a 3-year-old is seen to have unexplained bruises on her thighs.
   Is this physical abuse?
b A child brought to the surgery because of vaginal discharge says her 'sore tuppence' is due to 'Grandpa tickling me'.
   What should the general practitioner do?
c A girl aged 7 years is brought urgently to the evening surgery at the health centre because of a 'straddle injury' but her hymen is torn.
   Is this an accident and previous CSA? Or re-abuse? What urgency is there here?
d A health visitor asks for advice about an infant of 8 months who has not gained weight for 2 months and whose mother has puerperal psychosis.
   Is the mother becoming depressed again and neglecting her baby?
e An 8-year-old boy begins to wet and soil, his mother is an alcoholic and has a series of partners.
   Is this emotional deprivation/abuse?
f Twins of 10 months have had no immunisations, no weight checks for 7 months, no hearing test and have not been taken to the ophthalmology clinic for treatment of their squints: the health visitor cannot gain access.
   Is this neglect?

Answers

a   Probable physical abuse – get more information.
b   Suggest immediate referral to local paediatrician with an interest in child abuse.
c   Requires admission for possible surgery – further investigation at hospital.
d   See in 'failure to thrive clinic' as soon as possible.
e & f Sounds like neglect; suggest a meeting of professionals to improve the care of the children.

- Is the child adequately dressed and clean?
- How does the child relate to the carer?

If the examination (for example, of the genitalia) is not felt to be adequate, a note is made to that effect. If interpretation of the physical signs is difficult the notes are appropriately annotated to acknowledge this (these notes will assist the avoidance of legal argument). A note saying 'looks normal to me' might better read 'difficult, I need a further opinion' as the parent will not conclude 'that's OK then' and the further opinion will not have to correct the initial opinion, perhaps undermining the GP's position.

If any specimens (urine, blood, etc.) are taken, record and also enter the result. Date and sign the notes, and write your surname in capitals below your signature. Be prepared to write a Medical Report for social services (SSD) and a Police Statement (see below).

Care is needed in the interpretation of the history and examination. It is good practice to discuss findings and interpretation with colleagues. Unless you are appropriately trained in child protection (paediatrician or police surgeon), report as to fact rather than expert opinion.

Medical report. This begins with a description of the doctor's professional position, degrees and clinical interest. It records where the child was seen, when, who accompanied the child, and then gives a succinct history with relevant details of the examination. The opinion given should be sustainable given the individual's level of expertise.

Police Statement. This is written on a police reporting form. It is usual for doctors to write their own statement rather than sign one provided by a police officer following an interview. The statement starts with name, qualifications and relevant training and expertise and then continues as for a medical report. Indicate why the referral was made but do not report any hearsay evidence, i.e. information learned from a third party.

Sometimes the police or SSD need an immediate report, i.e. that day, because an adult is in custody or the SSD are going to court to apply for an Emergency Protection Order. The report may be brief but it should be typed and a copy kept. It should include a note to the fact that it is an interim report.

The doctor may be harassed by the police (or others) to give an instant opinion. It may be necessary to insist on having time to think and debate with colleagues before giving an opinion whilst appreciating that the police may themselves be under pressure and that the SSD have a responsibility to protect, for example, other siblings.

There is a standard fee for providing a Police Statement, and a fee is payable by the local authority for a report.

PHYSICAL ABUSE

Definition

The Department of Health in *Working Together* (1989) uses the definition 'actual or likely physical injury to a child, or failure to prevent physical injury (or suffering) to a child including deliberate poisoning, suffocation and Munchausen's syndrome by proxy'.

A more clinical definition would be 'any physical assault which results in injury' (bruising, laceration, burn, scald, fracture, etc.).

In the UK

- Parents are allowed to use 'reasonable force' in chastisement, which in practice means that children may be smacked but not bruised by their carers.
- Parents may also give a baby or childminder permission to hit their child as a form of discipline.
- Hitting is not allowed in nurseries, schools, children's homes or foster homes.
- There is evidence that most physical abuse begins as 'punishment...which then goes too far'.

In the UK, parents hit over 60% of 1-year-old children and over 95% of 4-year-olds. Hitting decreases with age, but if children are still hit at 11 years they are more likely to be delinquent at 16 years. Recent research found that most smacking was an 'irritated or angry response rather than a controlled one'. Nearly all children had been hit and '15% had experiences which could be categorised as severe'.

Physical violence is one reason children give for running away, and in adolescence teenagers may hit back. There is an association between partner violence, child physical abuse and CSA.

Bullying may be part of endemic violence in households, schools, the workplace and communities; it is difficult to eradicate given the prevalence of violence. Many schools now acknowledge that bullying exists; there are effective anti-bullying strategies and resource packs for schools.

Recognition of physical abuse

Points to note

Record the developmental stage of the child. A baby of 3 months cannot injure himself by hitting himself in the mouth with a dummy. Rolling is a 5–6-month skill—newborns cannot therefore roll across a bed and fall out 'the other side'. Rolling against cot bars does not inflict 4 parallel linear bruises, and 'bouncy cradles' cannot cause acute subdural haematomata.

History

- Does it make sense?
- Is it consistent?
- Who was there?
- Is there a history of pain (all injuries hurt)?
- Is there a history of loss of function (limb fracture)?
- Has there been a delay in asking for help?
- Has medical advice been ignored?
- Have there been previous injuries or abuse?
- Is the child's name on the Child Protection Register (CPR), are the family known to SSD, is the health visitor, midwife, GP concerned?

Patterns of injury

Bleeding disorders that may enter the differential diagnosis are listed in Box 17.4.

- Bruises always require explanation in immobile infants. Toddlers have bruises on the forehead, chin and nose. Older children have bruises over bony prominences, forearms and shins.
- Bruises in unusual sites—on the cheek (Figure 17.1), angle of jaw, ears (Figure 17.2), neck, upper arms, chest, abdomen, inner thighs—are of concern and need explanation (Table 17.1).
- Are the injuries consistent with the history? Are there too many, too severe, different colours (yellowing of bruise after 48 hours), two black eyes (unless there has been a blow to the forehead)?
- Examine the shape of the lesions (Figure 17.3):
  —finger-tip, round/oval, 0.5–1.5 cm

Box 17.4   Bleeding disorders

Idiopathic thrombocytopenic purpura
- Well child, with or without history of recent infection
- Usually self limiting disorder
- Low platelet count

Haemophilia
- Mild disease may present on walking
- Often known family history
- Prolonged PTT and low level factor VIII

Christmas disease
- As haemophilia but low level factor IX

von Willebrand's disease
- Well child, may present after surgery with 'oozing' from wound
- Family history
- Prolonged bleeding time, low level factor VIII

Notes:
1. PTT—partial thromboplastin time—reflects impaired clotting.
2. There are several disorders such as acute leukaemia, meningococcal septicaemia, and Henoch–Schönlein purpura where the child may appear 'bruised', but the child is ill and the diagnosis should be evident.

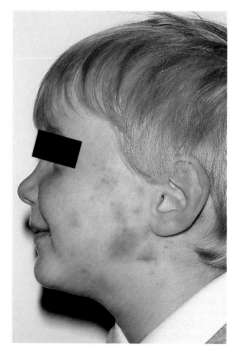

Figure 17.1   Physical abuse: boy of 4 years with multiple bruising on side of face and ear of different ages, notice finger nail scratches.

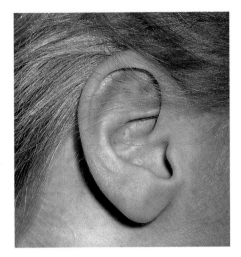

Figure 17.2 Physical abuse: girl aged 7 years with classic bruising of ear pinna.

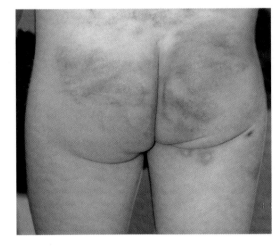

Figure 17.3 Physical abuse: boy of 6 years with badly beaten buttocks, note linear marks within bruising likely to have been caused by repeated hand marks.

Table 17.1 Differential diagnosis of bruising—is it abuse?

Differential diagnosis	Features/investigations
Mongolian blue spot	May be several similar lesions
Café-au-lait spot	Characteristic colour
Prominent vein	Does not change over time
Bleeding disorder (Box 17.4)	Bruising with minimal trauma, initially over bony points, later spontaneous
Collagen disorder, e.g. Ehlers–Danlos syndrome	Characteristic scars and inelastic skin
Ink, paint, felt-tip pen, shoe dye	Wash off

—implement, e.g. belt-shaped, buckle, stick
—contact burn, e.g. shape of grill.
• Repeated injuries are suggestive of abuse.

Specific injuries that suggest abuse

Torn frenulum (upper lip), especially in infancy.
Multiple injuries after a minor/moderate fall.

Fractures (see also p. 302):
Spiral fractures are caused by a pull and twist and are frequently the result of abuse. The humerus, femur and tibia are the long bones

Table 17.2 Fractures

Bone	Fracture	Abuse	Accident
Humerus	Spiral	+++	+
	Supracondylar	+	+
	Metaphysis	+++	Rare
Femur	Spiral/oblique	+++ < 2 years	+
	Metaphysis	+++	Rare
Tibia	Spiral	+ (+++ < 1 year)	+
	Metaphysis	+++	Rare

+ = level of concern
1. Skull fracture—wide, long, multiple, depressed, growing—associated with abuse.
2. Rib fractures—associated with crush injury as in RTA or shaking injury, not as result of cardiopulmonary resuscitation.
3. Toddler fracture—spiral fracture of tibia, but with history of running and twisting on falling.
4. Multiple fractures—think abuse?
5. Head injury and skull fracture in infancy—a shaking/impact injury?
6. Differential diagnosis—accident, bony disorder (osteogenesis imperfecta, metabolic bone disease, birth injury).

involved, and the risk of abuse is greatest in infancy (see Table 17.2). The 'toddler fracture' occurs when a child, usually 1H–3 years old, falls and twists his leg whilst running and suffers a spiral fracture of the tibia. Less commonly a femur may fracture in a similar way.

Metaphyseal (corner) fractures at the ends of long bones, usually the tibia and femur, are highly correlated with abuse in the absence of severe bone disease. They may be seen as part of a 'shaking injury' or a 'pull and twist'.

Skull fracture is uncommon after ordinary falls. Skull fracture with associated brain damage is highly suggestive of abuse in the absence of a fall of more than 3 metres or a road traffic accident (RTA).

Rib fractures. Apart from an RTA the usual trauma is a crushing/squeezing injury. They are not due to cardiopulmonary resuscitation and may be seen in association with subdural haematoma and other fractures.

Severe head injury occurring after a fall of less than 3 metres.

Retinal haemorrhages with or without subdural haematoma. This is the classic shaking injury and may present with 'apnoeic attacks', seizures, breathing difficulty, 'collapse', slow feeding/irritability, or an enlarging head. On examination there may be finger-tip bruises on the chest and upper arms. X-ray may reveal rib, metaphyseal and skull fractures. A CT brain scan is diagnostic and blood-stained fluid is seen on a subdural tap. An MRI scan may be useful to elucidate the damage and time the injury.

Burns and scalds (Box 17.5):

Box 17.5   Scald, burn or skin infection/disorder

Cigarette or impetigo?
Impetigo may blister, is superficial with a yellow crust, does not scar, responds rapidly to antibiotics.

Scald or nappy rash?
Nappy rash may blister and scar but its distribution is characteristic.

Scald or skin infection?
Scalds commonly become infected.

Note: inflicted burns are more commonly on the back of hand, dorsum of foot, and buttocks.

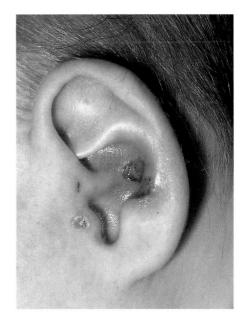

Figure 17.4   Physical abuse: infant aged 10 months with cigarette burn inside ear. This is an inflicted injury and there is an association with sexual abuse.

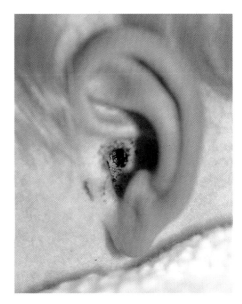

Figure 17.5   Physical abuse: healing cigarette burn in ear.

- Cigarette burns are round, 0.5–1.5 cm, cratered and heal with scarring (Figures 17.4, 17.5).
- Contact burns are found on the back of the hand, dorsum of the foot, and buttocks.

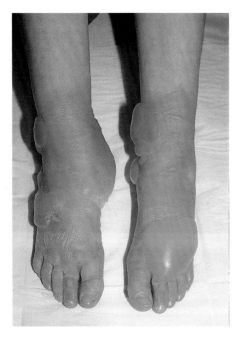

Figure 17.6 Physical abuse: girl of 3 years with forced immersion scald.

- Immersion scalds have a stocking and glove distribution (Figure 17.6).
- Repeated burns are worrying.
- All inflicted burns are sadistic, and there is a link with CSA.

Bites are usually inflicted by peers in the 1–3-year age group. A forensic orthodontist will help to interpret the findings and may identify the abuser by use of impressions.

Intra-abdominal injury from blunt trauma may cause a perforated gut, haematoma, etc., and has a high mortality because of late diagnosis.

Injuries should be photographed.

Investigations

1. Haematological:
   - Hb, FBC, platelet count and blood film
   - clotting screen (PT, PTT)
   - factor VIII and IX level as needed
2. Radiology:
   - if fracture is suspected
   - skeletal survey for children under 3 years with injuries (soft tissue or bony)

3. Further investigations to elucidate rarities, e.g. osteogenesis imperfecta, metabolic disorder
4. Microbiology to differentiate bullous impetigo from cigarette burn.

Other opinions

- Obtain an ophthalmological opinion in all cases of possible impact/shake injury.
- Paediatric radiologist.
- Consult a paediatric dermatologist if there are unusual skin lesions, e.g. self inflicted.

Differential diagnosis

This includes bleeding and skin disorders (see Boxes 17.4, 17.5, and Table 17.1).

Diagnosis

The diagnosis in physical abuse usually requires additional information from the police and SSD investigation:

- What does the child, carer, third party say?
- Has the child been abused before?
- Has there been any CSA or neglect?
- Is there a family history of previous abuse, or a schedule 1 offender in the household?

After all the information has been collected it is usually possible to have a clear opinion as to the probability of abuse or accident, and also whether the injuries are consistent with the given history.

POISONING, SUFFOCATION AND FICTITIOUS ILLNESS

Poisoning (Table 17.3), suffocation, fictitious illness and Munchausen's syndrome by proxy are related and potentially very dangerous forms of abuse.

Suffocation

This is uncommon and difficult to detect. In spite of the violence of the act there may be no signs of injury. Suffocation usually occurs in infancy and is uncommon over 3 years of age.

Table 17.3 Relationship between accidental, neglectful and deliberate poisoning

	Accident	Neglect	Deliberate
Age	2–3 years 6 years and older ?self harm*	2–3 years 6 years and older ?self harm*	Infancy–3 years Any age
History	Usually clear and makes sense, e.g. house move	Social chaos, no drug cabinet	None—ill child Recurrent episodes Previous 'accidental' poisoning
Symptoms	Uncommon < 15% < 1% intensive care Rarely fatal	Uncommon < 15% < 1% intensive care Rarely fatal	Seizures, drowsiness, coma, vomiting, diarrhoea, death
Substance	Drugs: analgesics medicine, iron Household: bleach, petroleum products	Drugs: anxiolytics, cough medicines, the 'pill' Household: detergent	Drugs: insulin, anticonvulsants, antidepressants, methadone Other: salt, corrosives
Past history	Nil	Repeated ingestions, accidents, SIDS, known to SSD	Other siblings ill/dead, previous SIDS, other abuses Mother 'ill'
Diagnosis	History equates with clinical picture	History may be vague, but largely accurate	History not compatible, THINK of poisoning, ask toxicologist

*Self harm must be taken seriously.

The presentation may be as 'near miss cot death' or the child may be dead. There may have been previous episodes of cyanosis or pallor thought to have been 'apnoea' or seizures. There may also have been previous unexplained deaths or illness, including SIDS, in the family.

Examination

• The infant may be well nourished and show no sign of injury.
• There may be signs of neglect, failure to thrive and physical abuse.
• The signs of suffocation are petechiae on the face (may be on eyelids initially).
• Bruises may be seen round the neck and on the upper chest and arms.
• Foreign material may be seen blocking the airways.
• There may be a family history of abuse or previous sudden death of a child.

Differential diagnosis

The main differential diagnosis is SIDS, and the investigations must be sensitive.

• In 'near miss' episodes respiratory, heart, and metabolic disorders and seizure must be consi-dered, as must significant gastro-oesophageal reflux.
• SIDS peaks at 3–4 months; 90% of victims are younger than 8 months.
• SIDS deaths have decreased in recent years but the association with social deprivation is established.
• SIDS is more common in abusing families and households where there is drug or substance abuse.

It is mandatory to discuss unexplained deaths with the coroner. A paediatric or forensic patho-logist should perform the autopsy. The autopsy may be non-contributory but can demonstrate recent or previous trauma.

Fictitious illness (factitious illness/ Munchausen's syndrome by proxy)

Definition

The condition is defined by:

• illness in a child which is faked and/or produced by the parent (carer)
• repeated presentation to different doctors, resulting in multiple investigations and opinions

- a denial by the perpetrator that she is the cause of the disorder(s)
- acute signs and symptoms that abate when the child is separated from carers.

Clinical features

These include:

- bleeding (haematuria, haematemesis)
- seizures
- drowsiness
- coma
- vomiting
- diarrhoea
- fever
- rashes.

Fictitious illness is as common in boys as in girls. The age at diagnosis is around 3 years, and length of the 'illness' may be many years. The mortality is around 10–20% and morbidity 10%. Other forms of abuse may occur: emotional in 100% of cases, physical in 1%, and failure to thrive in 1%. There may be a history of abuse in the siblings; the mother is usually the abuser and appears caring, capable and supportive.

An older child may collude with the induced 'illness' or show other signs of emotional distress.

Diagnosis

This may be difficult; it depends upon the physician realising the possibility of fictitious illness and then working out a strategy to establish the facts and ultimately to confront the carers. Early discussion with the SSD is recommended. Some cases are easier to recognise (but difficult to manage), e.g. when the child has mild asthma and does not respond to standard treatment but has no chest deformity or wheeze and always has a good peak flow rate. Recurrent hospital and clinic appointments ensue and there may be abuse of steroids. The mother gains a lot of attention but the child may be over-treated and restricted in physical activity, even 'invalidised'. It may be best to confront the situation gradually, as the child 'grows out of' the illness.

CHILD SEXUAL ABUSE (CSA)

Definition

CSA is defined in *Working Together* as 'actual or likely sexual exploitation of a child or adolescent'. The child may be dependent and/or developmentally immature. Another definition is the exploitation of a child for the sexual gratification of an adult.

Consent is a pivotal issue in CSA; a child or teenager cannot give consent to an activity that he does not fully comprehend. Sexual maturity does not confer understanding, as is evident for example if a teenager has learning problems or a 10-year-old girl reaches menarche.

Prevalence of CSA in the UK (Box 17.6)

The occurrence of CSA in the UK was confirmed in the *Cleveland Report* in 1988: 'We have learned during the Inquiry that sexual abuse occurs in children of all ages including the very young, to boys as well as girls, in all classes of society and frequently within the privacy of the family'.

The range of sexual abuse

- CSA covers a spectrum—from a stranger exposing himself in the park, to a child who is raped by his father several times a week.
- It includes CSA in the family (which accounts for most CSA in childhood), CSA in 'rings' (paedophile, ritual, other), CSA in foster care, children's homes, schools, hospitals, 'date' abuse and stranger abuse (more common in teenagers).
- The child's father is most frequently the abuser, followed by other 'father figures', e.g. uncle, grandfather, teenage brother, cousin, or baby-sitter.

Box 17.6 Estimated prevalence of CSA in the UK (from several studies)

- Female   12–59%
- Male   8–27%

Note: these prevalence studies employed different methodologies.

- Women are involved in 15–20% of CSA— either alone, with a partner, or as part of a ring. The relationship is as for male abusers.
- The younger the abuser the greater the chance that he was abused himself. Almost all girl abusers are victims of CSA.
- Whilst some abusers only abuse, for example, prepubertal boys (i.e. fixated paedophile), many fathers who abuse assault their sons and daughters.
- Children with disability are at greater risk of all types of abuse. The abuser may be a family member, taxi driver, escort, teacher, special needs assistant, nurse, respite carer, etc.
- Abusers may choose a career in child care. Paedophiles are often 'good with children'.
- CSA covers activities from exposure to masturbation (of child or adult); oral, anal, vaginal penetration; intracrural intercourse; enforced 'child to child' sex, and pornography (viewing or making).
- Anal and oral sex may occur from a very young age. Vaginal penetration is uncommon in girls under 7 years.
- 'Stranger' rape is more likely to be traumatic. In a city of 750 000 (Leeds) there is approximately one such rape of a young girl every 1–2 years, compared to 500–600 referrals annually to community paediatricians for possible CSA.

Presentation

Behavioural

The child may allege CSA but the description may be fragmented, partial and not repeated after disclosure to a trusted adult or friend. False allegations of CSA have been described in a very small percentage of child disclosures. They remain unlikely but do occur more often in older children or in custody disputes.

The child may behave in a sexually promiscuous or play in a sexually explicit way. Older children may be used in prostitution. Younger children may begin to masturbate obsessively. There may be changes in behaviour; for example the child may become weepy or sad, or start wetting or soiling. In other children the behaviour becomes aggressive and defiant (truancy, shop-lifting, substance abuse). The child may sexually assault other children and sometimes adults.

Teenagers may harm themselves, e.g. by wrist cutting, overdose, or substance abuse. The child may develop psychosomatic symptoms, such as abdominal pain or migraine.

Symptomatic

- Vaginal bleeding in a prepubertal girl is highly correlated with trauma, i.e. CSA or accidental injury (Box 17.7). Organic causes are rare but should be excluded (see Chapter 10).

Box 17.7 Accidental injury of the genitalia in girls

- The history is one of a sudden painful injury with immediate bleeding. In straddle injury there may be difficulty in micturition.
- Straddle injury is the most common injury, for example as the child falls astride a climbing frame. The injury is anterior and may be asymmetrical. Swelling and bruising affect the tissues trapped below the pubis—clitoris, urethra and anterior labia majora and minora. There may be a laceration, usually on the labia minora.
- Penetrative injury to the labia occurs in young girls, out of nappies, who fall astride toys. There is minor bruising and sometimes a short laceration to the labia minora which may bleed profusely. Suturing is rarely needed. The hymen is not penetrated.
- Forced abduction of the legs may cause a midline tear at the posterior fourchette. This is a very uncommon injury (e.g. gymnastics) and CSA must be considered.
- Tampon use may cause slight stretching of the hymenal opening.
- A foreign body inserted through the hymen is painful and is associated with a vaginal discharge and frequently CSA. Foreign body insertion in the urethra of boys or girls is uncommon and likely to be part of sexual assault.
- Seat-belt injury to the female genitalia has been described; the history must be that the child was forced astride the belt with considerable force, as in a road traffic accident.
- Self masturbation in girls does not cause injury unless the child is emotionally disturbed, when occasionally self mutilation is seen. (Masturbation in boys does not cause injury to the penis, except in teenagers who may cause injury to the frenulum or use appliances.)
- Female genital mutilation (circumcision is the least mutilating and infundibulation the most serious form) is illegal in the UK but widely practised worldwide. An anaesthetic is commonly unavailable and these children suffer extreme pain.

- Rectal bleeding, usually repeated, in the absence of constipation.
- Genital soreness, with or without vaginal discharge. This is relatively common in the 3--6-year age group; poor hygiene, excessive washing or sensitivity to bubble-bath or soap may be the cause but trauma, e.g. from rough masturbation, should be considered if the symptoms recur. Candidal infection is rarely a cause.
- Dysuria and frequency with no proven urinary tract infection.
- Sexually transmitted disease.
- Pregnancy.

Procedure for the physical examination

- It is up to individual doctors to decide whether they have the appropriate experience to differentiate normal from abnormal and trauma from organic disease, e.g. lichen sclerosus.
- Most practitioners would feel comfortable in examining a 3-year-old girl with urinary symptoms, but if the child has made disclosures of CSA many will request a second opinion.
- The advice of a consultant paediatrician or senior social worker (child protection) should be sought urgently if the assault was made in the previous 72 hours or if the child is considered to be 'at risk'.
- In some areas a police surgeon will be involved in the examination with the paediatrician.
- If the clinical picture is not clear, current practice is to hold a strategy meeting (doctor, health visitor, social worker) to decide how to proceed.
- Before older children are seen by the paediatrician, they should have opportunity to discuss the examination and, if possible, choose a doctor of their preferred gender.
- Children should be asked whom they want to be present at the examination.
- Consent for the examination and photography is required.
- Facilities should be child-friendly; a nurse to chaperone the doctor is essential. Ideally a colposcope should be available which pro-

vides good illumination, magnification and an integral facility for photography.

Forensic examination

Microbiological/sexually transmitted disease (STD) and forensic packs are available. The latter are used to look for evidence of semen, saliva, blood and pubic hairs which may be matched with the alleged abuser. Occasionally there are fibres (from clothing) or other trace evidence which will corroborate the child's allegation. 'Scene of crime' forensic scientists will also look for corroborative evidence. The forensic examination is helpful only if there has been an assault in the last 72 hours in prepubertal girls and boys, or 5 days in pubertal girls.

The 'chain of evidence' must be followed meticulously; this means that all samples taken by the doctor must be labelled, dated, signed and handed to the police officer who will in turn sign and date them before passing them to the laboratory.

Sexually transmitted diseases (STD)

A screen for STD is indicated if there are any signs or symptoms suggestive of STD, especially in 'stranger' abuse. Teenagers who have been sexually abused may be sexually promiscuous and are therefore at particular risk of STD including hepatitis and HIV infection.

STD is usually acquired sexually in children; sharing a bath or towel may be the proffered (but highly unlikely) route of infection. Vertical transmission from the mother during vaginal delivery is recognised—Chlamydia is the infection most commonly seen, while gonorrhoea is uncommon. Anogenital warts may be transmitted in utero (like HIV and syphilis) or at birth.

The probability of CSA as the route for infection varies with the child's age and the particular STD. Gonorrhoea, Trichomonas and Chlamydia occurring after the neonatal period are increasingly likely to have been sexually transmitted. Genital herpes is also usually transmitted sexually. Anogenital warts are the subject of much debate but, in children over 2 years of age, the probability of abuse increases. A schedule for an infection screen is available.

The physical examination (Box 17.8)

The physical examination is a complete review; it includes assessment of growth and should note any soft tissue injuries as well as trauma to the mouth, genitalia and anus.

The demeanour of the child should be noted during the examination (Box 17.9).

Girls

The genital examination in girls takes place in the supine, 'frog-legged' position. It is important to know the range of what constitutes normality (Figure 17.7). The stage of puberty should be noted. Although inspection alone is usually adequate in prepubertal girls, a digital examination is required at puberty.

Normal and abnormal genitalia are described in Boxes 17.10 and 17.11.

Boys

Boys who are sexually abused not uncommonly suffer genital injury. The range of injuries is listed

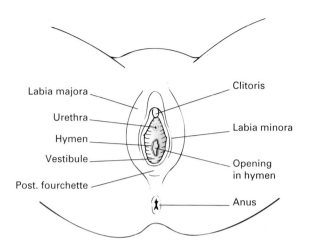

Labia majora — Clitoris
Urethra — Labia minora
Hymen —
Vestibule — Opening in hymen
Post. fourchette —
— Anus

Figure 17.7 Normal anatomy of prepubertal girl.

Box 17.8 Examination in CSA

- Detect traumatic or infective conditions which may require treatment
- Evaluate the nature of any abuse
- Reassure the child who may feel that serious damage has been done
- Start the process of recovery
- Include siblings of an index child
- Include any young abuser who may also be a victim

Box 17.9 Points to note on examination

- Was the child angry, sad, appropriately shy?
- Did he behave in a sexualised way, e.g. have an immediate, even sustained erection when he undressed?
- Did he start to masturbate?
- Why was he so sexually excitable?

Box 17.10 Normal genital findings in girls

1. The hymen is present.
2. The configuration of the hymen changes with age: sleeve, annular, and fimbriated are seen in girls up to the age of 3 years, when a crescentic shape becomes more common. A septate hymen is rare; check for duplex vagina and uterus.
3. In infancy the hymen is thick, under the influence of maternal hormones. As the influence of maternal oestrogen diminishes the hymen thins and fine blood vessels are visible. At puberty the hymen again becomes thickened and redundant. The blood vessels are no longer visible and there is a white, physiological discharge.
4. The hymenal opening in prepubertal girls is less than 4 mm. At puberty it is approximately 1 cm.
5. Vaginal ridges may give the appearance of a bump in the margin of the hymen where they meet.
6. Notches are not seen in the posterior hymen and are uncommon anteriorly; in a crescentic hymen shallow, symmetrical notches are normal.
7. Minor degrees of labial fusion, usually posterior, are common.
8. The hymen is very rarely imperforate.
9. The hymenal opening is usually closed on inspection and requires labial separation or traction to open it. The area of hymen appears greater than the opening, i.e. there is no loss of hymenal tissue as in attenuation.
10. There may be non-specific reddening and discharge.

Box 17.11   Signs associated with genital abuse in girls

1. *Tear of hymen—may extend to vaginal wall and posterior fourchette (Figure 17.8)
2. *Attenuation or loss of hymenal tissue
3. Enlarged hymenal opening. There is dispute about absolute measurements—a horizontal opening of 5 mm is unusual at 5 years; 7 mm is wide, and greater than 7 mm is rarely seen. At puberty 1 cm is usual, 1.5–2.0 cm is compatible with digital penetration, and 3.5 cm indicates penile penetration (5th finger tip, index finger and 2nd and 3rd fingers respectively).
4. Distorted or asymmetric hymenal configuration
5. *Posterior notch in hymen. Anterior notch must be distinguished from crescentic hymen, thus an asymmetric notch is more significant.
6. Irregular, thickened or rolled edge to hymen (if not related to vaginal ridge)
7. Scar at posterior fourchette
8. Labial fusion, particularly long, thick fusion in older girls
9. Erythema, with or without swelling of the hymen
10. Abrasions, laceration, burn, bruising, bite of genitalia, breasts
11. Dilated urethral opening
12. Vaginal foreign body
13. STD
14. Other signs of abuse: anal, physical, emotional, neglect, failure to thrive
15. Pregnancy
16. The child's demeanour during the exam: passive, frightened, flirtatious, angry

*A tear of the hymen and attenuation of the hymen are two signs highly correlated with abuse.

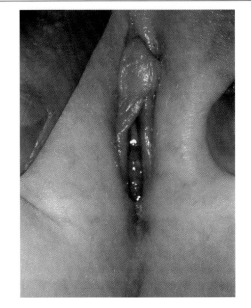

Figure 17.8   Sexual abuse: girl of 3 years with swollen, bruised genitalia and friable area of posterior fourchette following sexual assault by a 15-year-old boy.

Box 17.12   Signs associated with genital abuse in boys

1. Bruising, petechial haemorrhage of penis and scrotum
2. Swelling of scrotum/penis (sucking injury)
3. Torn frenulum (forced retraction of foreskin)
4. Incised wound to penis, usually proximal and dorsal but may be circumferential
5. Red, linear, circumferential mark due to ligature, hair
6. Burns or scalds
7. Damage to the urethral meatus from insertion of foreign body
8. STD
9. Signs of anal or oral CSA
10. Other signs of abuse: physical, emotional, neglect, growth disorder
11. Behaviour during examination: angry, passive, sexualised (erection, masturbation)

---

in Box 17.12 and the differential diagnosis in Table 17.4. The behaviour of the boy should be noted (Box 17.9). When examining the boy it is necessary to gently retract the foreskin to check any damage to the frenulum and also the urethra.

Any urethral discharge should be cultured as part of an STD screen. Forensic swabs for saliva may be useful if there has been oral sex.

Anus

The child is asked to lie on the left side 'curled in a ball'; the buttocks are parted and the external sphincter observed over 30 seconds. The physical signs associated with anal abuse are listed in Box 17.13.

Table 17.4   Differential diagnosis of genital abuse

Male	Female
Masturbation by child unlikely to cause injury, forced retraction of foreskin as part of CSA may lead to damage to frenulum	Masturbation by child does not cause signs unless 'excessive', as follows CSA or self mutilation in emotionally harmed child secondary to CSA
Skin disorder, e.g. bullous impetigo, may mimic burn	Skin disorder, e.g. lichen sclerosus, may mimic trauma
Accidental injury, e.g. zip; rarely toilet seat, bicycle crossbar	Accidental injuries: straddle injury is anterior, often unilateral and without signs of penetration. Hymenal damage. *Not* gymnastic or riding injury
Circumcision may be performed without anaesthetic and inexpertly leading to urethral stricture, partial or complete amputation—usually as a religious ritual	Circumcision and genital mutilation are illegal in UK (Prohibition of Female Circumcision Act 1985)
	Tampon use does not damage hymen but may cause slight stretching
Urethritis: caused by CSA?	Recurrent vulvitis/vulvovaginitis—non-specific infection or STD; occasionally thread worm infestation; contact, e.g. soap, bubble bath
	Rarities: urethral prolapse, caruncle, polyp, vascular lesion
	Bruise

Diagnosis

The diagnosis of CSA is built up as for physical abuse, the practitioner giving an opinion based on the available medical information (history, examination, laboratory tests) with additional input from the police and the SSD as to the probability or otherwise. Are the physical signs consistent with the history? If there are no abnormal physical signs do not conclude without careful thought that there is 'no abuse'; there may indeed be no signs of 'recent penetrative abuse' but healing may be rapid. Oral sex, masturbation, intracrural intercourse and even anal abuse (in adolescence) may leave no signs.

There is often a place in CSA for a further medical opinion, and it is good practice to discuss cases with colleagues, preferably with colposcope pictures.

Other forms of CSA

- Sex rings
- Ritual abuse
- Children used in prostitution
- Children used in pornography.
- These may, and often do, co-exist.

NEGLECT

Definition

The definition of neglect in *Working Together* (1991) is: 'The persistent or severe neglect of a child, or the failure to protect a child from exposure to any kind of danger, including cold or starvation, or extreme failure to carry out important aspects of care, resulting in the significant impairment of the child's health or development, including non-organic failure to thrive'.

Neglect is very damaging but is insidious and often goes unrecognised, although the number of children on CPRs because of neglect is increasing. Child poverty is increasing in the UK: 1 child in 3 is brought up in poverty.

Associations

Neglect is associated with:

- poverty, poor housing, unemployment, homelessness, large families, lone parent, parental alcohol or drug abuse
- high perinatal, infant and childhood morbidity and mortality
- incomplete immunisation and routine health surveillance

Box 17.13 Signs associated with anal abuse

1. Perianal erythema—a non-specific sign which may result from trauma, nappy rash, threadworms or poor hygiene.
2. Perianal bruising, superficial laceration, abrasions. Bruising is uncommon in CSA; scratches (from finger nails) need careful interpretation—does the child have an 'itchy bottom'?
3. Anal verge haematoma is rare and very significant with regard to CSA.
4. 'Tyre sign', i.e. superficial swelling in a ring round anal margin—reflects recent trauma
5. Venous congestion, N.B. observed over 30 seconds. This varies from a flat halo around the anal margin to segmental swelling (arc) to grossly dilated veins. This is the sign which may remain when healing is otherwise complete.
6. Fissures are caused by tearing of the lining of the anal canal. The tear extends over the anal margin and across the perianal skin. The usual cause is severe constipation—a single fissure at 6 or 12 o'clock is seen. In the absence of constipation, deep and/or multiple fissures are significant. A fresh laceration (Figure 17.9) or healed scar extending beyond the anal margin is diagnostic of abuse (RCP 1997). Superficial linear breaks in the skin are sometimes called acute fissures and are seen in nappy rash, candidiasis, eczema and diarrhoea.
7. Anal laxity is demonstrated when the buttocks are separated and the external sphincter gapes to reveal the anal mucosa which may appear to prolapse into the canal in young children. Laxity is also seen secondary to neurogenic bowel and in gross constipation.
8. Anal gaping occurs when the anus, on inspection, is widely open and remains open. It is an acute sign of anal penetration.
9. Reflex anal dilatation (buttock separation test) is demonstrated by observing the anus over 30 seconds. If the sign is present, the external sphincter relaxes, followed by the internal sphincter, giving a view into the rectum. The sphincters open and shut over seconds. The dilatation may be up to 2.5 cm but 1–1.5 cm is more usual. Lesser degrees of dilatation are seen during healing following abuse. The sign is seen when a child passes flatus or is ready to have his bowels open (re-examine after defecation). The sign has also been described in inflammatory bowel disease.
10. Chronic signs of anal abuse are: thickening of the anal verge skin with loss of skin folds, lax anal sphincter. Funnelling, i.e. a deeply placed anus, is seen in teenagers who are repeatedly abused; it is a controversial sign.
11. Scars are uncommon, occurring in less than 10%.
12. STD.
13. Other signs of abuse—genital, physical, emotional, growth.

Notes:
- Healing may be very rapid after abuse.
- Anal abuse in adolescents: in spite of penetration there may be no abnormal signs.
- Signs are usual in infancy and in younger children.

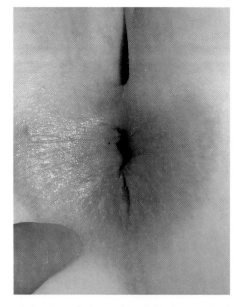

Figure 17.9 Sexual abuse: girl aged 7 years with some perianal reddening, gaping anus and recent extensive tear from anal penetration the previous night.

- poor growth and development, school failure
- accidents (in the home, on the roads, etc.).

Clinical features (Table 17.5)

Appearance. The child's appearance may demonstrate poor physical care. He may be dirty with ill fitting clothes, thin hair (sometimes with alopecia), nits, dirty nails, ingrained dirt on his body, or offensive body odour.

Growth. Serial measurements may show poor growth, stunting and obesity in adolescence.

Neglected medical conditions: squint, dental caries, asthma, undescended testes (usually with a history of failed clinic appointments).

Abuse. There may be signs of other forms of abuse.

Table 17.5 Signs of neglect and emotional deprivation/abuse

	Infant	Pre-school child	School child	Teenager
Physical	FTT recurrrent infection and admissions Nappy and skin rashes	Short ± underweight Microcephaly Unkempt, dirty	Short ± underweight Unkempt, dirty	Short ± underweight/obese Unkempt, dirty Poor general health, failed immunisation, visual/hearing difficulty
Development	General delay	Language delay Distractible Emotional immaturity	Learning delay Distractible Lacks confidence Immature	School failure Illiterate Lacks social skills and confidence
Behaviour	Attachment disorder: anxious, avoidant, unresponsive	Over-active Aggressive Impulsive Too 'friendly'	Over-active Aggressive Impulsive Withdrawn Low confidence Poor peer/adult relationships Poor school progress Wets/soils Destructive	School truancy Runaway Drink and substance abuse Steals, lies, self harm, sexual promiscuity, destructive to self, others and property

Development:

Motor skills are the least affected by neglect unless the child is kept in a cot or strapped in a buggy, but he may be clumsy and later have poor pencil skills.

Poor vision from amblyopic eye (neglected squint), broken/lost glasses.

Poor hearing because of glue ear, perforated ear drums and failure to keep audiology appointments.

Language delay is part of neglect; these children will not learn to listen and speak without attention.

Social skills are not developed, e.g. dressing, toileting, eating at a table.

Behaviour. In the clinic the child may be over-active, distractible, over-friendly or withdrawn, passive and silent (Figure 17.10).

Diagnosis

Neglect is diagnosed from the clinical picture and information from the health visitor, teacher, home care assistant, etc., about the attachment between the child and mother, the physical state of the child(ren) and the home, school/nursery attendance, behaviour, etc.

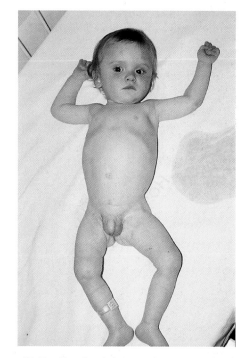

Figure 17.10 Emotional abuse and neglect: infant of 10 months showing frozen watchfulness and failing to thrive.

Management

Management initially consists of supporting the child and family whilst attempting to improve the parenting skills. The most difficult aspect is to judge when parenting is not 'good enough'.

Non-organic failure to thrive (FTT)

This is the description of a child who is growth retarded because of malnutrition. The term 'non-organic FTT' is used to differentiate the condition from FTT resulting from heart disease, renal disorder or malabsorption. In order to grow optimally a child needs an adequate diet but also to be loved and nurtured. Around 95% of cases of FTT are non-organic FTT. The consequences are developmental, especially language delay, emotional disorder and an impaired growth rate. The child's head circumference also grows at less than the expected rate; as most of the growth takes place during the first 2 years of life, severe FTT leads to a smaller head than expected and microcephaly.

Non-organic FTT is often seen in the context of multiple family and financial difficulties. The family may be very stressed, and other members may have eating problems.

Growth

Growth charts are essential in the recognition of FTT. Serial measurements give the growth rate (see Figures 17.11, 17.12).

The mid upper arm circumference (MUAC) is a useful measurement for children of 12–60 months:

- 14–15 cm—some concern
- < 14 cm—serious concern.

Patterns of growth which cause concern are:

- weight loss
- plateauing of weight
- dipping or 'saw-tooth' pattern
- steady weight on or below the 2nd centile—needs careful assessment as to whether this represents a poor growth rate or 'small normal'; always check parental height (remember that they may be growth retarded too)
- weight lies more than one major percentile below the height in infancy and two centiles at age 2 years and over.

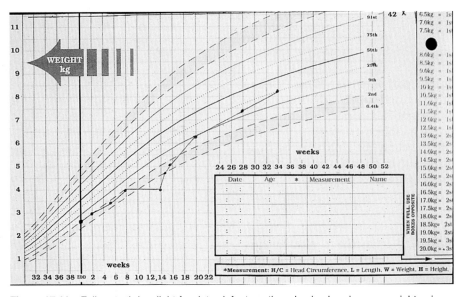

Figure 17.11   Failure to thrive: light-for-dates infant, mother abusing heroin, poor weight gain with plateauing until grandmother took over the care; the FTT was due to lack of calories (mother disorganised, no routine to feeding and 'unavailable' to baby because intoxicated).

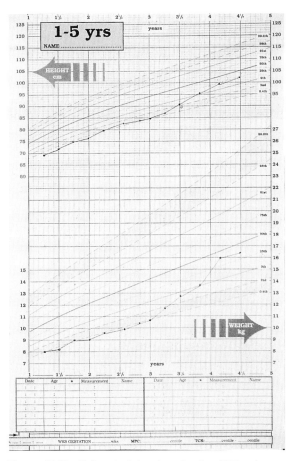

Figure 17.12   Failure to thrive: longstanding FTT, note poor weight gain, growth parallel to 0.4 percentile, until child physically abused; better growth rate evident when in good foster care.

Initial investigations

- A detailed history of eating behaviour
- A dietary history ± a 3-day diary
- Assessment of parent–child attachment
- Developmental screen
- Health visitor's report
- Physical examination including accurate measurements of growth (unclothed)
- Haemoglobin, ferritin level
- Observation of behaviour, language and social development.

Management

Management may consist of advice and reassur-ance, but some cases are more complex and benefit from a team approach including a paedi-atric dietician and child psychologist as well as the health visitor and paediatrician. Hospital admission may be required in the underweight infant to enable skilled observations by paedi-atric nursing staff. Food supplements are rarely needed. A regimen of small meals and snacks with reference to the child's current preferences and a minimum of adult pressure usually proves successful.

Social work input in the assessment and man-agement of more complex cases is needed and may provide other support such as home care, nursery and links to voluntary agencies such as Home Start. Child protection issues may lead to a Child Protection Conference and a formal plan of support.

Prognosis

The prognosis in severe FTT is worrying although many infants and children will improve with intervention. Learning and emotional disorders persist in the long term, reflecting the emotional abuse and deprivation which underlies much of this condition.

EMOTIONAL ABUSE

Emotional abuse is defined as: 'the habitual verbal harassment of a child by disparagement, criticism, threat and ridicule, and the inversion of love; by verbal and non-verbal means rejection and withdrawal are substituted'.

Emotional abuse and deprivation is the most damaging form of abuse. It is probably also the most widespread form, occurring in all social classes; it always involves emotional neglect and sometimes physical neglect. Failure to thrive occurs in the context of emotional deprivation; all sexually and many physically abused children are also emotionally abused (Figure 17.13).

Management

Problems with personal relationships within the family are ideally recognised by the health visitor

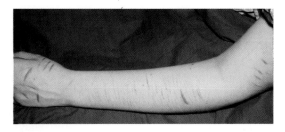

Figure 17.13 Emotional abuse: girl aged 14 with repeated slash marks on arm following childhood of emotional and sexual abuse.

or GP while the child is in its infancy. Work with the family is more likely to be effective before behaviour patterns become established and if the adults have some insight and wish to change their own behaviour rather than blaming the child.

Child protection issues are involved; referral to a child and family team incorporating a psychologist, psychiatrist and social worker enables assessment and treatment. The prognosis of children brought up in harsh, critical and unloving homes is poor, particularly in terms of their ability to form and sustain adult relationships.

THE MANAGEMENT OF POSSIBLE CHILD ABUSE

Early recognition of families who are having child rearing problems (Box 17.2) may allow the various family and child agencies to offer support to the family and, by reducing some of the pressures on the family, lessen the risk of abuse and neglect. It seems that this approach is not successful, however, in the prevention of CSA.

Early diagnosis of abuse may also prevent escalating violence. An example might be a 3-month-old baby with two small bruises on her cheeks. Violence towards infants is very dangerous, and a severe shaking injury may follow.

The medical assessment of abuse has been described above, under the various categories of maltreatment. An immediate assessment is necessary if a medical practitioner sees an infant with multiple bruises and failure to thrive. Informal discussions with the child's health visitor

and partners in the practice may be useful but the infant is at risk and the situation requires immediate hospital referral to a paediatrician interested in non-organic FTT and abuse.

The parents will usually co-operate and may be very worried about their wasted baby. If the parents are not co-operative the SSD should be contacted and will probably be able to negotiate with the family and accompany the parents to the hospital. The social worker will check to see if the child or any siblings are on the CPR or are known to the SSD.

On rare occasions the family may still be unco-operative; a decision must then be made, usually by a senior social worker, in consultation with the doctor and local authority legal department, as to whether an Emergency Protection Order is needed. This is obtained from the on-call juvenile magistrate.

Paediatric assessment

Throughout this assessment it is important that the parents are given time and that the staff are well informed and sensitive. Alienation of the family will have an adverse effect on the short and longer term management but may be unavoidable.

The paediatrician undertakes a detailed assessment and will explain more directly why investigations are needed. This is usually the responsibility of a senior doctor as the next step is to explain to the parents that the explanations for the bruising are not satisfactory and the SSD are to be informed (if not already involved).

A strategy meeting may be held in person or by telephone between the health professionals, the SSD and the police to plan the investigation. The police involved are usually from child protection units, have specialist training and are not in uniform.

The initial child protection conference

This is convened by the SSD and is chaired by an experienced social worker who does not have responsibility for the case. The parents, and

Box 17.14 A hypothetical case

An infant of 6 months is seen to have multiple bruises (face, chest) and is admitted to hospital. Investigation has not demonstrated any bleeding or clotting disorder but a skeletal survey shows that there are 3 healing posterior rib fractures and bilateral metaphyseal fractures of the lower end of the tibia. This appears to be a case of serious child abuse. In hospital the infant's bruises heal, she rapidly gains weight and becomes much more alert, and smiles more than on admission. The parents are infrequent visitors and they are both 'rough' and impatient with their baby. They have declined offers to be resident. There are two other siblings aged 2 and 3 years. They too have been examined and are underweight and overactive with poor language and social skills.

The SSD check the extended family; could the older siblings stay with Grandma while the assessment is completed? The dynamics within the family have been altered by the admission of the baby, and the older children may be at increased risk.

At the initial child protection conference it becomes evident that both parents are abusing heroin. The infant is placed on the Child Protection Register under the categories of physical and emotional abuse and neglect. The siblings are registered under emotional abuse and neglect. The parents are urgently referred to the Addiction Unit. The police seek the advice of the Crown Prosecution Service, and the SSD go to the Family Proceedings Court to initiate care proceedings. The Court appoints a guardian ad litem for the children and the case goes 'up' to the County Court.

The parents continue to abuse drugs and have to thieve and prostitute themselves to pay for the drugs. The grandparents seek a Residence Order and care for all three grandchildren. The children's names are removed from the CPR and social work becomes voluntary. Access of the parents to their children is made by arrangement with the grandparents.

---

sometimes teenage children, are invited, as are other relevant professionals (social worker, paediatrician, GP, health visitor, school nurse, police, probation, housing manager, etc.).

The tasks of the initial conference are:

- to share relevant information about the child and family
- to decide whether there has been abuse or neglect and if the child(ren) in the household are at risk of further abuse
- to place the child(ren)'s name(s) on the CPR if there is ongoing risk
- to seek legal advice if legal proceedings are likely
- to appoint a key worker to co-ordinate the case and core group who will work with the family (social worker, health visitor, GP, paediatrician, nursery worker, etc.) and provide the services that the assessment has found to be needed
- to arrange a child protection review conference, to be held no more than 6 months after the initial conference.

The Child Protection Register (CPR)

- The decision to put a child's name on the CPR is made at the initial child protection conference.
- The child must be at *ongoing risk of harm* and is registered under the applicable category or categories of abuse, e.g. physical abuse and neglect, sexual abuse, emotional abuse.
- A child protection plan is formulated.
- The child's name is removed following a review conference at which it is established that the factors leading to registration have changed.

The review child protection conference

This must be held at least every 6 months and monitors the effectiveness of the child protection plan. The conference should be attended by parents, older children and core group professionals.

Considerations:

- Is the child protected or is abuse continuing?
- Is there good interagency working?
- Should the child be de-registered?

Summary of the role of the primary health care team in child protection

- Pre-pregnancy health counselling is increasingly important. The family history and any drug or substance abuse may be discussed to prevent, as far as possible, intrauterine abuse.
- The family should be supported during the

antenatal period and referred to the SSD for support and a possible child protection conference if the welfare of the baby is likely to cause concern.

- Child health surveillance is now usually the responsibility of the GP and health visitor. Early attachment difficulties, FTT and other abuses may be recognised during routine visits, and early diagnosis may allow the prevention of escalating abuse.
- Unsatisfactory care needs to be recognised and the welfare of the child put first, despite the GP's difficulty in also having the care of other family members.

All professionals who care for children should be aware of the local Area Child Protection Committee (ACPC) procedures and the Department of Health publications such as *Working Together* and the addendum *Medical Responsibility*. Attendance at local multidisciplinary training will give health professionals understanding of local practice, e.g. when to refer and to whom, local facilities and prevention strategies (Box 17.15).

THE CHILDREN ACT 1989 (ENGLAND AND WALES)

The Children Act 1989 brought together legis-

Box 17.15 Prevention of abuse
- Talk to children about conflict resolution in schools: aggression, stress and bullying
- Educate all teenagers about parenthood: provide easy access to family planning clinics
- Raise awareness about violence amongst health professionals
- Primary health teams may recognise the onset of abuse behaviours and intervene effectively before the behaviours become entrenched
- Research the links between social deprivation, ill health and violence
- Invest in children and families to eliminate childhood poverty
- Provide support for adults and children who have been traumatised physically and emotionally by violence
- Acknowledge the place of alcohol and substance abuse in child maltreatment and neglect
- Insist that all perpetrators of CSA are assessed formally and offered appropriate therapy

---

lation concerning children in a comprehensive way to cover private law (such as custody, guardianship) and public law (where parents and the local authority may be in dispute). It covers most of the law relating to children.

Court structure was also changed so that all cases are now heard in specialised Family Proceedings Courts. Cases may begin in the former Magistrates' Court and be dealt with in that Court or, if the case is seen to be more complex, it may be passed to the higher Family Proceedings Courts (where cases may also be started). The courts presided over by a judge are the County Court, High Court and occasionally the House of Lords. Any practitioner who has been involved in any way with a child may be asked to write a Police Statement and may be asked to attend any of the courts, by use of a Witness Order if necessary. The court may also ask for sight of the relevant medical notes and they may enforce disclosure.

Criminal proceedings

Criminal prosecutions are not part of the Children Act (1989). Cases may be brought against the abuser(s) but less than 5% of cases of CSA are successfully prosecuted. The number of prosecutions in child abuse, especially CSA, is low (5–10%). The evidence in criminal cases must prove that the defendant is guilty 'beyond all reasonable doubt' compared with 'on the balance of probability' in civil cases. This lower standard of proof is needed if children are to be protected, but even so can be difficult to achieve. In a crime where the child's word may stand against that of an adult the difficulties are obvious. It is very stressful for children to give evidence in criminal cases in spite of the use of videotaped interviews and video-links in the court. The child has to be available for cross-examination, which may be very destructive.

Civil proceedings

The Children Act attempts to maintain the child's welfare as its paramount concern whilst being fair to parents, allowing them the right to quickly

---

> **Box 17.16** Factors to be considered in court proceedings
>
> 1. The wishes and feelings of the child
> 2. The child's physical, emotional and educational needs
> 3. The likely effect on the child of any change in circumstances
> 4. The child's age, sex and background including racial, religious and cultural characteristics
> 5. Any harm the child has suffered or is at risk of suffering
> 6. The capability of parents or carers in meeting the child's needs
> 7. The powers available to the court in the particular circumstances

---

> **Box 17.17** People who have parental responsibility
>
> - Both married parents (even if divorced or their child is 'looked after', i.e. in a voluntary arrangement with the local authority)
> - Single mother
> - Unmarried father, if he has the mother's written agreement or by applying to the court
> - Others (e.g. grandparents, cohabitee, local authority) by application to the court
> - Parental responsibility may be shared

---

challenge local authority actions and to avoid undue intervention into family life (Box 17.16). 'Children in need' should receive appropriate support from the local services in discussion with their families. Child maltreatment is considered in terms of 'significant harm' which the child has suffered or is at risk of suffering.

Definitions:

A **'child in need'** is the term used to cover the large group of children who have extra needs, as defined by the Act (see Box 1.18, p. 25). 'Development' includes physical, intellectual, emotional, social or behavioural development. The definition of 'health' is of physical or mental health.

'Significant harm' is the description used when parenting is not adequate or is abusive; the Act defines this as: 'any avoidable impairment of health and development in the child, attributable to an act or omission by the parent'. It is caused by ill treatment through neglect, physical abuse, sexual abuse or emotional abuse.

Delay is recognised to be prejudicial in the hearing of children's cases and the Act has attempted (but on the whole, failed) to minimise the time taken for cases to come before the court.

Parental responsibility is a basic principle of the Act (Box 17.17). Rather than the parents having rights over the children they have duties and obligations towards them. The context is, however, that the upbringing of children is primarily the responsibility of parents.

The **'no order' principle** is a continuation of the philosophy that the upbringing of children is the responsibility of parents; the role of the State is to help where necessary but otherwise not to intervene *unless* the conditions for an order are met *and* that making an order is better for the child than not making an order.

Partnership with parents. This gives the local authority the duty to provide services to families with children in need but in partnership with the parents, that is, by asking their views and working with them to meet the child's needs, within the home if possible.

Emergency protection of children
(Figure 17.14)

The majority of children who have been abused stay at home during the SSD investigation; of those who are removed, many return home within 2 weeks. The alleged abuser, rather than the child, may be asked to leave the home until the full investigation is completed and the situation is clarified.

The parents may agree to a voluntary arrangement with the SSD to accommodate the abused child rather than going to court.

Orders available in child protection

Emergency Protection Order (EPO):

- May be granted by any Family Proceedings Court.
- Lasts for up to 8 days.
- May be renewable, once, for a further 7 days.
- May be challenged in court after 72 hours.
- Applicants may be from SSD or NSPCC.

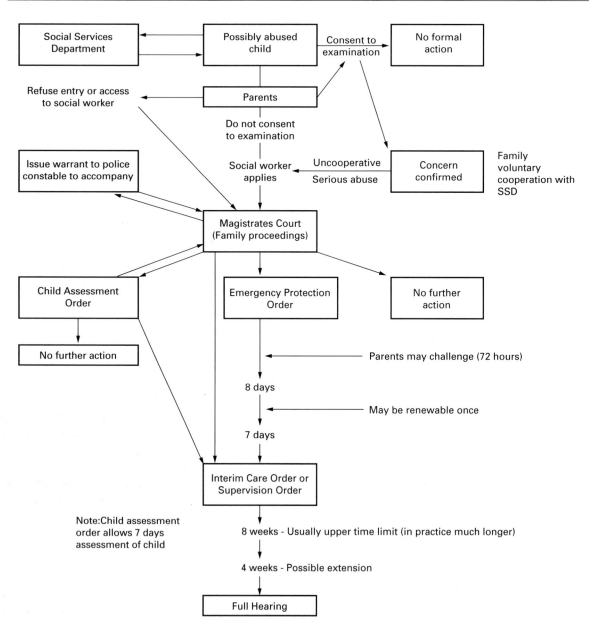

Figure 17.14 Organisation of child protection in England and Wales (Children Act 1989).

- The court has to be satisfied that there is reasonable cause to believe that the child is likely to suffer significant harm if he or she is not removed to accommodation provided by the applicant, or there is reasonable cause to suspect that the child is suffering or is likely to suffer significant harm or that access to the child is denied and is required as a matter of urgency.

Police protection. A police officer, with permission from a senior police officer, may remove children on a Police Protection Order or prevent their removal from a safe place, e.g. a hospital, *without* a court order for up to 72 hours, where the officer has reasonable cause to believe that the child is likely to suffer significant harm.

Child Assessment Order. This order allows for assessment, but by notice to the carers, with pre-arranged appointments (for example, for paediatric assessment).

- Enables the assessment of a child's health and welfare where concern exists but there is doubt whether emergency removal is justified.
- Only the NSPCC or the SSD may apply to the court.
- The grounds are that the applicant believes that the child is suffering or is likely to suffer significant harm and an assessment is unlikely to be allowed (by the parents) without an order.
- Lasts for up to 7 days.

Care Order (CO) and Supervision Order (SO):
The court may make a CO or SO only if it is satisfied that the child is:

- suffering or likely to suffer significant harm *and*
- the harm or likelihood of harm, is attributable to the standard of care being below that which could be reasonably expected

or

- the child is beyond parental control.

Care Order:

- The SSD (local authority) or NSPCC may apply.
- The conditions, as above, must be satisfied.
- Parental responsibility lies with the SSD and is shared with parent(s).
- The child may be placed with foster parents, in a children's home or with parents.
- Lasts until the child is 18 years old or until revoked by the court.

Interim CO (ICO):

- Allows a child to be placed in care while there is a full investigation.
- Parental responsibility is shared between the SSD (local authority) and parent(s).
- Lasts for up to 8 weeks with extensions of 4 weeks.

Supervision Order:

- The conditions, as above, must be satisfied.
- Lasts for 1 year, with a maximum of 3 extensions of 1 year each.
- The child remains at home.

Education Supervision Order:

- The applicant is the education authority.
- A CO may not be granted on educational grounds alone.

Section 8 Orders (Private Law Proceedings)

Residence Order:

- Determines with whom the child should live, e.g. grandparents, foster parents.
- Gives parental responsibility.

Contact Order:

- Defines any form of contact (personal, letter, telephone, etc.).
- Places an obligation on the person with whom the child lives to allow such contact.

Specific Issues Order. This is used to solve particular problems, for example if those with parental responsibility disagree on the need for medical treatment.

Prohibited Steps Order. This defines acts which the person with parental responsibility is forbidden to undertake, e.g. take the child out of the country.

Consent

Consent before examination is sought from the child's parent or whoever has parental responsibility (Box 17.17).

- In an emergency a baby-sitter or neighbour, for example, may act to get medical help and the medical practitioner may rely on his clinical judgement.
- Older children may give or refuse consent themselves if they understand the nature of the examination, that is, they are Gillick competent, even if the court has authorised the examination.

- If consent is denied, the High Court may authorise assessment or treatment if this is in the best interests of a child under 18 years.
- Repeated medical and psychiatric examinations for forensic purposes, if court proceedings have started, require authorisation by the court or they may be disallowed in court.
- If in doubt the doctor should seek legal advice.

Confidentiality

In the context of child abuse the General Medical Council authorises disclosure of information to 'an appropriate responsible person or statutory agency, in order to prevent further harm to the patient', but also warns that disclosure may later require justification.

Other advice (Child protection: Medical Responsibility) warns against promises of secrecy and makes clear the expectation that information may be shared on a controlled 'need to know' basis in the interests of the child.

Knowledge that a child is or may be being abused or neglected is an 'exceptional circumstance' and will invariably justify a doctor making disclosure to an appropriate person or officer of a statutory agency.

CHILDREN IN CARE

The phrase 'children in care' refers to children who are the subject of care proceedings, whereas if there is a voluntary agreement with the parents they are 'looked after or accommodated' by the local authority. Parents may remove their child when accommodated at any time and they continue to have parental rights.

'Out of home care'

The emphasis in child and family policy in the Children Act 1989 is on the importance of the natural family and the duty of the local authority to support 'children in need' and their families. Clearly, a balance has to be struck; the Department of Health advised: 'The Act seeks to protect children both from the harm that can arise from failures within the family and the harm which can be caused by unwarranted intervention in their family life'.

Children may be:

- adopted
- fostered
- cared for in children's homes.

Adoption (Box 17.18)

When a child is adopted the legal rights and duties concerning the child pass from the natural parent(s) to the adopters. The adoption is legally irrevocable and is permanent. The child takes the adopters' surname and inherits in the same way as a natural child.

Adoption in England and Wales peaked in the late 1960s when, in 1969, 27 000 children were adopted; 75% of these were infants placed with non-relatives. Since then the numbers of available infants has fallen because of better contraception, access to abortion, and different attitudes and support for single parents. Older children, children with special needs, and children adopted by a step-parent now constitute the majority of children available for adoption.

In 1991 only 7000 children were adopted, of whom 900 were infants.

The current position in adoption. Whilst there

Box 17.18 Adoption in practice

- Adoption, unless by a close relative or the child comes from abroad, is managed by an adoption agency, e.g. local SSD, Barnardo's, National Children's Home
- Applicants must be 21 years old
- Adopters may be single, married (and adopt jointly) or the natural parent
- Before making an adoption order the court must be satisfied that the parent(s) understand and agree to the adoption
- The court may dispense with parental agreement, for example in cases of child abuse, by dispensing a freeing order
- A mother may not agree to an adoption until the infant is 6 weeks old and the child must be with prospective adopters for 13 weeks before an Adoption Order can be made
- An adopted child may have access to his original birth certificate at the age of 18 years

are very few healthy infants available for adoption, there are thousands of older children with special needs, physical disability, learning and emotional problems who could be placed. Much effort is directed towards placing children in a home with a cultural and ethnic background similar to their own.

Adoption panels operate according to the Adoption Regulations (1977, 1983, 1997), which have recently been changed to make their workings more accessible and accountable by including at least three independent members, a quorum of six (to include a social worker and chair or vice-chair) and limiting the time spent as a panel member apart from the medical advisor to a period of not more than two consecutive periods of 3 years. The medical advisor, who is usually a senior community paediatrician, evaluates the medical information available about the child, birth parents and prospective adopters, and advises the panel as to its significance. The nature of the work is shown by a review of 151 children referred for medical opinion between 1990 and 1993:

- 19% were under 1 year old but 50% had potential or actual health problems—disability, a family history of schizophrenia, or a sibling with a disability.
- 56% of the whole group had a medical, behavioural or learning problem or substantial family history risk. Examples given include profound deafness, achondroplasia, Down's syndrome, fetal alcohol syndrome, abuse (all types), schizophrenia (one or both parents), and incest.

Long-term follow-up of children with special needs by the medical advisor and other professionals may be helpful in supporting the adoptive placement. 10–20% of adoptive placements break down, although this is rare with normal infants.

Foster care and children's homes

Children may be looked after in foster homes or children's homes, but the numbers have fallen from 60 000 children in 1991 to 49 000 in 1995. The percentage of children in foster care rather than children's homes rose from 58% to 65%.

Once in care, 20% of children do not return home and of those that do 38% suffer a breakdown of the placement. The rate of foster care breakdown is:

- 1 in 4 by the age of 8 years
- 1 in 2 by 12 years
- 1 in 2–3 15–16-year-old teenagers run away from care.

Children may be 'looked after' at the request of their parents, and of these children about 40% will, in time, become the responsibility of the local authority.

Approximately 40% of children are admitted under statutory orders (Care Order) because of abuse. Other children are admitted under the guise of 'social problems' such as maternal illness, housing problems, abandonment and parental imprisonment. The family background of children in care compared with the general population shows that 6 times as many had a lone parent, 5 times as many families were on income support, and 3 times as many were in rented accommodation. The usual picture is therefore of poverty, unemployment, large families and single parents.

45% of the children in foster care are 9–15 years old; many are in long-term placements and unable to go home because of the harm they suffered or were at risk of suffering. The physical needs of children in care are usually met but their educational and emotional needs are often complex, and foster parents and residential workers are not trained to cope with such disturbed, demanding and abusive children.

An additional risk is abuse and emotional deprivation in care. This may occur in foster care or residential units. The overall rate is not known, although it is recognised that much 'care' is unsatisfactory.

The medical responsibility for children in care

Children who have been abused or neglected may:

- have failed to grow physically, intellectually and emotionally
- have difficult and disordered behaviour
- have unrecognised or partially treated

medical problems—squint, glue ear, dental caries, asthma, incomplete immunisation.

In recognition of the deficiencies in previous medical provision, children in the care of the local authority are subject to Boarding Out Regulations (1988) under which a doctor examines the child, provides a report, and the child (2–18 years) is reviewed annually (infants 6-monthly). These reviews may be very useful in checking the emotional as well as physical well-being of the child in care and in recognising when the child and carers need further support. A swift, repeated physical examination without consideration of the wider needs of the child and carer is of little value and is likely to be resented by older children.

Runaways

Runaways are usually very disadvantaged children who have been in care, but the pattern of running usually starts while the child is at home and begins with school truancy (Box 17.19).

CHILDREN AND CRIMINAL RESPONSIBILITY

Under the law in England the age of criminal responsibility is 10 years—younger than in most European countries. In Scandinavia it is 15 years, in Portugal and Spain 16 years; the only country where it is lower is Scotland, at 8 years.

In law the performance of an act does not constitute guilt unless there is a guilty intention. This may obviously be difficult to establish in childhood—was the child a mischief, performing a childish act rather than a criminal one? This difficulty has been recognised in common law in the presumption that children between 10 and 13 years

---

Box 17.19 Characteristics of runaways

- Equal numbers of boys and girls run; most stay locally with friends or relatives
- Boys are more likely to be 'pushed out of home' and girls to run; around 50% give maltreatment as the reason for running
- The peak age is 14–16 years but 10% are under the age of 12 years
- Many children begin by truanting, staying away during the day; the behaviour escalates, most returning after a few days, but 30% of children run more than 5 times and may stay away
- 25% of runaways have school problems: on average they are 2 years behind in school work
- Drug, alcohol and solvent abuse is prevalent
- Criminal activities increase the longer the child stays away
- 50% of runaways are from care, mainly children's homes. Running from home is probably under-reported

---

are *doli incapax*—they are assumed not to know the difference between right and wrong (this means seriously wrong, morally wrong or evil).

In the UK this presumption, which gives partial immunity from prosecution to 10—13-year-olds, has been abolished. The prosecution currently has the onus of showing beyond all reasonable doubt that, in the particular case, the child did know the difference in right from wrong in the required sense.

'Doli incapax' makes allowance for the fact that the child is still developing in terms of understanding, knowledge and powers of reasoning. In addition, responsibility for the child's behaviour lies with parents and society who promote moral development: locking up children in punitive institutions will not allow normal social development or produce educated, caring adults. Antisocial children are usually in need of care rather than punishment.

FURTHER READING

Department of Health 1989 An introductory guide for the NHS to the Children Act. DoH, London

Department of Health, BMA 1995 Child protection, medical responsibilities. Conference of Medical Royal College. HMSO, London

Department of Health, Welsh Office 1995 Child protection: clarification of arrangement between the NHS and other agencies. HMSO, London

Hobbs C J, Wynne J M 1995 Physical signs of child abuse. W B Saunders, London

Hobbs C J, Hanks H, Wynne J M 1998 Child abuse and neglect: a clinician's handbook, 2nd edn. Churchill Livingstone, Edinburgh

Meadow R (ed) 1997 ABC of child abuse. BMJ Publishing, London

Royal College of Physicians 1997 Physical signs of sexual abuse in children. Report of the Royal College of Physicians, London

Working Together under the Children Act 1991 HMSO, London

Internet address

http://www.nspcc.org.uk

INTERNET ADDRESSES

Accidents
http://www.rospa.co.uk

Cerebral palsy
http://www.scope.org.uk

Child Health Informatics Consortium
http://www.capita-ec.com/childinf

Child protection
http://www.nspcc.org.uk

Congenital disorders
http://www.uab.edu/pedinfo/DiseasesCongenital.html

Development
http://www.luhs.org/health/topics/chil/index.htm

Diabetes
http://www.idi.org.au/frameset6.htm

ENT disorders
http://icarus.med.utoronto.ca/carr/manual/outline.html

Environmental health
http://www.cehn.org

Epilepsy
http://bay.ion.bpmf.ac.uk/nsehome/open.html

Genetics
http://www.vh.org/Providers/Textbooks/ClinicalGenetics/Contents.html

General medical search engine
http://www.omni.ac.uk

General paediatric search engines
http://www.pedinfo.org
http://www.mc.vanderbilt.edu/peds/pidl/index.htm

Growth
http://www.cgf.org.uk

Haematology
http://edcenter. med.cornell.edu/CUMC_PathNotes/Hematopathology/Hematopathology.html

Infectious diseases
http://hopkins-id.edu

Nephrology
http://www.mc.vanderbilt.edu/peds/pidl/nephro/index.htm

Neurology
http://www.ninds.nih.gov/healinfo/nindspub.htm

Paediatric cardiology
http://www.tc.umn.edu/nlhome/m475/bjarn001/stuff/abstract.html

Paediatric surgery
http://home.coqui.net/titolugo/index.htm

Poisoning
http://www.peds.umn.edu/divisions/pccm/teaching/acp/poison.html

Respiratory disease
http://hebw.uwcm.ac.uk/respdis/index.html

Royal College of Paediatrics and Child Health link site
http://www.rcpch.ac.uk/visitors/links.htm

SIDS
http://dspace.dial.pipex.com/fsid/

The newborn infant
http://silk.nih.gov/SILK/Cochrane/Cochrane.htm

UK infectious disease statistics
http://www.phls.co.uk

UK national statistics
http://www.doh.gov.uk/public.stats1.htm

Index